Rheumatic Disorders in Childhood

POSTGRADUATE PAEDIATRICS SERIES

Under the General Editorship of

JOHN APLEY
CBE, MD, BS, FRCP

Emeritus Consultant Paediatrician,
United Bristol Hospitals

Rheumatic Disorders in Childhood

BARBARA M. ANSELL
MD, FRCP

Head of Division of Rheumatology, Clinical Research Centre,
Northwick Park Hospital, Harrow, Middlesex
Consultant Physician, Canadian Red Cross
Memorial Hospital, Taplow

BUTTERWORTHS
London - Boston
Sydney - Wellington - Durban - Toronto

United Kingdom London	**Butterworth & Co (Publishers) Ltd** 88 Kingsway, WC2B 6AB
Australia Sydney	**Butterworth Pty Ltd** 586 Pacific Highway, Chatswood, NSW 2067 Also at Melbourne, Brisbane, Adelaide and Perth
Canada Toronto	**Butterworth & Co (Canada) Ltd** 2265 Midland Avenue, Scarborough, Ontario, M1P 4S1
New Zealand Wellington	**Butterworths of New Zealand Ltd** T & W Young Building, 77–85 Customhouse Quay, 1, CPO Box 472
South Africa Durban	**Butterworth & Co (South Africa) Ltd** 152–154 Gale Street
USA Boston	**Butterworth (Publishers) Inc** 10 Tower Office Park, Woburn, Mass. 01801

First published 1980

ISBN 0 407 00186 7

British Library Cataloguing in Publication Data
Ansell, Barbara M
Rheumatic disorders in childhood. – (Postgraduate paediatrics series).
1. Rheumatism in children
I. Title II. Series
618.9'27'2 RJ482.R48 80-40275

ISBN 0 407 00186 7

Typeset by Butterworths Litho Preparation Department
Plates made by Adroit Photolitho Ltd, Birmingham
Printed and bound in England by W. J. Mackay Ltd, Chatham

Preface

There has been a steadily increasing interest in rheumatic disorders of childhood in recent years and an increasing realisation of how widespread they are. The Medical Research Council's Rheumatism Unit at Taplow, under the direction of Professor E. G. L. Bywaters was a focal point for paediatric rheumatology, attracting workers from all parts of the world. My interest stems from joining him as a registrar in the 1950s, at what was then the Special Unit for Juvenile Rheumatism. Subsequently, after my appointment there as a consultant in 1962, I took an active role in many clinical and collaborative laboratory research projects. Professor Bywaters was a superb teacher, always questioning, but with much wisdom, and encouraging his staff to do likewise. Since moving to the Clinical Research Centre at Northwick Park Hospital, I have tried to continue the meticulous assessment of clinical data impressed on me in my earlier years.

The overall popularity of the subject today has been highlighted for me by the frequency with which one is asked to lecture and to help in organising symposia relating to some aspect of rheumatic disorders in childhood, as well as the numbers of doctors attending the basic courses held at the Clinical Research Centre, Northwick Park Hospital in 1978 and 1980.

Rheumatic disease in childhood has come to mean something very difference since the days when rheumatic fever was common in Western countries; that has become rare (though this may change again) but other childhood rheumatic disorders are being recognised more frequently, both in hospital and in general practice. The idea behind this book was to put together information on rheumatic problems likely to confront paediatricians and rheumatologists, as well as family community doctors, while at the same time indicating some of the current thoughts on chronic arthritis in childhood, and the rarer connective tissue disorders. The common disorders are discussed in some detail, but attention is also drawn to rarer ones that are likely to cause difficulty in diagnosis. It is hoped that the many illustrations that are included will appeal to doctors in active clinical practice. The book is essentially a practical guide, focusing predominantly on diagnosis and treatment. No attempt is made to cover every aspect, and the bibliography aims to be useful and up to date rather than exhaustive.

From the outset of this venture Dr. John Apley, Editor-in-Chief, has been a constant source of support, and to him I owe an enormous debt of gratitude for his criticism and encouragement. A book of this nature is, of course, dependent on the help and goodwill of many people, and it would be impossible to name all of them. I am indebted to the many doctors who have referred cases and readily allowed me to quote them, and also to my colleagues in rheumatology and paediatrics, many of whom have come to work with us from different parts of the world, who have helped in patient care and in numerous studies. I am especially grateful for the many valuable comments I have received while preparing this book, in particular from Dr. Martin Barrett from the Hospital for Sick Children, Great Ormond Street, Mr. George Arden and Mr. Malcolm Swann, the orthopaedic surgeons attached to the Taplow Unit, and Mr. Jack Kanski, the ophthalmologist. I must also thank Sarah Hartwell, Pat Spencer and Lesley Bentley for their secretarial help, and Jean Tyler for her excellent photography, as well as my family and friends for their forebearance during its production. Finally I must record my gratitude to the publishers, Butterworths, for their help throughout the time-consuming task.

BMA

Contents

CHAPTER 1

Aches and Pains

Limb pain in childhood is not uncommon, but serious rheumatic diseases are rare. A long history of pain with no abnormal physical signs, and no deterioration in general health, is unlikely to be the fore-runner of a serious rheumatic illness. Indeed, pain is often attention-seeking, i.e. the equivalent of saying 'Will you read me a story?'. A child rapidly comes to realise that complaints of pain in an arm or leg gain far more notice than other tried devices. At times he or she may just be copying some other member of the family. It can be an expression of tension.

However, should a child look unwell, be anaemic, lose weight or have other constitutional symptoms, then the onset of aches and pains should be regarded as more serious. These pains can result from infiltration in bone, as in leukaemia or neuroblastoma or from occult neoplasms.

Cramps occurring at rest, the commest type in childhood, are rarely due to underlying muscle disorder. However, cramps relating to exercise and relieved by rest usually point to a muscle disorder. They can be the presenting feature in some of the rare metabolic myopathies such as myoglobinuric syndromes and occasionally muscular dystrophy (Dubowitz, 1978). Very occasionally pain localised to one site may be due to a bone disease such as an osteoid osteoma, osteochondroma or Osgood–Schlatter disease.

A careful history from both parents and the child is essential. This will include, not only details of the pain in the limbs, but also pain in other sites such as the head or abdomen. It is important to have a good family history in view of the increased incidence of 'rheumatic' disorders of all types, including limb pains, in the families of children with limb pain; the frequency of emotional disturbances in such families also appears to be above average. Provided care is taken in questioning the parents and the child, the distinction between limb and joint pain is usually straightforward; it is particularly helpful to get a relaxed child to point to where it hurts.

RECURRENT LIMB PAIN (*Table 1.1*)

Limb pains, often previously referred to as 'growing pains', are more common than any other form of rheumatic disorder in childhood. Apley and Naish (1955) noted a frequency of 4.2 per cent in schoolchildren of all ages. This affects both sexes and is most common between six and 13 years. In two-thirds of affected children the pains will occur only in the legs, while in the remaining third they may be in the arms, trunk and legs, either at the same time or at different times; it is most unusual to have pain only in the arms. The limb pain is usually described as aching or heavy, tending to come on during the day time or evening; in about a quarter, pains are predominantly nocturnal. Usually the pain is localised to the shins or deep in the calves or thighs; it does not seem to be a typical cramp. It is severe enough to wake the child out of sleep, appears to be eased by rubbing and will pass off after a short time, when the child falls asleep again. It can however, occur several nights in succession. Nocturnal pain appears to be entirely restricted to the legs. On examination, even during an acute episode, there are no abnormal signs in the limbs. Growth in height and weight is unaffected and developmental progress is normal. The ESR (erythrocyte sedimentation rate) is normal, as is the haemoglobin and white cell count. It is common

TABLE 1.1
Features of psychogenic recurrent limb pain

Features of psychogenic recurrent limb pain
Both sexes, 6–13 years
Predominantly lower limbs
Sometimes only nocturnal
No deterioration in health
Family history common

for pain at other sites to have brought the child to the doctor's attention previously.

Emotional disturbances also tend to be commoner in this group of children. It is important to investigate impacts of everyday life, such as difficulty in keeping up or bullying at school, lack of friends, nightmares and domestic differences between parents, all of which can cause a feeling of insecurity. As already indicated, there is a high family incidence of 'rheumatic complaints' and in the study by Apley and Naish (1955), the family pattern seemed to determine, in most cases, whether the child's pains were predominantly diurnal or nocturnal. The emotional disturbances in the families of such children will vary from one member to another and from time to time in any one person. It is important that tension states are recognised early, otherwise dissension can arise between the family and the doctor saying that he 'can find nothing wrong and the blood tests are all normal' and the mother constantly asserting that the child is in pain and therefore 'there must be something wrong'. The term 'growing pains' is probably entirely incorrect, but parents will accepts this as a benign condition. As Apley (1976) pointed out: 'Physical growth is not painful, but emotional growth can hurt like hell'.

HYSTERIA

Hysteria is a curious pain disorder which can involve just one limb or one joint. The child appears to be unable to straighten or move the limb, but on examination it appears normal. In such children very simple manoeuvres such as getting the child, who claims to be unable to flex a hip, to sit up normally, or who claims to be unable to move the elbow, to stretch it to pick up an object, can often convince the parent and child that the lesion is functional rather than organic. It may be a true conversion hysteria or a prolongation of previous illness. Hysterical prolongation of symptoms originally part of an organic disease are particularly difficult to diagnose and treat (Creak, 1969). The initial illnes is often a sore throat, or fever associated with myalgia or arthralgia, in a child who rarely has a background of psychological abnormality. The diagnosis can usually be made on the bizarre character of the gait, the severity of the torticollis (*see* p. 15) or the disproportion of disability to any objective evidence of muscle weakness, but it is not always apparent why the child seems to need to continue 'the sick role situation'. It is important to recognise this, so as to avoid over-investigation. Management includes the reassurance that the condition has a good prognosis and it is helped by the institution of a well-planned programme of physical activities. Any important precipitating or aggravating psychological stresses in school or at home should be dealt with as quickly as possible by the most appropriate means, whether it be by using the social worker, or by using the whole psychological team (Dubowitz and Hersov, 1976).

HYPERMOBILITY OF JOINTS

Generalised joint laxity is a feature of a number of hereditary connective tissue disorders such as the Marfan and Ehlers–Danlos syndromes, while several rare disorders of amino acid metabolism such as homocystinuria and hyperlysinaemia may also be associated with marked joint laxity. Criteria of joint hypermobility have been defined (Carter and Sweetnam, 1958) and it is only when the range of motion is in excess of the accepted normal in most joints that the subject is considered to have generalised hypermobility. The normal range of joint movement varies considerably according to age, sex, race, body build and possibly also training.

The term '*hypermobility syndrome*' has been coined to describe a situation in which the isolated finding of generalised joint laxity, in otherwise normal subjects, is associated with musculoskeletal complaints (Ansell, 1972). In young children, this syndrome is observed equally in both sexes but towards puberty it predominates in girls. The discomfort tends to come after exercise and is particularly common during phases of rapid growth. Symptoms are most usual in the lower limbs, although hypermobility can also be demonstrated in the upper limbs. The knees are the most frequent sites of joint complaints, but occasionally ankle symptoms predominate. Adolescents, who are usually exceptionally good at sports, can present wih knee effusions or soft-tissue swelling of one or both ankles. Histologically, there is no evidence of serious inflammation, the whole picture being compatible with trauma. The synovial fluid has a high viscosity, contains few cells and has a low protein content. Episodes of traumatic synovitis affecting the knees and ankles are not severe enough to warrant enthusiasts giving up their favourite sport. In examining for hypermobility the features to look for are: passive opposition of the thumb to the flexor aspects of the forearm (*Figure 1.1*); passive hyperextension of the fingers, particularly the fifth; the ability to extend the elbows and knees more than 10 degrees; and an excessive range of passive dorsiflexion of the ankle, with eversion of the foot (*Table 1.2*).

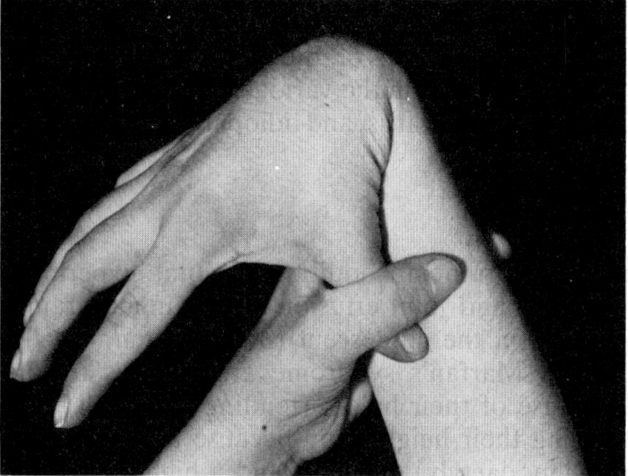

Figure 1.1. Hypermobility syndrome. Passive opposition of the thumb to the flexor aspect of the forearm in a girl of 13, who presented with pain in the knees and ankles which usually occurred in the evenings after sport at school

Many questions remain to be answered. Is joint hypermobility a discrete entity, or is it a graded trait? The fact that some patients with generalised hypermobility of joints get premature osteoarthrosis, while others continue in jobs (such as being contortionists) without any problems, suggests differences in the basic defect which are probably due to different genes. It has been suggested that hyperextensile joints result from a defect in collagen formation, but to date, in the absence of well-defined evidence, it has not been possible to demonstrate any structural or metabolic change. However, there is little doubt that there is a strong familial tendency to this syndrome. There is also a close association with a number of orthopaedic conditions, including

TABLE 1.2
Joint hypermobility

(1) Passive opposition of thumb to forearm
(2) Passive hyperextension at metacarpophalageal joints of 5 to 90 degrees or more
(3) Hyperextension of elbows by 10 degrees or more
(4) Hyperextension of knees by 10 degrees or more
(5) Excessive range of passive dorsiflexion of ankle

Three of five required for diagnosis

familial dislocation of the patella, recurrent shoulder dislocation and congenital dislocation of the hip (although there may be different factors at work in the various types of hip dislocation), as well as talipes equinovarus and idiopathic scoliosis.

Marfan's syndrome

In Marfan's syndrome in addition to joint hypermobility with episodes of pain and joint effusion after minimal trauma, pain is not uncommon in the adolescent (Sinclair *et al.*, 1960). Patients suffering from Marfan's syndrome are obvious by the time of puberty because of their height (tending to be tall but with their span exceeding their height) and because they have long slender fingers (arachnodactyly) and toes and a high-arched palate. The most commonly associated skeletal abnormalities are scoliosis, talipes equinovarus and slipped epiphysis. In addition, up to 30 per cent have eye defects, most commonly ectopia lentis and some 20 per cent have cardiovascular anomalies, septum and conduction defects and aneurysms, particularly of the aorta.

Turnover of collagen appears increased and fibroblasts in tissue culture accumulate excess hyaluranate, suggesting a complex abnormality involving both collagen and glycosaminoglycans.

A disease which can be confused with Marfan's syndrome but manifests in addition, mental deficiency and osteoporosis, is homocystinuria (caused by a genetically determined deficiency of cystathionine synthetase) (Brenton *et al.*, 1972).

Ehlers–Danlos syndrome (Beighton, 1970)

In the Ehlers–Danlos syndrome hypermobility of joints with recurrent effusions and dislocations are common, but it is rare for these to be the presenting features. The hyperextensible skin with easy bruising and tell-tale scars will usually aid diagnosis. Type III (Pope and Nicholls, 1978) is the most likely to give rise to problems as it is so mild that it may not have been recognised when the child presents with joint symptoms (Jimenez and Lálly, 1979).

INTERCURRENT INFECTIONS

Infections, whatever their nature, can at the time of the fever, be associated with muscle and joint pain. However, there does appear to be a group of children, who, every time they get a sore throat, develop limb and joint pain out of all proportion to the severity of their intercurrent infection. At times there is evidence of a streptococcal aetiology, either from a throat swab or rising ASO titres. This pain comes *with* the sore throat rather than at some distant time. There is no swelling or limitation of movement of the joints and no carditis. At the time of the sore throat the ESR may be raised but settles rapidly in one to two weeks. A proportion of these children have been shown to have a low IgA. The importance of recognising intercurrent infection is, firstly, to distinguish it from rheumatic fever and, secondly, to control repeated streptococcal infections with appropriate antibiotics. Should this be unsuccessful, tonsillectomy may need to be considered.

Up to a week following upper respiratory infections or an influenza-like illness, severe myalgia with weakness of the muscles can develop. At the time the white blood cell count and platelets may be low and the CPK raised. Intercurrent infection is distinguished from polymyositis by the rapid spontaneous resolution occurring after a few days (McKinlay and Mitchell, 1976).

RICKETS

Infantile rickets has been well described in the immigrant population both from India and Pakistan (Benson *et al.*, 1963). The adolescent form occurs particularly in Pakistanis, who are well-nourished when they present, complaining of pain around the knees often aggravated by exercise. The ESR is normal and if the diagnosis of rickets is not considered, the symptoms are often thought to be psychogenic (Ford *et al.*, 1972).

IDIOPATHIC JUVENILE OSTEOPOROSIS

Previously healthy children approaching puberty present with pain at the ankles and knees or sometimes in the back. In contrast to limb pains described previously, this pain tends to be referred to the joints, more closely mimicking an arthritis. At this stage, with the ESR normal, it is not uncommon for these pains to be dismissed as psychological. A metaphyseal fracture with periosteal reaction just above the epiphyseal line at the knees or ankles is the diagnostic feature of idiopathic juvenile osteoporosis (Brenton and Dent, 1976). Histological and biochemical analyses are usually normal, apart from a negative calcium balance in severely affected patients who can get acetabuli protrusio.

COLD SENSITIVITY

In cold weather complaints of pain in the feet and ankles, affecting boys more than girls, are not unusual. Frequently, the child has been walking through puddles or standing around watching a football match, often in wet socks, and even though he changes later, he complains of persistent aching. There is considerable variation in patient susceptibility, some having mild, others having severe pain in the feet, ankles and legs.

PAINFUL FEET

Restriction with too tight socks and shoes can lead to discomfort and ultimately deformity. Ingrowing toenails, particularly of a great toe, often mean an ill-fitting shoe; claw toes are not uncommon and are aggravated by poor-fitting shoes. Avascular necrosis of the head of the second metatarsal (Freiberg's disease), occurs particularly in adolescents. There is usually a period of pain localised to that site. The pain subsides, although some distortion of the metatarsal head can be detected on palpation. Radiology is useful in differentiating this condition from others, as it is in pain localised to the tarsus due to avascular necrosis of the navicular. Again, this usually settles with time. Painful heels may be due to plantar fasciitis, which can be traumatic. Repeated episodes, and particularly the development of a calcaneal spur radiologically, should lead to the suspicion that the child, often a boy, may go on to suffer from juvenile ankylosing spondylitis (*see* p. 106). Fatigue or pain after weight-bearing can occur when a true flat foot deformity is present. In children with true flat feet the heel is everted, and the forefoot twists, so that the line of weight-bearing is directed on to the first metatarsophalangeal joint (Gross, 1977).

'PULLED' ELBOWS

This is most common between the age of one and three years, and considering how frequently mothers urge loitering children along by a sharp pull on the arm, it is relatively unusual. Pain is usually in the elbow, but can be referred to wrist and shoulder. The 'pulled' elbow is equivalent to 'radial head' dislocation and needs appropriate treatment (Illingworth, 1975).

BACK PAIN

Back pain is uncommon in children. Indeed, in an infant this condition has to be inferred from the parent's story of the child not wishing to be picked up, or being unwilling to stand or walk. In a child under the age of ten years, the presence of persistent back symptoms, often with muscle spasm and loss of movement, although rare, usually means a serious underlying pathological process which will, of course, include tumours (*Table 1.3*).

TABLE 1.3
Tumours which can cause back pain

Benign	*Malignant*
Aneurysmal bone cyst	Ewing's tumour
Osteoid osteoma	Osteogenic sarcoma
Osteogenic fibroma	Metastatic lesions
Eosinophilic granuloma (Histocytosis X)	Leukaemia Neuroblastoma Lymphoma
Benign osteoblastoma	
Vertebral giant cell tumours	

Persistent low back pain in older children (ten years and upwards), without disturbance of the general health, can be associated with spondylolisthesis (Blackburne and Velikas, 1977) which should be detected by adequate radiological assessment. As the age gets into double figures, back pain, while still unusual, does become somewhat more frequent (*Table 1.4*). Injury at sport probably constitutes the most common presentation to the general practitioner. This injury is usually short-lived, although, with an increasing number of young people tending to take up various forms of sport and athletics, it is beginning to cause relatively more problems. Indeed, in a number of teenagers who are not good at sport a minor injury is aggravated so that they can withdraw from the sport with honour.

Psychological back pain tends to 'hurt everywhere', is not relieved by any of the usually tried measures and has an absence of positive physical, laboratory or radiological findings. As with limb pains, this type of pain tends to run in families and contact with a parent or grandparent who has a similar complaint is not uncommon. Before assuming back pain is psychological, physical disease should be excluded, some idea of emotional disturbance should be sought and it is important to be reasonably certain that there is no underlying physical problem. It should be remembered that typical intervertebral disc compression syndromes do occasionally occur in teenagers, while, very rarely, juvenile ankylosing spondylitis (*see* p. 106) can present with back pain and very little in the way of abnormal laboratory or radiological findings initially.

TABLE 1.4
Some causes of back pain in adolescents

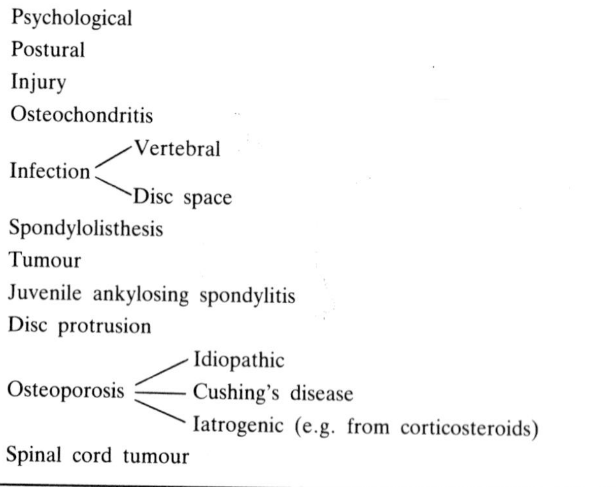

Cause	
Psychological	
Postural	
Injury	
Osteochondritis	
Infection	Vertebral
	Disc space
Spondylolisthesis	
Tumour	
Juvenile ankylosing spondylitis	
Disc protrusion	
Osteoporosis	Idiopathic
	Cushing's disease
	Iatrogenic (e.g. from corticosteroids)
Spinal cord tumour	

As in all types of rheumatic illness a good history is essential. This will need to be taken from the parents in the case of a young child, but teenagers should be encouraged to describe their own symptoms with verification from the family. The physical examination should include evaluation of posture, stance and gait as well as an examination of the back, legs, abdomen etc.

Postural pain

Faulty posture characterised by drooping of the spine, trunk, increased lumbar lordosis and forward drooping shoulders, rarely causes back pain until the second decade. It is important to look for causes which will vary from obvious ones such as unequal length of legs, to lack of sleep or poor lighting when reading. Treatment with purposeful exercises and corrective posture in recumbency is important if serious postural backache is to be avoided in later life (Hayden, 1967).

Scoliosis

Scoliosis rarely gives rise to pain although, particularly in adolescence, it can give rise to severe mental anguish. Some types of scoliosis can be easily explained, e.g. congenital malformation of vertebrae or an asymmetrical muscle paralysis, but the vast majority of types are idiopathic, with little known about aetiology and pathogenesis. Scoliosis is not rare: it has been suggested that as many as four in 1000 adolescent girls can be affected although in adolescent boys the incidence is only a tenth of this (Keim, 1976).

Osteochondritis of the spine

Osteochondritis of the spine is also known as Scheuermann's disease or juvenile kyphosis, and occcurs in teenagers. The thoracic region, particularly the lower part, is the most common site for this disease, although it can affect the lumbar region. The aetiology is unknown. It would appear that the initial abnormality is due to minor herniation of disc material related to the presence of multiple weakened areas within the cartilagenous plate, possibly on a congenital basis.

Clinically, the usual presentation is with pain together with localised tenderness, but at times kyphosis is the initial feature. Radiographic abnormalities include irregular vertebral outline, single or multiple radiolucencies within the vertebral body, often with sclerosis, and narrowing of the anterior vertebral body (*Figure 1.2a* and *b*). Discovertebral trauma due to a compression injury may also be associated with cartilagenous herniation, although in this instance there is usually more irregularity of vertebral body shape; indeed, the subsequent sclerosis may make this difficult to distinguish from infection. Ischaemia of the cartilagenous end plates occurs in sickle cell anaemia and produces a characteristic central indentation, the typical H appearance (*see Figure 7.3*, p. 220); this is asymptomatic unless secondary infection occurs (*see* p. 220).

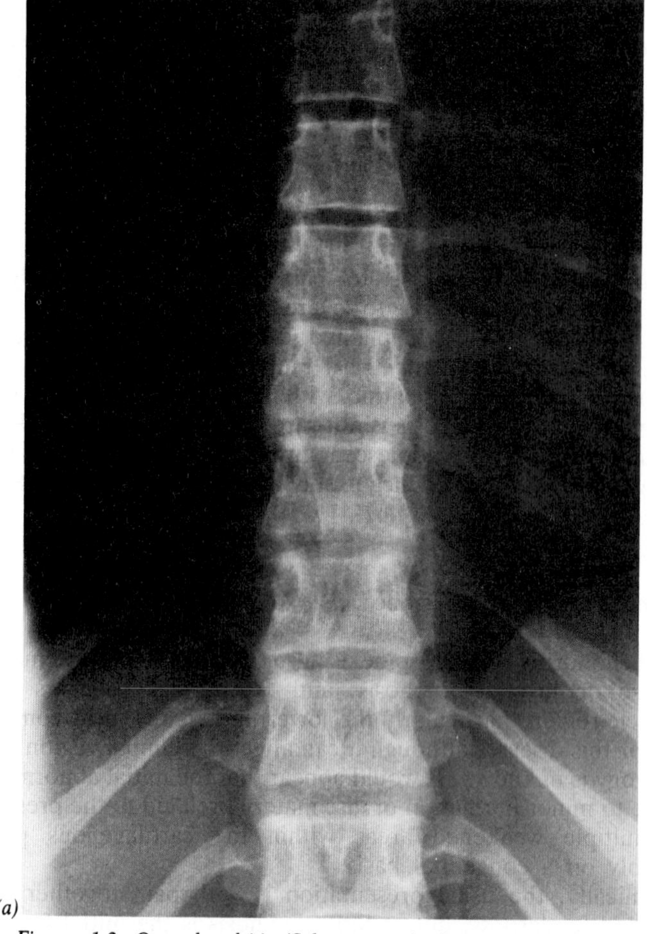

Figures 1.2. Osteochondritis (Scheuermann's disease or juvenile kyphosis). (a) A 12 year old girl with episodes of pain in the thoracic region for six months and now developing a mild kyphosis

Juvenile spondyloarthrosis or discitis

Juvenile discitis was at one time considered to be always due to infection as the radiological features closely resemble those of known infective conditions. However, Alexander (1970) has suggested that a non-infective cause is more likely in the majority of cases of juvenile discitis. He has suggested that it is due to partial dislocation of the epiphysis during the vulnerable period before the development of the protective metaphyseal changes

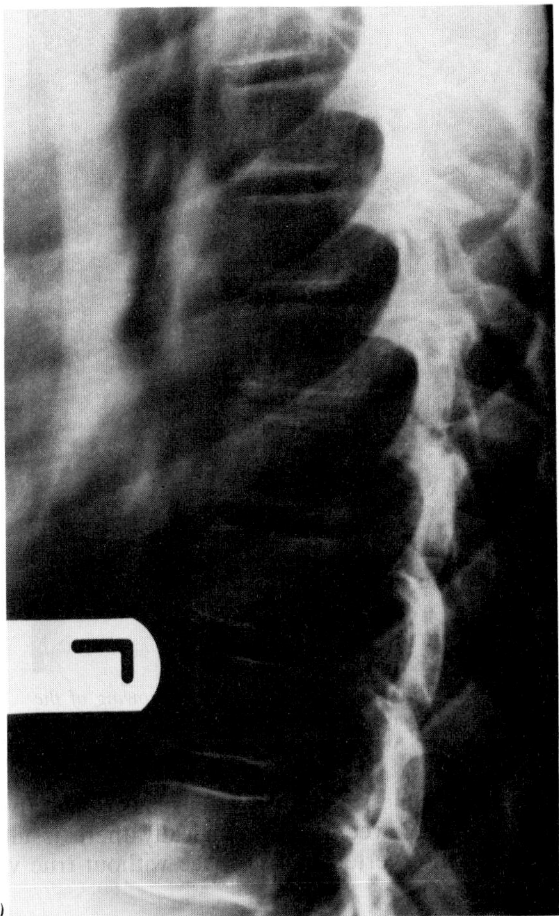

(b)

Figure 1.2(b). Note the disc space narrowing at D6/7 with irregularity of the opposing vertebral margins and slight loss of height at the right side of D6, all consistent with osteochondritis

which start about the age of eight years. The third to the fifth lumbar vertebrae, the most common site of involvement, are at the maximum stress on forward flexion and at maximum mobility on lateral flexion. The condition is rare above the tenth dorsal vertebra, at which range lateral flexion is much less. There is not uncommonly a history of minor trauma before the sudden onset of pain in the back. There is relatively little disturbance of general health, certainly no systemic illness and the ESR is usually normal.

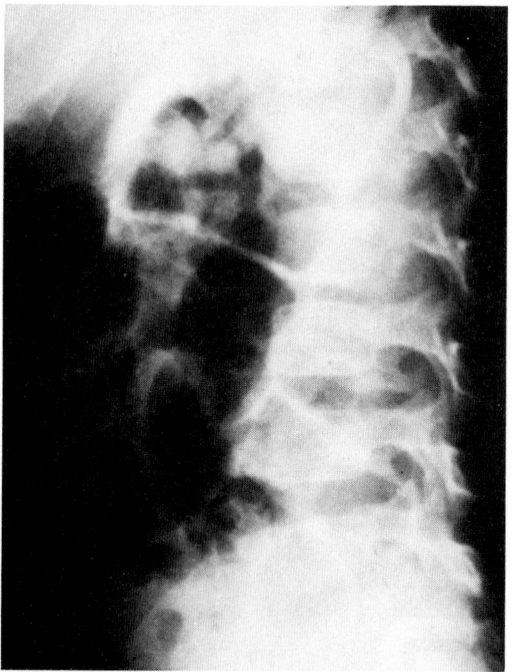

Figure 1.3. Juvenile discitis. Note the narrowing of the lumbar disc space, which was obvious some months after the acute symptoms

The duration of the illness is short-lived, usually two to five weeks but can last up to 12 weeks. Radiologically there is ultimately narrowing of the intervertebral disc space without true vertebral erosion (*Figure 1.3*).

Infections

Vertebral

Acute osteomyelitis is uncommon but can occur at any age. It is usually due to *Staphylococcus aureus*, but can be caused by other organisms including the *Brucellae*. The onset is acute with fever, toxaemia, and back pain which is often fairly well localised but can radiate to the chest and abdomen. Investigations and management are as for osteomyelitis (*see* p. 240).

Tuberculosis is now rare. It should, however, be borne in mind, particularly in Asian children and when there is a history of contact with tuberculosis. The symptoms of pain and stiffness with loss of movement usually develop gradually over weeks or months. A cold abscess can develop which in the lumbar region points as a psoas abscess, but in the thoracic region may give rise to paraplegia (*see* p. 27).

Intervertebral disc space infection

This infection is relatively more common particularly in children under ten years as the blood supply to the intervertebral disc present during the first decade allows haematogenous spread. It is also thought that the infection may arise as a sequel to a very small intervertebral abscess. Intervertebral disc space infection is most common in the upper lumbar region. The usual onset is of acute pain in the back associated with fever and a raised ESR. In those children under five years there is relatively little complaint about the back, but more of abdominal pain and sometimes there is difficulty in walking. At other times the infection can present as a vague lower limb pain. On examination there is local tenderness, spasm of muscles and loss of movement. At presentation, routine radiology is likely to be normal, but bone scanning with technetium is valuable in localising the lesion (Wenger *et al.*,1978); ultimately disc space narrowing does occur. Every effort should be made to identify the organism present. This should be treated as any infection in any other site (*see* p. 260).

NECK PROBLEMS

Torticollis

An infant who presents with torticollis requires a neurological, ophthalmological and radiological assessment before it can be assumed that torticollis is due to unilateral shortening of the sternomastoid muscle. Acute transient torticollis may be the result of trauma, be seen in association with swelling of lymph nodes after throat infections or occur apparently spontaneously after thoat infections. In older children, therapy with drugs such as phenothiazine, haloperidol and methodopramide may be associated with spasm of muscle (Boltshauser, 1976). Psychogenic torticollis needs to be differentiated from that due to trauma or disease (*see* p. 64). Very occasionally juvenile chronic arthritis can present as torticollis, which is due to subluxation of C2 on C3, predominantly unilateral apophyseal joint involvement or atlanto-axial subluxation (*see* p. 63).

Calcification of intervertebral discs

Transient calcification of a cervical intervertebral disc space usually C6/7 in a child aged five to ten years is associated with a severe neck pain and often fever. Its aetiology is unknown but occasionally appears to follow intercurrent infection. Spontaneous resolution usually occurs over six to ten weeks but very occasionally spinal cord compression warrants surgical treatment (Swick, 1975). Histologically, well developed hyaline and fibrocartilage is seen with several stages of calcification recognisable in Swick's two cases. Very occasionally, asymptomatic calcification is found in multiple discs, usually in the thoracic spine, when one or more cervical ones may also be affected.

REFERENCES

Alexander, C. J. (1970). The aetiology of juvenile spondyloarthritis (discitis). *Clinical Radiology,* **21,** 178–187

Ansell, B. M. (1972). Hypermobility of joints. *Modern Trends in Orthopaedics*, **6**, 25. London; Butterworths

Apley, J. (1976). Limb pains with no organic disease. *Clinics in Rheumatic Diseases*, **2**, 487. Philadelphia; W. B. Saunders Co Ltd

Apley, J. and Naish, J. M. (1955). *Modern Trends in Psychomatic Medicine.* London; Butterworths

Beighton, P. (1970). *Ehlers–Danlos Syndrome.* London; Heinemann

Benson, P. F., Stroud, C. E., Mitchell, N. J. and Nicholaides, A. (1963). Rickets in immigrant children in London. *British Medical Journal*, **1**, 1054

Blackburne, J. S. and Velikas, E. P. (1977). Spondylolisthesis in children and adolescents. *Journal of Bone and Joint Surgery*, **59B**, 490

Boltshauser, E. (1976). Different diagnosis of torticollis in childhood. *Schweiz. Med. Wochenschr.*, **106**, 1261

Brenton, D. P. and Dent, C. F. (1976). Idiopathic juvenile osteoporosis. In *Inborn Errors of Calcium and Bone Metabolism*, p. 222 Lancaster; MTP Press

Brenton, D. P., Daw, C. J., James, J. I. P., Hay, R. L. and Wynne Davies, R. (1972). Homocystinuria and Marfan's Syndrome: a comparison. *Journal of Bone and Joint Surgery,* **54B,** 277

Carter, C. and Sweetnam, R. (1958). Familial joint laxity and recurrent dislocation of the patella. *Journal of Bone and Joint Surgery*, **40B**, 664

Creak, M. (1969). Hysteria in childhood. *Acta Paedopsychiat. (Basel)*, **36**, 269–274

Dubowitz, V. (1978). Muscle disorders in childhood. *Major Problems in Clinical Paediatrics*, **16**. Philadelphia; W. B. Saunders Co Ltd

Dubowitz, V. and Hersov, L. (1976). Management of children with non-organic (hysterical) disorders of motor function. *Developmental Medicine and Child Neurology*, **18**, 358

Ford, J. A., Colhoun, E. M., McIntosh, W. B. and Dunnigan, M. G. (1972). Rickets and osteomalacia in the Glasgow Pakistani community 1961–1977. *British Medical Journal*, **2**, 677

Gross, R. H. (1977). Foot pain in children. *Paediatric Clinics of North America*, **24**, 813

Hayden, J. W. (1967). Back pain in childhood. *Paediatric Clinics of North America*, **14**, 611

Illingworth, C. M. (1975). Pulled elbows: a study of 100 patients. *British Medical Journal*, **2**, 672

Jimenez, S. A. and Lally, E. Y. (1979/80). Disorders of collagen metabolism. *Bulletin of Rheumatic Diseases,* **3–4,** 1016

Keim, H. A (1976). *The Adolescent Spine*. (Modern Orthopaedic Monographs Series) New York; Grune and Stratton

McKinlay, I. A. and Mitchell, I. (1976). Transient acute myositis in childhood. *Archives of Diseases in Childhood*, **51**, 135

Pope, F. M. and Nicholls, A. C. (1978). Molecular abnormalities of collagen. *Journal of Clinical Pathology*, **30**, suppl. (Royal College of Pathology) **12**, 95

Sinclair, R. J., Kitchin, A. H. and Turner, R. W. (1960). The Marfan Syndrome. *Quarterly Journal of Medicine*, **29**, 19

Swick, H. N. (1975). Calcification of intervertebral discs in childhood. *Journal of Pediatrics*, **86**, 364

Wenger, D. R., Bobechko, W. P. and Gilday, D. L. (1978). The spectrum of intervertebral disc space infection in children. *Journal of Bone and Joint Surgery*, **60-A/1**, 100

CHAPTER 2

Monarticular arthritis

Any child with pain and/or swelling of a single joint, presents problems in diagnosis, prognosis and treatment which differ in many respects from those of polyarthritis (*see* Chapter 3). These problems are therefore considered in this separate chapter.

The onset of monarticular arthritis may be sudden or insidious. Presentation will vary according to the age of the child and the cause. In a young child, the parents may notice swelling of a joint, disinclination to use a limb, or screaming on being stood up, while the older child will often complain of pain and difficulty in using a joint. When a child has swelling, of even a single joint, it is important to establish the diagnosis and begin appropriate treatment at the earliest possible moment, as delay can lead to irreparable harm with lifelong consequences. A synovial joint is an extremely sensitive structure. The main features of monarticular arthritis are pain, swelling and deformity, and loss of function of the joint in varying proportions. It should always be remembered that a single joint can be involved as part of a generalised process or as the precursor of polyarthritis (*Table 2.1*).

History

The history of onset is of paramount importance; it should be taken meticulously from the patient when old enough, as well as from the parents. It should include specific questions relating to other possible joint involvement. Clues may be immediate, such as a recent infection or a background of haemophilia. Alternatively, clues can be hidden and leading questions will be needed to bring

TABLE 2.1
Causes of monarticular arthritis

Causes
Trauma
Mechanical derangements
Infections
Juvenile chronic arthritis
Arthritis associated with other disorders, e.g. psoriasis, ulcerative colitis and regional enteritis
Blood dyscrasias
Synovial anomalies
Neoplasms – local or generalised

out relevant symptoms such as a transitory rash or an earlier episode of similar trouble, perhaps affecting another joint. Children are prone to injury and this is probably the commonest cause of a single painful swollen joint. However, trauma should not be assumed unless the history can be fully substantiated by the child or a witness. Minor repetitive incidents can produce a simple traumatic synovitis which will mimic the signs of a more serious pathological process. It should also be remembered that minor injury or excessive use can provoke a reaction in a joint already the site of any early pathological process.

Examination

Examination should be conducted with all the child's clothes removed at some stage. It is essential that all reachable joints are examined to make certain that the doctor is dealing with a truly monarticular arthritis. Special attention should be paid to the general condition of the child; an overall examination is required to look for other physical abnormalities, such as cervical lymphadenopathy suggesting a previous upper respiratory infection, or a patch of psoriasis suggesting a possible cause of chronic arthritis. From the general examination of the child, it will be determined if fever is present, and whether there is generalised or localised wasting, as well as the state of the affected joint.

Investigations

The following haematological investigations will need to be considered (*Table 2.2*). As far as possible, all necessary studies

TABLE 2.2
Investigations which may be necessary (*see text*)

Haematological
ESR, Hb, WBC with differential. Platelets
Blood cultures
Antibodies to *Brucella, Salmonella,* etc.
Bleeding and cloting times
Antinuclear antibodies
Rheumatoid factor
Serum store for viral antibodies, etc.
Radiological
X-ray of affected and opposite joint
Anterior/posterior and lateral views
Tomography
Bone scan
Other
Synovial fluid analysis and culture
Synovial membrane histology and culture
Tuberculin tests

should be planned before blood is taken in order to avoid multiple venepunctures. These studies may include blood culture, agglutinations to *Salmonella, Brucella* etc., antinuclear antibodies and rheumatoid factor. It is also advisable to store a small sample of serum in case viral antibodies or further studies are required at a later date. Usually, agglutination tests for IgM rheumatoid factor (i.e. Latex, SCAT) are negative, but the presence of antinuclear antibodies, particularly in high titre, will suggest that the condition is juvenile chronic arthritis (Still's disease) (*see* p. 87).

It is important to x-ray the affected joint and the opposite one, as it is only by comparison that minor radiological changes can be appreciated. The films should be accurately centred to include the epiphyseal and metaphyseal region on either side of the target joint; it is essential to see the anterior/posterior and lateral views, particularly in joints like the knees, elbows and hips, as certain features may be defined in one view but not in another. For instance, a minimal slip of the femoral epiphysis may be recognised only in the lateral view. In special circumstances, oblique or specially angled views will be necessary to identify a lesion, e.g. the tunnel or intercondylar view of the knee for osteochondritis dissecans. Whenever possible, the joint of the opposite limb should be x-rayed on the same film as the affected side. This will enable minor differences such as osteoporosis, epiphyseal overgrowth from hyperaemia (*Figure 2.1*) as well as differences in soft tissue shadows to be detected. Tomography and bone scanning are occasionally helpful when the bone itself contains a lesion which is ill-defined on standard radiographs. Even when the x-rays are normal at first presentation, it may be necessary to repeat appropriate x-rays at a later date if joint symptoms persist.

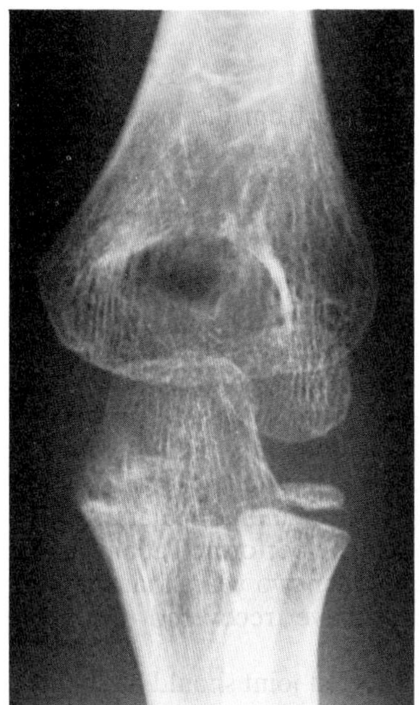

(a)

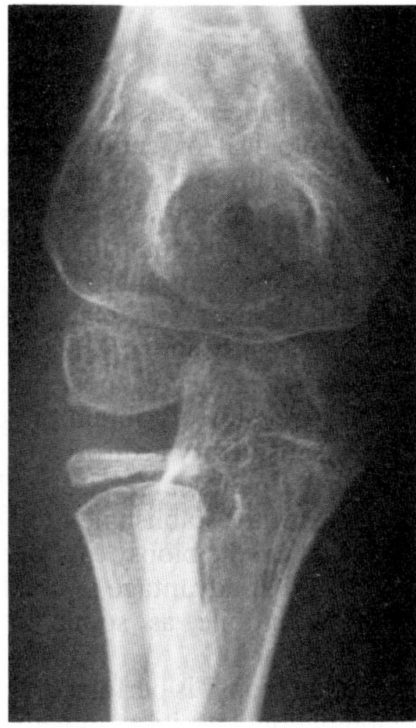

(b)

Figure 2.1a and b. Monarticular arthritis of the elbow. Showing osteoporosis, a periosteal reaction and overgrowth of the epiphyses of the left elbow as compared to the right. Biopsy confirmed juvenile chronic arthritis

Aspiration of synovial fluid

Synovial fluid for investigation is essential in suspected cases of infection and at times helpful in the rheumatic conditions. Aspiration of a swollen joint requires a full sterile procedure. In an older child it may be possible to do this under local anaesthesia but in a frightened restless ill younger child, not only is it kinder to give a general anaesthetic but it is more likely that satisfactory information will be obtained from the material so obtained. The fluid can be clear, turbid, or blood-stained. Examination for the type and number of cells and organisms will give clues, e.g. to infection. The protein content is also helpful (*see* Appendix, p. 280). It is essential that the fluid is cultured; if there is any suspicion of tuberculosis being the cause of the swollen joint a guinea-pig inoculation must be performed. Under such circumstances, chest x-ray and a Heaf or Mantoux test are essential.

Biopsy

Biopsy will be necessary to obtain tissue from the involved joint for histological or cultural examination when other procedures have not allowed a diagnosis to be made. Two methods are available – open or needle biopsy. The knee is the most commonly affected joint in monarthritis: an open biopsy can lead to loss of movement or contracture, particularly in young children, so every effort should be made to avoid open biopsy. The newer techniques of needle biopsy and arthroscopy are extremely valuable; using the latter, a good view of most parts of the joint can be obtained, so that it is possible to obtain the biopsy from a selected site. In our hands, satisfactory arthroscopy can be done in a child as young as two and a half years. This is the ideal method of doing a knee biopsy for the establishment of diagnosis in monarticular arthritis.

Closed needle biopsy can, of course, be performed at any age; it has the great advantage in children under two years that they can be fully mobile as soon as they have recovered from the anaesthetic.

If open biopsy is performed the affected joint should be splinted in a functional position immediately following surgery to prevent a contracture being induced by the procedure; then as soon as possible the joint can be fully remobilised. It will, of course, be necessary to do an open biopsy at sites other than the knee, with the possible exception of the elbow, where a needle biopsy is feasible.

Principles of management

Inflammation in a single joint is frequently associated with muscle spasm leading to the joint being held in a postion of comfort; this is usually flexion. If the inflammation is untreated, the danger is in the development of a flexion contracture, so that when the muscle spasm is relieved the flexion deformity remains. This deformity is produced by the shortening and later fibrosis of the capsule and ligaments.

When a patient is admitted the affected joint should be rested in a position of useful function. An affected hip is best controlled by traction with some abduction; extension strapping is applied to the skin and weight transmitted to a pulley at the end of the bed. The weight should be 0.5 kg for every 5 kg of the patient's weight. In preventing a flexion contracture the patient should, of course, be nursed flat on his back.

A swollen knee is held straight by a posterior splint, conventionally made from plaster of Paris, while the foot and ankle are maintained at a right-angle to the leg by a similar method. If these splints are held in place by a light crepe bandage, regular access and inspection of the joint can continue.

If the arthritis is in the shoulder, the shoulder is supported by a sling; if in the elbow, by a collar and cuff (which holds the joint at a right-angle) or a plaster shell; while the arthritic wrist should be in a cock-up splint with the fingers and thumb flexed over a roll of bandage in the palm.

Once the diagnosis is established, appropriate therapy is instituted.

SEPTIC ARTHRITIS

Infection should be suspected if a joint is hot, tense and swollen and with all movement rigidly guarded in a child who is febrile, toxic and in severe pain. These symptoms will most usually be the result of septicaemia or bacteraemia, the source of which may not be obvious. They can follow undeclared penetrating injuries, while the issue may be further confused by the fact that infection can reach the joint cavity from osteomyelitis in an adjacent bone. This fact is of particular importance in the hip where the femoral metaphysis is intracapsular. During examination, the doctor should look for a mark on the skin over the joint and bruising around it, as well as an infected focus such as a paronychia or an open sore elsewhere. The most valuable clinical sign of osteomyelitis is persistent localised bone tenderness in the metaphysis.

In infancy

Septic arthritis in infancy requires separate consideration because of the special features which occur when the disease arises in the first year of life. The most striking feature is the rapid destruction, due to the vulnerability of cartilage and the lack of a metaphyseal barrier. There is frequently immunodeficiency characterised by a subdued clinical response to infection (Lloyd Roberts and Ratliff, 1978). The most usual site of infection is the hip, with *Staphylococcus aureus* the usual invader, although a wide range of bacteria have been described. Presentation can be that of a baby who appears very ill, flaccid, rejects or vomits feeds, is icteric, cyanosed or convulsing. On the other hand, the baby may be relatively unaffected by this severe illness, presenting as a mild unexplained fever, feeding difficulty or failure to thrive.

Local examination can fail initially to reveal the true nature of the problem,particularly if antibiotics have already been given. There may be little more than a disinclination to move the joint or a pain reaction on passive movement. The hip will, however, soon adopt a flexed and adducted position while oedema affecting particularly the adductor region and genitalia gradually appears. Ultimately, signs of an abscess and of hip displacement develop; by this time destruction will probably have proceeded beyond the stage of potential recovery. In contrast to the older child, periostitis around the proximal femoral shaft may appear in the infant within a few days of onset.

The compromised host

In patients with immune deficiency, either primary or induced (as in leukaemia and its therapy) and less commonly, in juvenile chronic arthritis, systemic lupus erythematosus and regional enteritis, joint infection may not only be masked but may also be due to less common organisms such as *Mycoplasma pneumoniae* (Webster *et al.*, 1977), *Haemophilus influenzae* or haemolytic streptococcus. Its recognition requires alertness. A change in the joint state or unusual signs or general deterioration in health, development of a low grade fever, etc. warrant investigation.

X-ray and other investigations

Early radiological examination is of little help as it takes a week or more from onset for raising of the periosteum or mottling of the bone to be seen; before that, all that is seen is capsular distension. Technetium scanning, however, may be of use in demonstrating a hot spot (*Figure 2.2*). While the ESR is usually raised and there is frequently a polymorph leucocytosis, these are not necessarily present and are non-specific. *It is therefore important in any case of suspected infection to take blood for culture and aspirate the joint before giving antibiotics.*

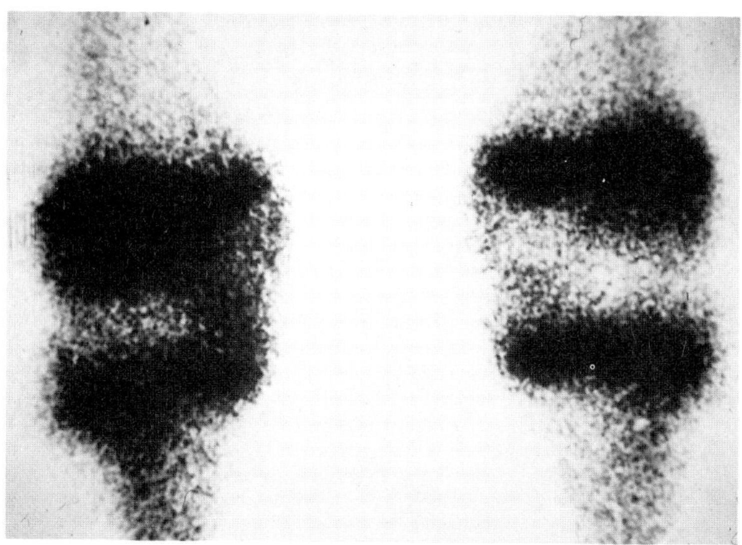

Figure 2.2. Monarticular arthritis due to infection. Technetium scan in a seven year old boy with three days of increasing pain and difficulty in extending the right knee. The plain x-ray was normal, but on technetium scanning there is increased uptake on the affected side. Blood culture grew Staphylococcus aureus

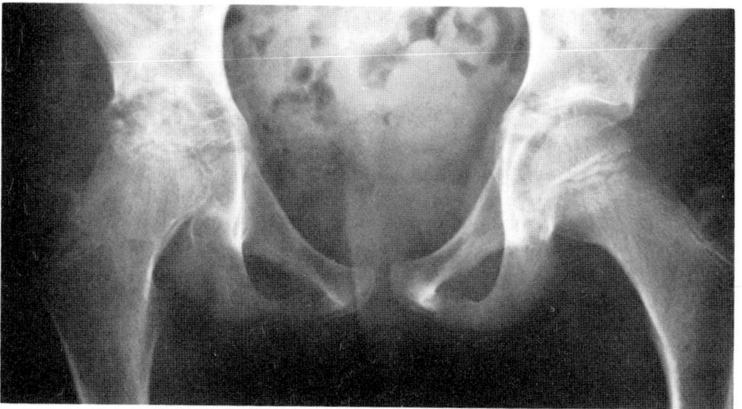

Figure 2.3. Monarticular septic arthritis of the right hip. Gross destruction where the diagnosis of septic arthritis had been delayed

While a turbid fluid, with a white count of 100 000 or more (polymorphonuclear cells predominating) suggests infection, the presence of organisms in the joint fluid presumes a diagnosis of septic arthritis. If the organisms cannot be identified, osteomyelitis must be reconsidered as the epiphyseal plate presents a barrier with the joint effusion a secondary symptom, rather than a primary one indicating direct infection. The importance of recognising infection early and treating it is based on the serious consequences if therapy is delayed (*Figure 2.3*) (Howard *et al.*, 1976). Should antibiotics have been given already, the diagnosis may be extremely difficult as the child is not particularly ill, the joint does not necessarily appear hot and tense, and cultures of both blood and synovial fluid will often be negative. Under such circumstances, a high ESR and high anti-staphylolysin titres are helpful, while ultimately on x-ray the ossific nucleus of bone may be seen to be speckled and can ultimately disappear.

Management

As soon as appropriate samples for diagnosis have been taken the affected joint is rested either in plaster or by traction in a position of function, and antibiotics are then commenced. Blockey and McAllister (1972) suggest fusidic acid microsuspension together with erythromycin, in appropriate dosage for the age of the child, until such time as cultures and sensitivities become available when, if necessary, these can be changed to more appropriate antibiotics according to sensitivities. If the child is under two years of age, the likelihood of *H. influenzae* is high so ampicillin is probably the drug of choice until confirmation of the organism is made (Clarke, 1978).

There are no indications for urgent surgical intervention in either septic arthritis or osteomyelitis (Nade, 1977). If there is still joint swelling at 48 hours all the infected effusion is aspirated. Reaccumulation of any effusion may warrant repetition of the procedure, when, if it is considered desirable, antibiotics can be put into the joint.

Only if there has been delay in diagnosis and pus is too thick to be withdrawn adequately with a wide bore needle, or there has been a failure to improve, will surgical drainage need to be considered.

This is also true for osteomyelitis, when failure to gain clinical improvement,as shown by persistent fever, increasing local tenderness after immobilisation, fluid replacement and adequate antibiotics will surgical drainage be required (Nade, 1977).

Antibiotics will need to be continued for six to 12 weeks according to the speed with which therapy was instituted and the response to it, with the ESR a useful guide.

As the infection subsides, the traction or splints are removed daily for gentle exercises. Once all spasm has passed, the limb may be left free so that muscle function can be encouraged by the performance of appropriate exercises. In the case of the lower limb, it is important to make sure that muscle function is adequate, prior to allowing weight bearing; thus after a knee infection the quadriceps should be strong enough to allow the child to hold the leg in the air and count to 50.

In compromised hosts, e.g. those with leukaemia or hypogammaglobulinaemia, it may be very difficult to control infections and high doses of antibiotics are essential. These high doses need to be continued for a minimum of 12 weeks, and sometimes up to a year, particularly if there has been a previous episode of infection which was difficult to treat. In bacteraemic shock or in patients on corticosteroids, corticosteroids are given in increased doses for two to three days.

TUBERCULOSIS

Typically, this causes a chronic, insidious, monarticular arthritis, with knee, hip and wrist the most common sites. In the UK and the USA it is now rare, but does still occur and the child from Asia and Africa appears to be at particular risk. Dactylitis or tendon sheath effusion at wrist or ankle has also been noted as the presenting sign in such children. The most frequent presenting symptom is pain, especially on movement, together with marked swelling. There is usually considerable muscle wasting. There may be general deterioration in health with loss of weight and low grade fever while other sites of infection, e.g. chest or renal tract, are occasionally found. Initially the only radiological abnormality is osteoporosis. Every effort should be made to establish a diagnosis before erosive changes have occurred (*Figures 2.4a* and *b*). The ESR is usually raised and the tuberculin skin test is positive. Confirmation of diagnosis is made by the identification of organisms in the synovial fluid or membrane.

Combined chemotherapy with immobilisation of the affected joint is generally successful. If there is severe persistent synovitis, synovectomy or even debridement may need to be considered.

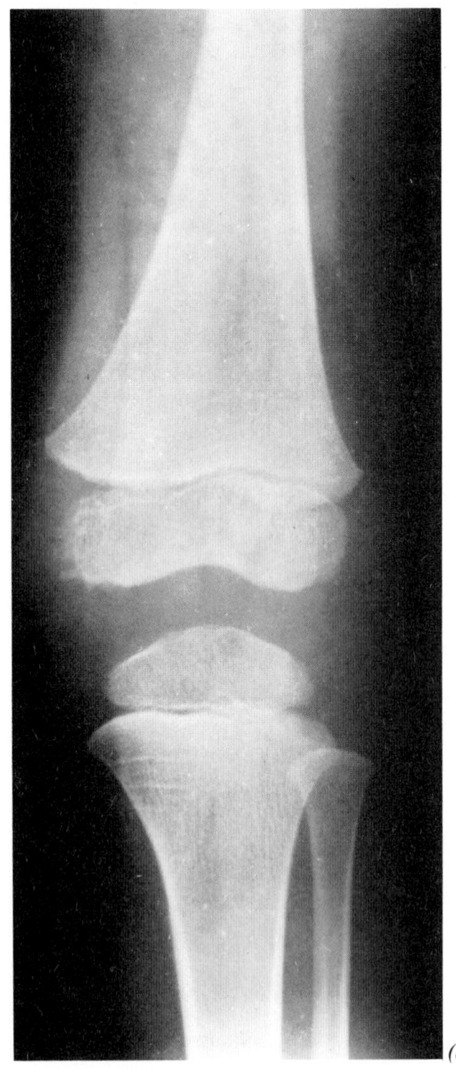

(a)

Figure 2.4a. Tuberculosis arthritis. Eight year old girl with swelling of the right knee of some ten days duration; no definite abnormality seen and trauma suspected

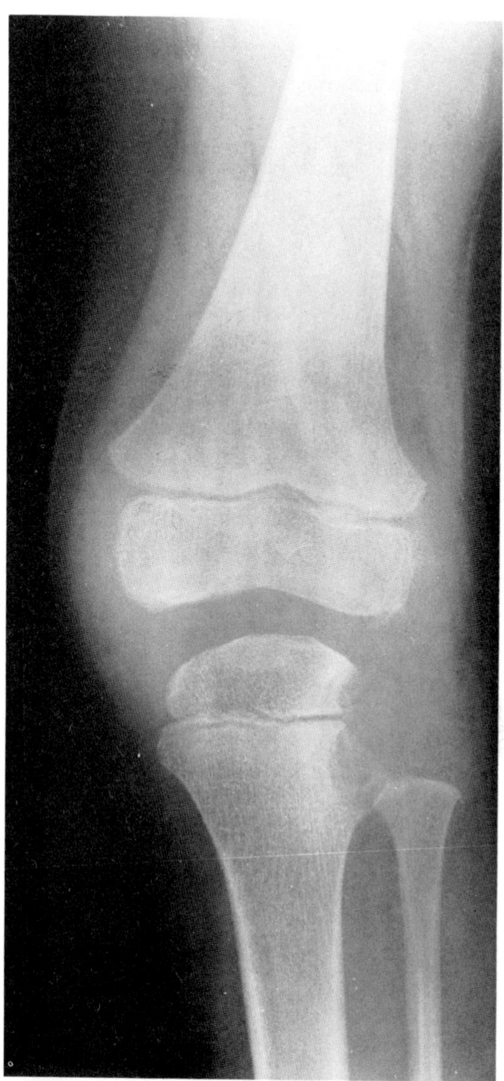

(b)

Figure 2.4b. Eight months later after persistent swelling of the knee gross erosion of the epiphysis and metaphysis. At this stage, the synovial biopsy was typical of tuberculosis and organisms were obtained from the synovial fluid and membrane

Other rare infections

The decline in tuberculosis and the increasing use of drugs which compromise the host make it important to consider atypical mycobacteria as a cause of monarticular arthritis. Fungal arthritis, coccidiomycosis, blastomycosis and sporotrichosis are also seen under such circumstances but often affect more than one joint (Goldenberg and Cohen, 1978).

JUVENILE CHRONIC ARTHRITIS (STILL'S DISEASE) (*See* Chapter 4)

Although juvenile chronic arthritis is generally considered polyarticular, Cassidy *et al.* (1967) reported a monarticular onset in 31 per cent of their cases, while in the author's experience this has been of the order of 12 per cent. Although any joints can be affected singly, the most usual are the knee and ankle, followed by the wrist. There is usually little disturbance of general health, the ESR is often normal, rheumatoid factor negative, although occasionally the presence of antinuclear antibodies will give a

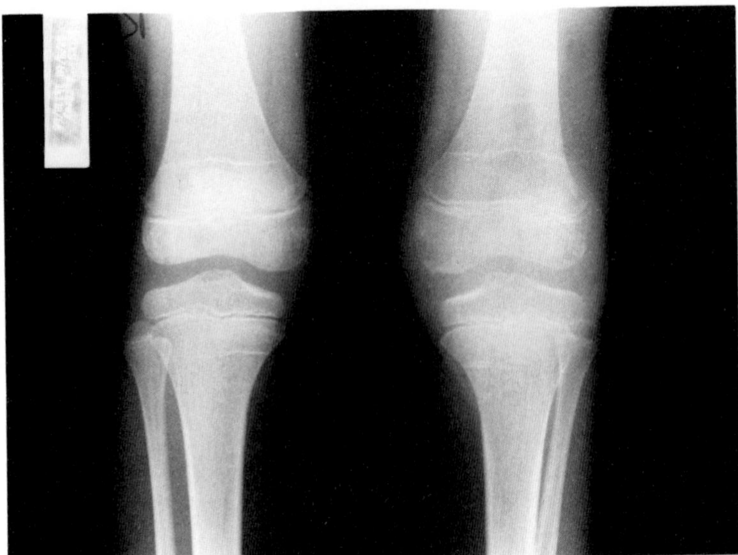

Figure 2.5. Juvenile chronic monarticular arthritis of the left knee after 11 months in an eight year old boy; note the osteoporosis with increased growth of the epiphyses and overgrowth of adjacent long bones on the affected side

diagnostic clue. Radiological changes consist of osteoporosis early, and, after about six months, accelerated epiphyseal maturation and overgrowth of long bones adjacent to the affected joint (*Figure 2.5*) occurs. Biopsy of the synovial membrane will provide a characteristic histological appearance. This substantive evidence is essential or ongoing diseases may be overlooked.

SYNOVIAL DISORDERS OTHER THAN TUBERCULOSIS AND JUVENILE CHRONIC ARTHRITIS

Haemangioma

The commonest site for haemangioma is the knee. Symptoms consist of episodes of acute swelling, often associated with minimal trauma; at times internal derangement may be suspected because of episodes of catching or locking. Examination in an acute phase reveals only an effusion with varying degrees of tenderness. Very occasionally, and particularly between acute episodes, a tender mass is felt. After several episodes overgrowth of the epiphyses and, occasionally the metaphyses occur. Aspiration may reveal almost pure blood, blood-stained synovial fluid or a deep yellow fluid with a high bilirubin content. The presence of cutaneous angiomata, particularly on the affected leg, epiphyseal overgrowth in the absence of persistent overt synovitis and the history of recurrent knee swelling with over-use are suggestive of the disorder but diagnosis is frequently not made until arthroscopy or arthrotomy. In the presence of cutaneous lesions, angiography will demonstrate the severity of the lesion.

Villonodular synovitis

This type of benign proliferation of synovial tissue is rare but must be differentiated from a malignant synovioma. Although it can affect any joint, or even a tendon sheath, the knee has the highest incidence of this disease. Symptoms include swelling from synovial thickening, discomfort and episodes mimicking mechanical derangement of the joint. Examination may reveal thickening, particularly of the suprapatellar pouch, and an effusion into the joint. In some 20 per cent of patients, radiographs will show subarticular cysts and, as in a single haemangioma, repeated bleeding into the joint will be associated with overgrowth of epiphyses radiologically. Occasionally, subarticular cysts and erosions are also seen. The synovial fluid is frequently blood-stained or deep yellow with a high bilirubin content. Needle biopsy will reveal characteristic histology consisting of hyperplasia, synovial cells often containing haemosiderin as well as increased vascularity and macrophages stuffed with products of erythrocyte degradation. If an arthrotomy is performed, brown hypertrophic grape-like lobulated processes are seen projecting into the joint space.

Malignant synovioma

Malignant synovioma is excessively rare and can only be differentiated from other causes of synovial proliferation on histology.

Transient synovitis of the hip

This term is used to describe a condition which is somewhat ill-defined and for which no definite cause has been established; it is also referred to variously as coxalgia fugax, irritable hip and observation hip. The last emphasises the fact that it is only by exclusion that patients fit into this category. Transient synovitis will need to be distinguished from a number of conditions as indicated in *Table 2.3*. This does not, however, stop it being the commonest cause of hip pain in children under the age of ten, with boys being more commonly affected than girls. The onset is

TABLE 2.3
Differential diagnosis of transient synovitis of the hip

Single episode	*Recurrent*
Infection of joint	Following streptococcal infections
Perthes' disease	In 'allergic' children
Slipped femoral epiphysis	Juvenile ankylosing spondylitis
Rheumatic fever	
Juvenile chronic arthritis	
Juvenile ankylosing spondylitis	
Leukaemia	
Gaucher's disease	
Osteoid osteoma	

usually abrupt but can be insidious with a complaint of pain in the hip and/or pain in the knee on the affected side. Loss of function varies from a limp to complete inability to take weight on the affected leg.

Examination will reveal a healthy child, and the degree of loss of movement of the hip will vary from acute spasm with loss of all movement to mild restriction. There is no evidence of muscle wasting. At times there is a low grade fever and, while the ESR can be raised, it is usually normal. It is rare for the haemoglobin or white blood cell count to be abnormal. Radiologically, there is usually no abnormality though occasionally there may be slight widening of the joint space on the affected side.

If there is a real doubt that infection could be present, e.g. in a child with a fever and acute spasm around the hip, the condition should be treated as such pending the result of investigations rather than waiting for two or three days. In general, this is a benign condition in which there is no good evidence for a viral infection and trauma remains the most frequent explanation. Very occasionally Perthes' disease appears to follow an episode of transient synovitis; long-term follow-up has occasionally revealed coxa magna on the affected side. Although occasionally a second episode of transient synovitis of the hip occurs on the opposite side, repeated episodes should lead to re-evaluation. This may be the precursor of juvenile ankylosing spondylitis (p. 106) particularly in older boys, while other causes include infiltration, as in leukaemia (p. 230) and osteoid osteoma (p. 34). Of interest also are the recurrent mild episodes after streptococcal infections and those conditions seen in allergic children, which carry a good prognosis.

Thorn synovitis

The frequency of foreign body synovitis due to penetration of a joint is not unknown and may well be commoner than the literature would suggest (Sugarman *et al.*, 1977). All the cases reported by these authors resulted from penetration by palm thorn. However, we have seen a similar picture in children following the penetration of rose thorns and other splinters of wood. The clinical presentation is that of an acute synovitis. It usually affects the knee but has been seen in a metacarpophalangeal joint. Tests reveal no evidence of infection and the condition develops into a chronic arthritis of the involved joint. Histologically there will ultimately be a granulomatous synovitis.

Absolute diagnosis is made by identifying the penetrating object, but this often requires polarised light microscopy. Management is by excision of the affected synovium.

In the initial diagnosis, a history of trauma or evidence of a puncture wound over the affected joint may be helpful. It is, however, usually necessary to consider arthroscopy and biopsy for diagnosis. It should also be remembered that any type of foreign body penetrating a joint can also give rise to infection, so even when there is a clear-cut history of injury and evidence of a penetrating wound, one should not omit the search for an infecting organism.

MECHANICAL DERANGEMENTS

Osteoid osteoma

When an osteoid osteoma is near a joint the presentation often suggests arthritis. As there is a predilection for the trochanteric area, recurrent acute or sub-acute pain and loss of movement of the hip is common. Radiologically, the tumour may be difficult to detect. There can be widespread osteoporosis, local sclerosis or a translucent area with a nidus in it; oblique projections, tomography and bone scanning are useful aids in diagnosis (Sim *et al.*, 1975).

Other benign bone tumours which can mimic arthritis include simple solitary cysts, aneurysmal bone cysts, localised fibrous dysplasia and localised eosinophilic granuloma; while in the older child of 12 or more, malignancy in the form of osteogenic sarcoma, chondrosarcoma and Ewing's tumour occasionally mimic a joint problem. Radiology will suggest the diagnosis and biopsy confirm it.

Perthes' disease

Perthes' disease is an ischaemic necrosis of the upper femoral epiphysis which, as it is an intracapsular bone, presents as a hip lesion (Catteral, 1970; Lloyd Roberts and Ratliff, 1978). The commonest age of onset of the disease is between the ages of four and nine but it may occur throughout childhood and adolescence. Boys are affected four times as often as girls and the disease can be bilateral in as many as 15 per cent. The presenting feature in Perthes' disease is usually a limp in a healthy child; this may be persistent or variable, often associated with some degree of pain felt in the groin and the knee. At times the child presents with a painful knee. On examination the child is generally fit and the physical signs are limited to the hip with loss of movement to a varying degree, particularly flexion, abduction and internal rotation. Haematological examination will be normal, but by the time of presentation epiphyseal changes are usually sufficiently advanced to allow an immediate diagnosis to be made radiologically (*Figure 2.6*).

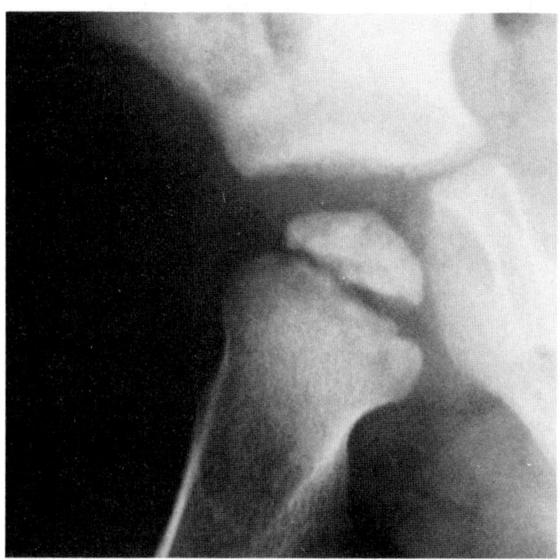

Figure 2.6. Perthes' disease in a five year old child with an intermittent limp over six months

Slipped upper femoral epiphysis

Slipped upper femoral epiphysis affects boys more commonly than girls and is prevalent particularly between the ages of 11 and 15 (Lloyd Roberts and Ratliff, 1978). The disorder appears more likely when there is some disorder of puberty and is seen particularly in the type of short fat child with delayed puberty or with normal puberty but excessive skeletal overgrowth. The slip may be sudden, producing acute symptoms, or slower, causing insidious symptoms over several weeks. The presenting features are pain, often referred to the knee, and a limp. On examination the hip is held in flexion, adduction and external rotation and with some loss of movement, the degree of loss of movement dependent on the severity of the slip. This curious affection of the capital epiphysis, which slips backwards, downwards and medially, may not be readily discernible on the anterior posterior films so a

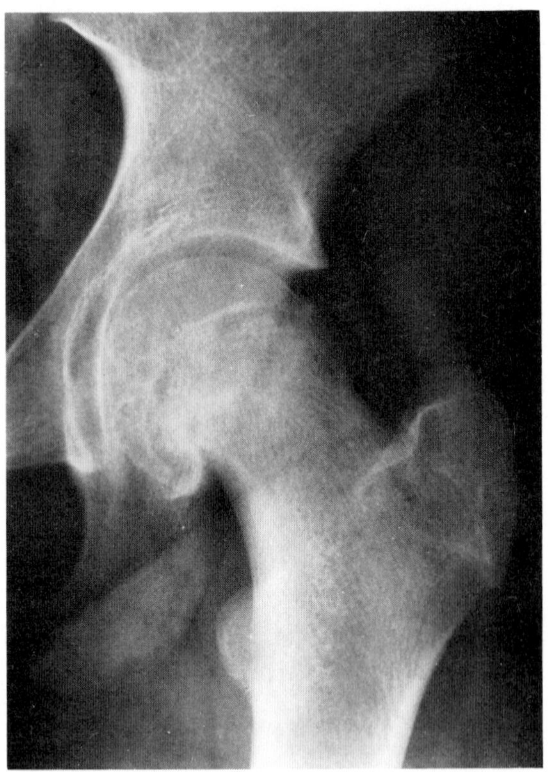

Figure 2.7. Slipped femoral epiphysis in a plump 14 year old who presented with a limp and pain

lateral view is mandatory (*Figure 2.7*). The contralateral hip should be included for comparison, but it must be recognised that up to 25 per cent of patients have a bilateral slip, although both sides may not be affected at the same time.

Osteochrondritis dissecans

Osteochrondritis dissecans is most common in teenage boys. The knee is the most usual site although the elbow, ankle and rarely the hip, can be affected. The symptoms are usually insidious and include discomfort in the joint, swelling and insecurity. Occasionally the presentation is acute, as a fragment of cartilage may become detached and form an intra-articular loose body with locking, swelling and severe pain. At such a time examination will reveal a painful swollen locked knee or elbow. An x-ray will elucidate the diagnosis, the characteristic areas affected are; in the knee, in the infero-lateral part of the medial femoral condyle (*Figure 2.8*), in the capitellum of the elbow, in the supero-medial aspect of the talus at the ankle, and in the superior articular aspect of the femoral head in the hip. When the lesion remains *in situ* there is a dense nidus of bone surrounded by an area of rarefaction in the sub-articular region; while if a fragment of bone has separated a loose body will be revealed.

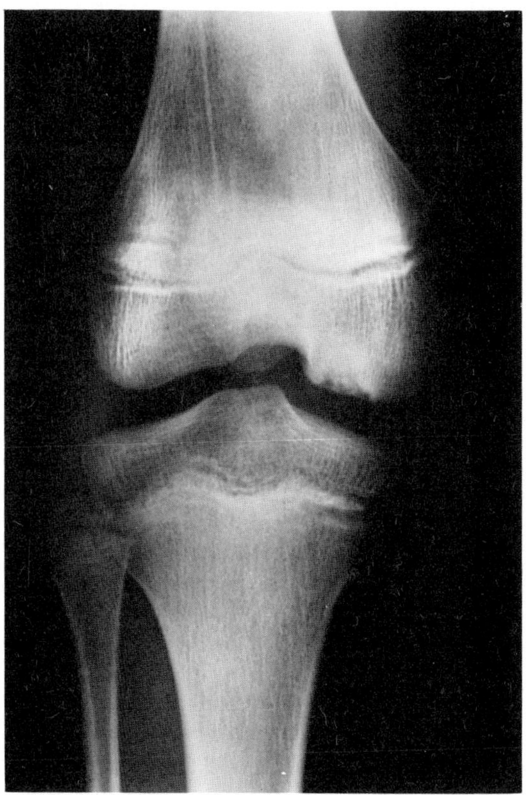

Figure 2.8. Osteochondritis dissecans in a boy of 12 with aching and locking of the knee

Chondromalacia patella

Chrondromalacia patella predominantly affects teenage girls, presenting with a slow onset of symptoms in one or both knees. It is characterised by generalised aching in the front of the joint, and is aggravated by exercise, particularly climbing stairs. The knee may catch but not lock and at times there is a complaint of creaking or grating from the joint which feels insecure and has a tendency to give way. On examination there is retropatellar tenderness and crepitus; there is occasionally a small effusion in the joint but there is no evidence of synovitis and marked wasting of the quadriceps muscle. The aetiological factor is believed to be injury, with contributory causes being an abnormal shape of the patella or femoral condyle and recurrent subluxation or dislocation of the patella. Initially radiographs are completely normal but ultimately, particularly using special skyline views, some 20–30 per cent will reveal sub-articular erosions.

Recurrent subluxation of the patella

While recurrent subluxation of the patella can arise spontaneously, it is more common following trauma. Recurrent subluxation can be easily overlooked as the cause of a painful swollen knee, and the situation may be compounded by the onset of secondary chondromalacia patella; many of the patients exhibit some degree of ligamentous laxity.

Only occasionally is there a clear history of the patella moving laterally and producing an obvious deformity with the knee locked in partial flexion. It is more usual for the history to suggest instability of the knee with 'giving way'and recurrent effusion. Examination will indicate tenderness on the medial side of the patella where the tissues are stretched. If the patient is guarding the knee due to apprehension, minor degrees of lateral hypermobility may be difficult to demonstrate. Radiologically, it may be possible to demonstrate that the patella is smaller and higher than normal and at times laterally disposed.

Infrapatellar lesions

Other lesions of the quadriceps apparatus may produce symptoms and signs simulating a monarthritis of the knee. This is particularly common in teenagers. At its distal attachment to the tibial

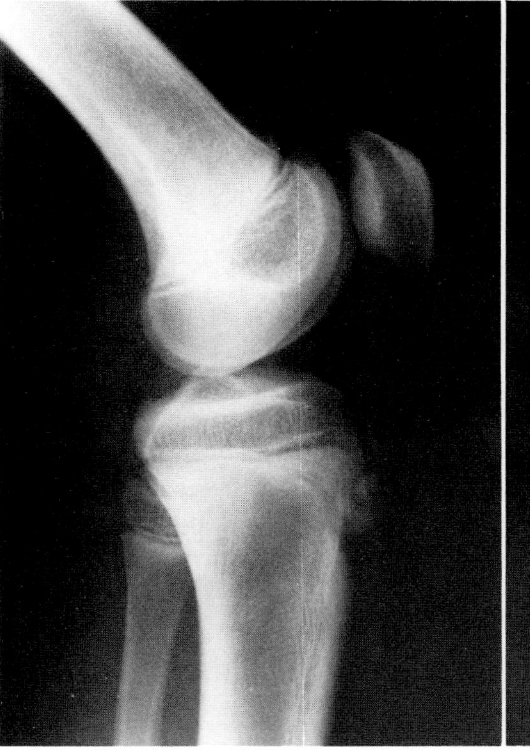

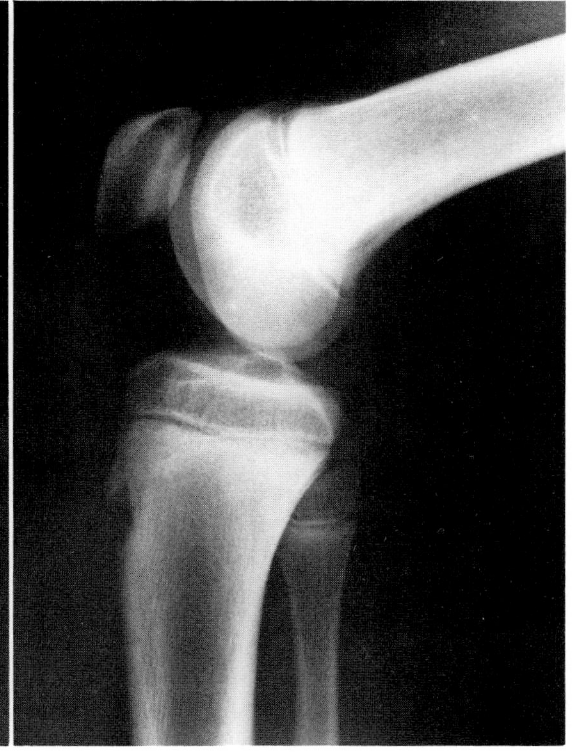

Figure 2.9. Osgood-Schlatter disease in a 12 year old boy with pain in the knee

tuberosity the patella tendon can be traumatised where the localised pain of Osgood–Schlatter disease may be confused with a lesion of the knee itself. Osgood–Schlatter disease (*Figure 2.9*) previously more common in boys than girls, appears to be coming more frequent in girls with the increased indulgence by them in athletics. Careful palpation with identification of the site of maximum tenderness helps in diagnosis. Particularly in plumpish teenage girls, infrapatellar discomfort is common. The retro-patellar fat pad crosses on either side of the patellar tendon and hangs partly into the joint where it is covered by synovial membrane; the fat pad is vulnerable to minor trauma, when it becomes oedematous and inflamed. The symptoms and signs simulate chondromalacia although careful palpation will define the lesion.

For the management of the knee problems discussed, the reader may consult Swann (1976); and for the hip lesions, Lloyd Roberts and Ratliff (1978).

REFERENCES

Blockey, N. J. and McAllister, T.A. (1972). Antibiotics in acute osteomyelitis in children. *Journal of Bone and Joint Surgery*, **54B**, 229

Cassidy, J. T., Brodie, D. L. and Martell, W. (1967). Monarticular juvenile arthritis. *Journal of Paediatrics*, **70**, 867

Catteral, A. J. (1970). The natural history of Perthes' disease. *Journal of Bone and Joint Surgery*, **52B**, 186

Clarke, J. T. (1978). Infectious arthritis – antibiotic therapy. *Clinics of Rheumatic Diseases*, **4**, 133

Goldenberg, D. L. and Cohen, A. S. (1978). Arthritis due to tuberculosis and fungal microorganisms. *Clinics in Rheumatic Diseases*, **4**, 211

Howard, J. B., Highgenboten, C. L. and Nelson, J. D. (1976). Residual effect of septic arthritis in infancy and childhood. *Journal of the American Medical Association*, **236**, 932

Lloyd Roberts, G. C. and Ratliff, A. H. C. (1978). Hip disorders in children. *Postgraduate Orthopaedic Series*. Edited by A. Graham Apley. London; Butterworths

Nade, S. (1977). Choice of antibiotics in the management of acute osteomyelitis and acute septic arthritis. *Archives of Diseases of Childhood*, **52**, 679

Sim, F. H., Dahlin, D. C. and Beabout, J. W. (1975). Osteoid osteoma – Diagnostic problem. *Journal of Bone and Joint Surgery*, **57A**, 154

Sugarman, M., Stobie, D. G., Quismorio, F. P., Terry, R. and Hanson, V. (1977). Plant thorn synovitis.*Arthritis and Rheumatism*,**20**, 1125

Swann, M. S. (1976). Monarthritis. *Clinics in Rheumatic Diseases*, **2**, 386

Trevers, S., Khettry, J., Biohe, F. H., Wilkinson, R. H. and Watts, H. (1976). Osteomyelitis; early scintographic detection. *Pediatrics*, **57**, 173

Webster, A. D. B., Taylor-Robinson, D., Furr, P. M. and Asherson, G. (1977). Mycoplasma septic arthritis in hypogammaglobulinaemia. *British Medical Journal*, **1**, 478

CHAPTER 3

Polyarthritis

Polyarthritis occurs in a variety of disorders. It may be transient, as in viral infections; or it may be associated with serious involvement of organs other than joints, as in rheumatic fever or systemic lupus erythematosus. It can complicate an underlying disorder, as in immunodeficiency or haemophilia. It may progress to a chronic, potentially crippling state, as in juvenile chronic arthritis. Because prognosis and therefore management will vary according to aetiology, precision of diagnosis, although difficult, is desirable.

History

In the history, it is important to know about the child's general health, e.g. whether he is suffering from any other disorder, such as ulcerative colitis or a blood dyscrasia. It is necessary to enquire about preceding events including infections, particularly those of the upper respiratory and gastro-intestinal tract, as well as accidents and previous illness.

Particularly in those who present with a frank arthritis, the family history is important for two reasons. Firstly it may help in diagnosis e.g. psoriasis, ankylosing spondylitis or familial Mediterranean fever may be present in a relative. Secondly, most families have at least one distant relative with some sort of rheumatism and one can often relieve their natural anxiety at the first consultation by excluding the same disorder in the child.

The age of the child is very important. The most common age of onset of systemic juvenile chronic arthritis is before the fifth birthday, whereas rheumatic fever tends to occur in the older child, eight or nine years old or upwards, and Henoch-Schoenlein purpura from about the age of three or four throughout schooldays. By contrast, psoriatic arthritis and juvenile ankylosing spondylitis tend to develop in children aged nine and upwards.

The pattern and severity of joint involvement may be difficult to ascertain as young children sometimes demonstrate arthritis solely by loss of function of a limb or an apathetic immobility. Older children, however, can often give a good account of their joint symptoms, and they should be encouraged to do this, particularly as they get towards adolescence, although parental confirmation is important.

Examination

In the general examination it will be possible to confirm the presence of a rash, to note its type and distribution and to look for lymphadenopathy. Small glands in the cervical region may denote previous infection, whereas a generalised lymphadenopathy affecting all sites may be helpful in differentiating infections, such as infectious mononucleosis, and systemic juvenile chronic arthritis from other forms of arthritis. Hepatosplenomegaly is similarly helpful in this respect.

The presence of pericarditis is not particularly useful diagnostically, as it can occur in systemic juvenile chronic arthritis, rheumatic fever or systemic lupus erythematosus. However, the presence of endocarditis as manifested by a soft mitral or aortic diastolic murmur is more suggestive of rheumatic fever (*see* Chapter 5) while knowledge of a previous murmur will make one think towards bacterial endocarditis. In this condition other features, such as petechiae, splinter haemorrhages, microscopic haematuria, and splenomegaly will also be contributory.

INFECTIONS

Viral

Arthropathy due to viral infection tends to be mild, resolving spontaneously in a few weeks. In contrast to bacterial infections, viral arthropathies are usually polyarticular and have been

TABLE 3.1
Viral infections that may be associated with arthropathy

Rubella
Mumps
Chickenpox
Glandular fever (Epstein–Barr virus)
Cytomegalic virus
Hepatitis B
Adenovirus – particularly 7
Influenza
Arbovirus

described with a number of well recognised diseases (*Table 3.1*). It is thought that the synovitis is due to immune complex deposition. Thus in arthritis due to infection with hepatitis B antigen and adenovirus, low serum values of C_3, C_4 and CH_{50} are obtained which return to normal during convalescence; immune complexes have been detected in both serum and synovial fluid (van H. Souter and Utsinger, 1978).

Rubella

Rubella is the best known viral infection; arthritis may accompany, precede or follow the rash. It can occur at any age, but usually tends to affect girls in the early teens. The occurrence of a rubella epidemic or contact in the family, as well as the clinical features of the rash and occipital lymphadenopathy, are all helpful diagnostic points.

The polyarthritis affects the hands and knees particularly; it can be migratory. Tenosynovitis is not uncommon in the hands, and it causes severe pain. Carpal tunnel syndrome has been seen as early as seven years when it causes intense pain at night.

The white blood count may well show a lymphocytosis, the ESR is usually raised and Turk cells may be present in the peripheral blood; occasionally the latex test is positive. A more definitive diagnosis can be made by finding a rising titre against rubella in the serum.

In children receiving rubella virus vaccines, the incidence of arthritis has been extremely variable, varying from 1 to 20 per cent. One vaccine, HPV-77DK12, has subsequently been withdrawn because of its high incidence of associated arthritis. The arthritis tends to occur three to six weeks after vaccination, lasting for about two weeks. Occasionally, however, knee synovitis, in particular, has persisted for several months. Carpal tunnel syndrome may also occur in arthropathy following rubella vaccination.

Following recovery from the arthritis it is not uncommon for the patient to have arthralgia for some time afterwards, and this is irrespective of whether the arthritis follows natural rubella or the inoculation.

Mumps

Mumps arthritis affects boys more commonly than girls and usually in the older age group, although it can be seen in young children. The arthritis tends to affect large joints and has a migratory pattern; because it is very occasionally accompanied by pericarditis, it can sometimes closely mimic rheumatic fever. However, features such as parotitis, abdominal pain or meningitis may also be present. One can suspect the diagnosis of rheumatic fever because of contacts but if parotitis is not witnessed a rising titre against mumps is essential for correct diagnosis.

Chickenpox

In young children of both sexes, a transient self-limiting, often pauci-articular arthritis develops with chickenpox at the same time or immediately after the rash.

Infectious mononucleosis (glandular fever)

Particularly in adolescents, glandular fever with widespread lymphadenopathy, splenomegaly, hepatomegaly with mild dysfunction, fever and rash can mimic systemic juvenile chronic arthritis or rheumatic fever. However, the arthritis usually comes on a few days after the sore throat, the rash tends to be larger, raised and does not recur as often as in systemic juvenile chronic arthritis. The presence of mononuclear cells in the blood and a positive Paul Bunnell test, or the more specific titres against EBV (Epstein–Barr Virus) confirm the diagnosis. In younger children cytomegalic virus infection can cause a very similar illness (Ginsburg *et al.*, 1977).

Infective hepatitis

Acute viral hepatitis, particularly Type B (formerly called serum hepatitis) which is related to Australia antigen, is not uncommonly associated with a serum sickness-like syndrome in the acute stages. This is marked by fever, malaise, loss of appetite, rashes, urticaria, maculopapular or erythematous eruptions, angioneurotic oedema and arthralgia in some 50 per cent of patients; arthritis is less common (Alarcon and Townes, 1973). Joint disturbances can also be prominent in anicteric cases (Schumacher and Gall, 1974). The small joints of hands, knees, wrists, ankles and feet tend to be involved in an additive pattern. Joint and skin symptoms are particularly associated with depressed levels of the C_3 component of complement in the serum; circulating immune complexes composed of anti-HBs Ag immunoglobulin, HBs Ag and complement are often present.

This type of arthritis is rare before adolescence. Loss of appetite and the variety of rashes should make one carry out liver function tests, which are usually abnormal even if the liver is not palpable and tender on examination. Hb Ag is usually positive. Rheumatoid factor and antinuclear antibodies can also be demonstrated, setting a trap for the unwary, but the clinical features as well as abnormal liver function tests will suggest the diagnosis.

Adenoviral arthritis

Arthritis associated with adenovirus upper respiratory infection (usually type 7) is now well documented (Utsinger, 1977). Several days after the onset of fever, coryza and pharyngitis, patients, usually about three to five years of age, develop a maculo-erythematous rash and a symmetrical arthritis. The most commonly involved joints are the knees, wrists and ankles. The arthritis is usually self-limiting requiring only palliative treatment with aspirin before it subsides within six weeks. One patient reported by Rahal *et al.* (1976) developed pharyngitis, pericarditis and a purpuric maculopapular rash with adenovirus 7 isolated from the pericardial fluid. She improved on prednisone and, two months later, a second self-limited episode of pericarditis occurred. Nine months later she developed fever, rash and a symmetrical polyarthritis which persisted for one month; 11 months later she had a further episode and subsequently recovered. She was classified as juvenile rheumatoid arthritis caused by adenovirus 7, but it is probable that this was in fact just a viral infection.

The work of Utsinger (1977) in identifying cryoprecipitate in the serum containing IgA, IgM, IgGl, IgG3, C_3 and C_4 and intact adenovirus virion provides evidence of the immune complex nature of the disease.

Other infections

Other infections, such as those with influenza, other adenoviruses, all the group of arboviruses and *Mycoplasma pneumoniae*, can all cause fever, rashes of many types and transient arthropathy.

In rat bite fever arthritis is common when infection is due to *Streptobacillus moniliformis* (Haverhill fever). While more common in the USA, rat bite fever is seen here, usually referred as systemic juvenile chronic arthritis. Up to two weeks after being bitten by a rat or eating food contaminated by rat excreta, the patient has a sudden fever and influenza-like illness, followed by polyarthritis which can be widespread or just affect the knees and elbows. Lymphadenopathy is confined to the site of the bite. The ESR is raised as is the white blood cell count; blood or synovial fluid culture will confirm the diagnosis. Treatment with penicillin and streptomycin causes rapid improvement (McGill and Martin, 1966).

Previous epidemiological studies of unclassified forms of polyarthritis have also suggested that many patients have short-lived illnesses that might well be related to viral diseases. This is further supported by the characterisation of a group of patients in Lyme, Connecticut (Steere *et al.*, 1977). These patients, usually children, developed a skin lesion which began as a red macule or papule expanding to form a large rind with central clearing (erythema chronicum migrans) and followed by the development of fever, headache, stiffness, monarticular or oligoarticular arthritis tending to last for about one week but occasionally persisting for some months. So far no organism has been identified but cryoprecipitates were detected in the serum together with increased levels of IgM.

This type of infection can be suspected on grounds of clustering. The presence of neutropenia with a relative lymphocytosis will suggest a viral infection while alterations in complement etc. support an immune complex mechanism. Absolute identification of the virus or evidence of infection by antibody titre rises may, however, be difficult.

Bacterial

In contrast to viral infections, bacterial infections are more likely to cause osteomyelitis or a monarticular arthritis (p. 23). However, there are two bacterial infections which warrant short comment as they can be associated with polyarthritis.

Meningococcal arthritis

Meningococcal arthritis usually occurs some five or more days after the onset of the acute infection at a time when the septicaemic stage is coming under antibiotic control (Larson *et al.*, 1977). It may affect two or three of the larger joints or only one, often a knee. It is rare to isolate the meningococcae from the affected joint. Allergic complications such as cutaneous vasculitis may be present. The arthritis is thought to be due to immune complex disease rather than persistent infection (Whittle *et al.*, 1973).

Gonococcal arthritis

Although primarily a disease of adults it is occasionally seen in adolescents, often female, in the UK and somewhat more commonly in the USA. The onset may be acute with fever and rigors and such patients will have a positive blood culture. The polyarthritis is often migratory, mimicking rheumatic fever. The joints most commonly involved are knees, ankles, wrists, tarsi and metatarsophalangeal joints.

Skin rashes occur in about one third of patients and consist of erythematous macules which may become petechial; very occasionally they become vesicular or pustular with a dark necrotic centre developing in the pustule. At the time of presentation, the skin lesions may differ in size and appearance due to the age of the lesion. It is rare for there to be any genital symptoms although direct questioning may reveal a vaginal discharge or history of recent exposure.

Diagnosis should be made only when gonococci have been cultured. This can be done from the blood, synovial fluid or tissue, genito-urinary tract or skin; the cultures need to be performed with particular care as they need special media preparations.

In management, penicillin is still the drug of choice and provided dosage is adequate there is a satisfactory response in four to six days, the arthritis regressing without residua. If therapy is not initiated quickly, as with any other septic arthritis (p. 26) joint destruction will occur (Munoz, 1978).

OTHER CAUSES OF ACUTE POLYARTHRITIS

The differential diagnosis between rheumatic fever and systemic juvenile chronic arthritis (Still's disease) used to be one of the most difficult. The decline in rheumatic fever (Chapter 5) which 30 years ago was the commonest cause of childhood arthritis with fever, has highlighted the importance of considering other conditions (*Table 3.2*). At a Workshop on the Care of Rheumatic Children held under the auspices of the WHO and the European League Against Rheumatism in 1977 (EULAR Monograph) the problem of nomenclature and classification of childhood arthritis

TABLE 3.2
Differential diagnosis of systemic juvenile chronic arthritis (Still's disease, juvenile rheumatoid arthritis)

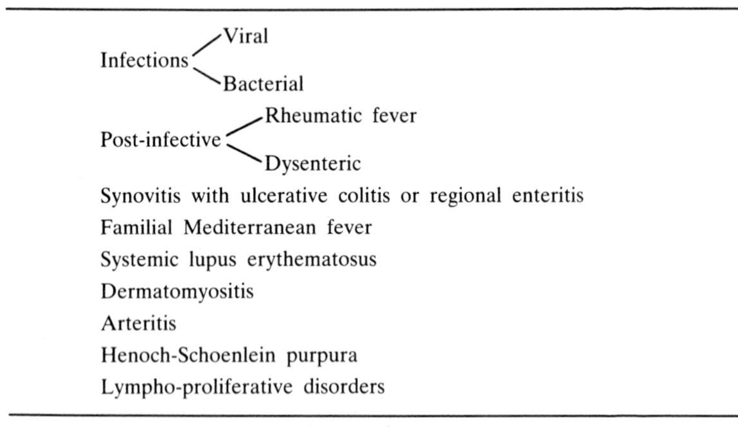

Infections — Viral / Bacterial
Post-infective — Rheumatic fever / Dysenteric
Synovitis with ulcerative colitis or regional enteritis
Familial Mediterranean fever
Systemic lupus erythematosus
Dermatomyositis
Arteritis
Henoch-Schoenlein purpura
Lympho-proliferative disorders

TABLE 3.3
Criteria for diagnosis of juvenile chronic arthritis (EULAR/WHO, 1977)

Onset	– under 16 years
Duration	– minimum three months
Classification by onset	
	Systemic illness
	Polyarthritis
	Pauci-articular (four or fewer joints)

TABLE 3.4
Exclusions from diagnosis of juvenile chronic arthritis

(a) *Arthropathies with characteristic specific features*	*(b)* *Distinct conditions of the musculo-skeletal system*	*(c)* *Specific diseases which can cause problems in diagnosis*
(i) Infectious	(i) Polymyositis and dermatomyositis	(i) Acute rheumatic fever
(ii) Non-rheumatological immunological disorders	(ii) Systemic sclerosis	(ii) Systemic lupus erythematosus
(iii) Haematological disorders	(iii) Keratoconjunctivitis sicca	(iii) Post-infectious arthropathies
(iv) Neoplasm	(iv) Mixed connective tissue disease	
(v) Psychogenic	(v) Vasculitis (Henoch-Schoenlein purpura, etc.)	
	(vi) Behcet's syndrome	
	(vii) Non-rheumatological conditions (chondromalacia, synovitis of hip, etc.)	

was reviewed. The American rheumatism criteria for juvenile rheumatoid arthritis (Brewer *et al.*, 1977) have been modified frequently and have not yet received universal acceptance. In particular, the term 'rheumatoid' was deplored as this implies a relationship with adult seropositive rheumatoid arthritis and this was not considered to be the case. Juvenile chronic arthritis was the term accepted by the European League Against Rheumatism who realised that it is still a generic descriptive term with considerable heterogeneity within this category. The criteria for diagnosis are shown in *Table 3.3* together with the sub-grouping suggested; the exclusions are given in *Table 3.4*. This nomenclature will now be used to discuss further the differential diagnosis of polyarthritis in childhood.

Systemic juvenile chronic arthritis (Still's disease, juvenile rheumatoid arthritis)

To make the diagnosis of systemic juvenile chronic arthritis, persistent fever of an intermittent type which is associated with at least one other typical feature is required. This could be the characteristic maculopapular rash, generalised lymphadenopathy, splenomegaly and hepatomegaly, or pericarditis.

The most common age of onset of the disease is under five years, when boys are affected as frequently as girls; but the disease can be seen throughout childhood and indeed, even into adult life. Later (i.e. five years old and onwards) girls are more commonly affected than boys by the disease.

Clinical features at onset

The fever is high and most often the fever pattern is quotidian or with one or two daily temperature spikes. Children under five years usually appear toxic, listless and are often very irritable. Older children may appear unwell at the height of the fever but in between times are often quite well and ready to be up and running about. Very occasionally, when the fever is prolonged or recurs it may become periodic. The pattern of this fever is very helpful in distinguishing juvenile chronic arthritis from some other forms of inflammatory arthritis (*Figure 3.1*).

In the majority of cases a rash is seen during the febrile course. In approximately half of the patients this will be the typical

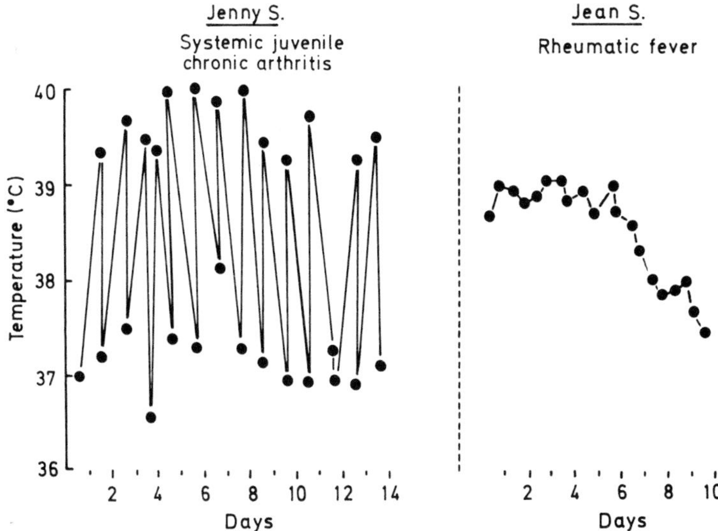

Figure 3.1. Systemic juvenile chronic arthritis. Fever pattern — comparison with rheumatic fever

maculopapular eruption which is a coppery-red colour (*Figure 3.2a* and *Plate 1*); at other times the rash is more confluent (*Figure 3.2b*) and is most florid where the skin has been rubbed or subjected to mild trauma-like pressure of underclothing; this response is known as the Kurbner phenomenon and may be very helpful in bringing out the rash by making light scratch marks along a susceptible site. After several minutes linear chains of macules or maculopapules appear that persist from hours to a day or so. Another way of bringing out the rash is to warm the child artificially in a warm bath or wait till the next spike of temperature. Very occasionally the rash is of an itching character and in these cases it is often slightly larger than usual (*Figure 3.2c*). The absence of any rash should make one wonder about the diagnosis; reactive arthropathy can be associated with a similar type of fever chart, as can ulcerative colitis with arthritis, while in older patients, a febrile onset of spondylitis (Kinsella *et al.*, 1978) or even psoriatic arthritis can occur.

Generalised lymphadenopathy, particularly of epitrochlear and axilliary nodes may be so prominent as to suggest lymphoma. Abdominal pain or distension due to either enlarged mesenteric nodes or serositis suggests an acute surgical abdomen. Splenomegaly is somewhat less common than lymphadenopathy but is also extremely helpful diagnostically. This may be associated with enlargement of the liver (*Figure 3.3*), though very occasionally, hepatomegaly occurs alone. In such circumstances it is important to check liver function as less common systemic features, and extremely serious ones, include hepatitis (Schaller *et al.*, 1970).

Pericarditis (*Figure 3.4*) is seen in a proportion of cases, the

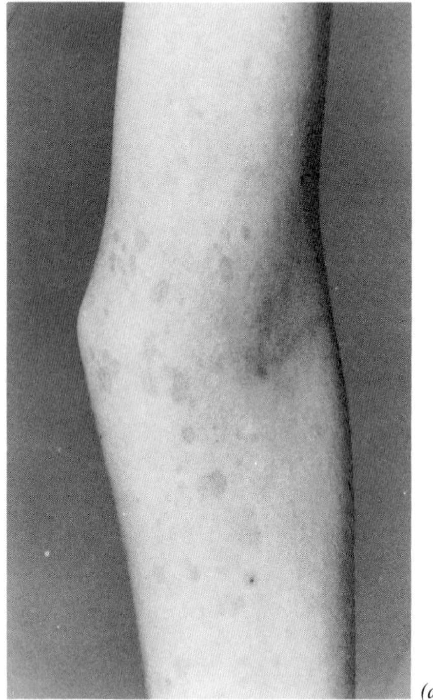

(a)

Figure 3.2. Systemic juvenile chronic arthritis. Rash; (a) typical (see Plate 1)

incidence possibly reflects how carefully one looks for it. Using echocardiography, it can be demonstrated more easily than by previous methods (Bernstein *et al.*, 1974). It is not uncommon for pericarditis to be associated with pleuritis and very occasionally pneumonitis. A rare problem is myocarditis which can go on to cardiac failure (Miller and French, 1977).

Another uncommon manifestation during the systemic phase is hepatitis (Schaller *et al.*, 1970). Initially there may be no joint symptoms, minor arthralgia, intermittent bouts of joint swelling or a severe arthritis; very occasionally presentation with acute neck pain suggests meningitis. Ultimately, the majority of these children do develop arthritis. The most usual sites are knees, wrists and carpi followed by ankles and tarsi (*Figure 3.5*). Flexor tendon involvement in the hand (*Figure 3.6*) which causes splinting of the metatarsophalangeal joints and loss of movement at proximal interphalangeal joints, is common after a few weeks; at times there will be associated swelling of proximal interphalangeal joints. Other joints are less commonly involved early.

Laboratory data

The Westergren ESR is usually high, 100 mm or more. There is a polymorphonucleocytosis often as high as 95 per cent, of a 25 000

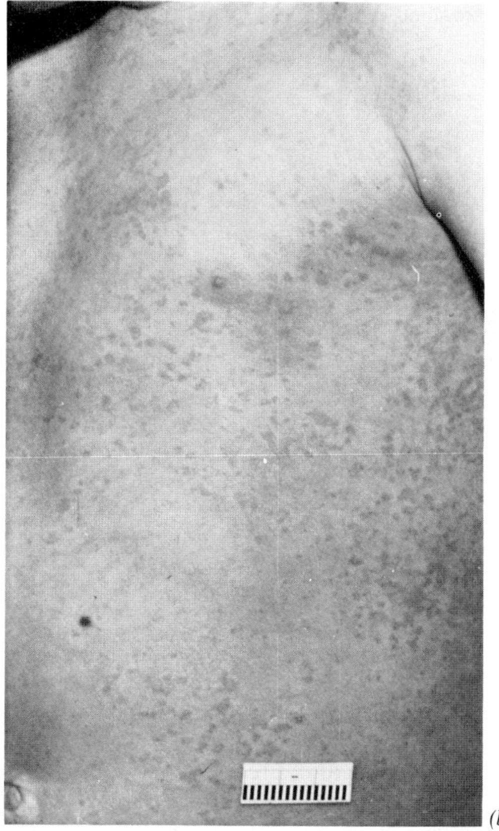

(b)

Figure 3.2. Systemic juvenile chronic arthritis. Rash; (b) confluent

or 30 000 white cell count, while the platelets may also be raised with counts of 750 000 or more not uncommon. The haemoglobin falls early, initially to 10 G or thereabouts, but it rarely goes very low in the early diagnostic stage; this fact is useful in distinguishing systemic juvenile chronic arthritis with hepatosplenomegaly, lymphadenopathy and general deterioration in health from malignancy and, in particular, leukaemia. All the immunoglobulins are

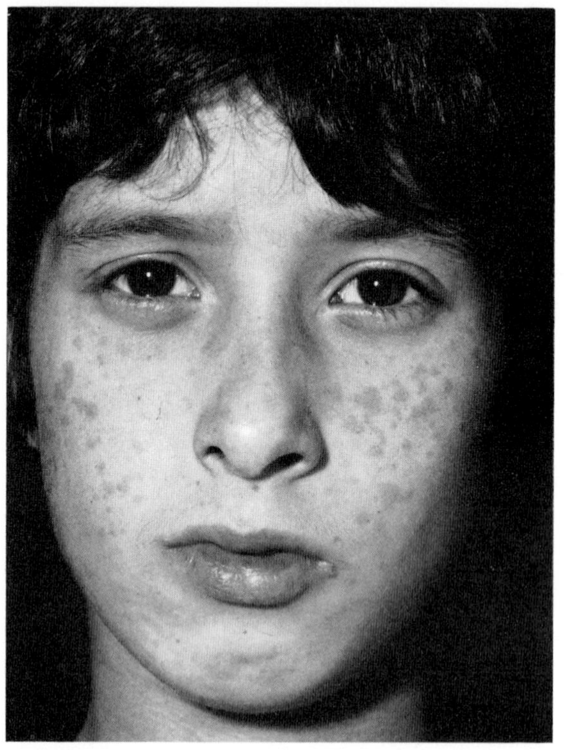
(c)

Figure 3.2. Systemic juvenile chronic arthritis. Rash; (c) on face

frequently raised while immune complexes using both $C1_q$ techniques and that of Levinsky (Moran *et al.*, 1978) can be detected relatively commonly in systemic illness (Rossen *et al.*, 1977). However, immune complexes are non-specific because by using the $C1_q$ technique they can also be detected in seropositive rheumatoid arthritis at all ages, the acute stage of dermatomyositis, systemic lupus erythematosus and various types of vasculitis, etc. (*see* Appendix). IgM rheumatoid factor is not usual in the serum although at times very small amounts of anti-IgM are

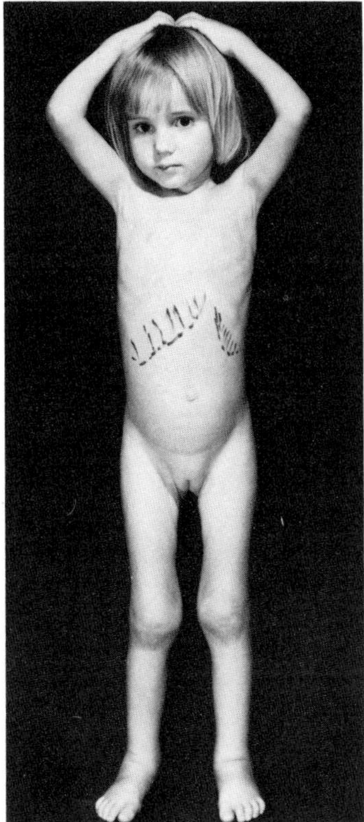

Figure 3.3. Systemic juvenile chronic arthritis. Hepatosplenomegaly and lymphadenopathy in girl of three and a half; note also arthritis of knees and ankles

present as shown by a weakly positive latex test; this is of no diagnostic significance. Similarly, it is rare to find anti-nuclear antibodies in systemic illness. As yet, no correlation with any genetic markers has been detected in this sub-group.

Diagnosis remains clinical, with the active exclusion of infections on the one hand and neoplasia on the other.

Differential diagnosis (see Table 3.2 p. 48)

In the first few days it can be very difficult to distinguish systemic juvenile chronic arthritis from a *viral infection*, but the persistent spiking fever and recurrent maculopapular eruption, together with

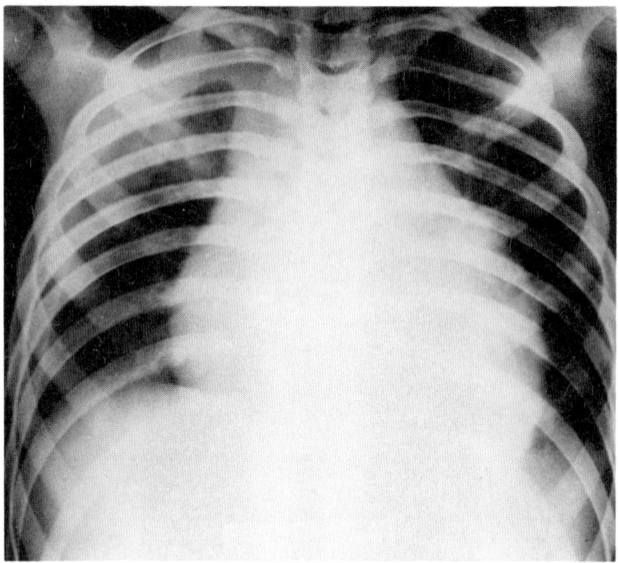

Figure 3.4. Systemic juvenile chronic arthritis. Pericardial effusion in a boy with systemic juvenile chronic arthritis; the straight left border of the cardiac silhouette is characteristic

the rising white blood count are helpful. Rarely bacterial infections give rise to confusion, as occasionally *osteomyelitis* (p. 25) is multifocal, while *septicaemia* can be associated with general limb pain. The doctor should beware of a single severely involved joint! Other important infections which need to be differentiated include *leishmaniasis*, where the low white blood count is helpful, *rocky mountain spotted fever* (Castleman *et al.*, 1973) and *Mycoplasma pneumonia* (Jones, 1970).

TABLE 3.5
Clinical comparison of rheumatic fever and systemic juvenile chronic arthritis

	Rheumatic fever	*Systemic juvenile chronic arthritis*
Fever	Sustained	Intermittent
Rash	Marginate	Macular
Lymphadenopathy	0	+
Hepatosplenomegaly	0*	+
Endocarditis	+	0
Pericarditis	+	+

*Except in cardiac failure

The most difficult differential diagnosis used to be *rheumatic fever* (p. 152), but this has now become so rare in Western countries, that it is often not even considered! The occasional case does still arise so it is important to remember some of the distinguishing features (*Table 3.5*), including the sustained fever which then drops over a few weeks and the rash, erythema marginatum (*Plate 2*).

The rash of *erythema multiforme* (*Figure 3.7*) needs to be differentiated from erythema marginatum. The former is fixed and raised, the latter marginate and moving. Although affected children are covered in rash, they are usually well, and there is

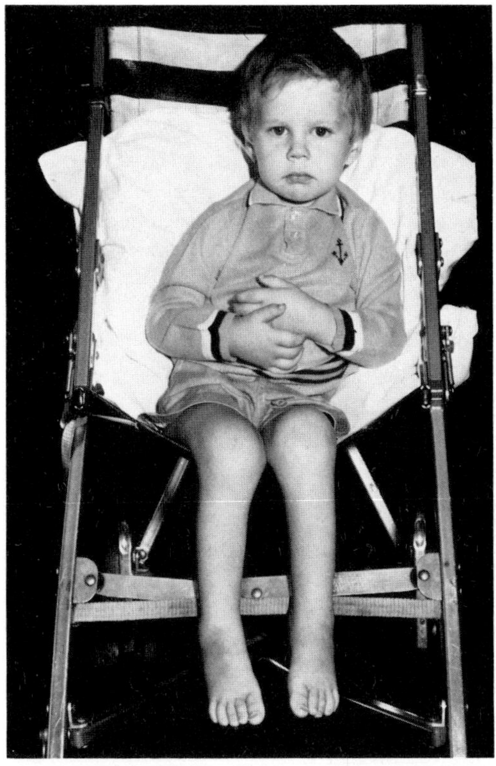

Figure 3.5. Systemic juvenile chronic arthritis. This boy, aged four, presented with fever, rash, hepato-splenomegaly and pericarditis four months earlier. Now he has severe arthritis of wrists and carpi, proximal interphalangeal joints (with flexor tenosynovitis) knees, ankles and tarsi

often a preceding sore throat in the few days prior to the rash – or there may be a history of drug ingestion. Arthralgia rather than arthritis can accompany the rash. Any fever that occurs is usually low grade.

By contrast, in *Stevens–Johnson syndrome* (erythema multiforme exudivatum) there is fever and systemic prostation as well as the lesions of the skin and the mucous membranes. Stevens–Johnson syndrome is most usually seen in young adolescent males; it often follows an upper respiratory infection, particularly with *Mycoplasma pneumonia* (Sonthelmer *et al.*, 1978), while a number of drugs have been implicated including Septrin, isoniazid, methotrexate etc. The skin lesions consist of erythematous papules which enlarge by peripheral expansion and usually go on to

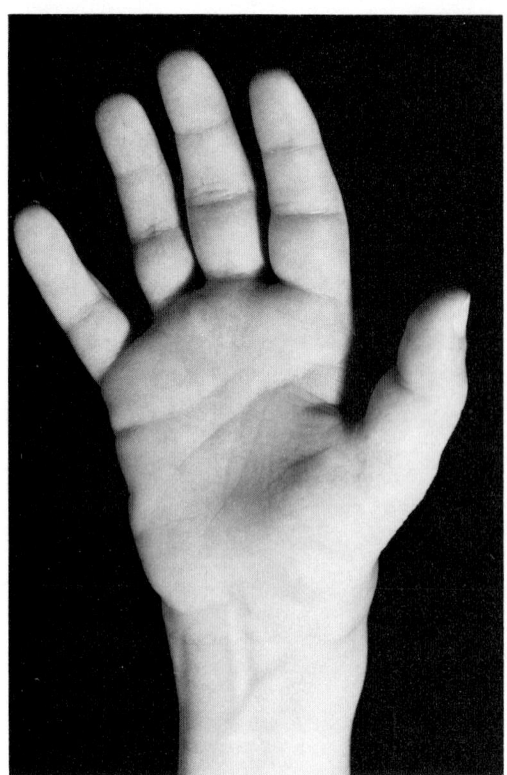

Figure 3.6. Juvenile chronic arthritis. Acute flexor tendon synovitis causing marked swelling over the proximal phalanges of all fingers, including thumb, which extends into the palm

vesicular formation. Any cutaneous area can be affected and ultimately vesiculobullous lesions occur on the mucous membranes at all sites, which include conjunctivae (*Plate 3*), mouth with appalling stomatitis, the anal/rectal junction, urethra and the vulva. Periarticular swelling occurs in association with the skin lesions. This is an extremely serious illness with a high mortality.

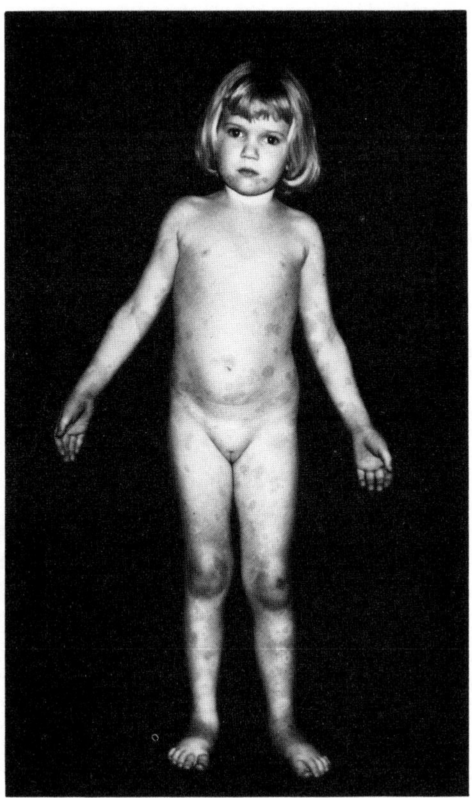

Figure 3.7. Erythema multiforme

Early recognition is essential if appropriate management measures are to be introduced. These measures consist of strict isolation and asepsis, replacement of fluids, high dosage corticosteroids and prompt treatment of any infection that occurs (Rasmussen, 1976).

Post-dysenteric Reiter's syndrome or alone arthropathy (p. 78) can be associated with the spiking fever but not the typical Still's rash. In both ulcerative colitis and regional enteritis (p. 74) the fever can be spiking or sustained, and various rashes have been noted, so that unless there is good evidence for infection, any diarrhoea needs investigation.

Familial Mediterranean fever (p. 81) must also be considered in children whose original symptoms are appropriate.

In 1948 Reimann drew attention to a group of patients with periodic high fever, together with other features, arthralgia and serositis resembling familial Mediterranean fever but with no genetic background and unusual rashes. More recently, children diagnosed as having *periodic syndrome* have been noted to have complement defects (Reimann *et al.*, 1970). There may well be other anomalies yet to be discovered; one such child referred to us as systemic juvenile chronic arthritis appears to produce excessive histamine. Between attacks, the patients are well and grow normally. Residual problems have not yet been noted. In some children such episodes appear to follow intercurrent infections. Attacks can frequently be aborted by the prompt administration of indomethacin.

In *systemic lupus erythematosus* (p. 168) the presence of multisystem involvement and typical rash in a child with a maintained, though not necessarily high, fever should give rise to suspicion. In *dermatomyositis* (p. 177), although fever with joint presentation can occur, the typical rash and muscle weakness usually develop quickly. Similarly, *arteritis* of any type can be associated with fever like that of juvenile chronic arthritis and limb pain. Similarly the oedema of a hand or foot with fever and rash in the early stage of *Henoch-Schoenlein purpura* (p. 206) has to be differentiated; this is usually easy because of the characteristic rash.

An uncommon cause of joint symptoms with fever in adolescents is *acne arthralgia* (Windour *et al.*, 1974). This usually occurs in a boy with severe acne conglobata who suffers episodic attacks of pain, usually in the large joints, particularly hips and knees, often with fever. The ESR and white blood cell count are raised, while C_3 is sometimes low. The acne should be vigorously treated including the use of tetracycline. The general manifestation usually settles on treatment with aspirin but occasionally corticosteroids are warranted.

It is in this age group that *Sweet's syndrome* (Gunawardena *et al.*, 1975) has also been seen. The relationship between this and the whole family of leucocytoclastic angitides has recently been discussed by Trentham *et al.*, (1976). The clinical features are episodic arthritis with fever and various skin ulcerating lesions as well as subcutaneous nodules. Histologically, one recent case

(Hollingworth, 1979) showed vasculitis of small vessels at the dermoepidermal junction with fibrin thrombosis and polymorphonuclear infiltration with leucocytoclasis in the surrounding vessels.

Lympho-proliferative disorders may also be difficult to distinguish (Emkey *et al.*, 1973). In our experience *angio-immunoblastomic lymphadenopathy* (Frizzeria *et al.*, 1975) has been a particular problem but the rash was not characteristic of juvenile chronic arthritis and the lymph nodes were remarkably large and rather firm. Parotid and submandibular swelling were the clues in one case, a second lymph gland biopsy being required for diagnosis. In leukaemia and neuroblastoma (Chapter 7) bone pain with relatively little synovitis of joints but severe pain on using the limb, and tenderness along the bone shaft, together with severe anaemia have been useful guides.

An unwillingness to make an absolute diagnosis unless the characteristic clinical picture of systemic juvenile chronic arthritis is present prevents premature conclusions. For this reason somewhat fuller descriptions of some of these syndromes follow (p. 167).

Polyarthritic onset juvenile chronic arthritis (Still's disease, juvenile rheumatoid arthritis)

Polyarthritis, which is defined as involvement of five or more joints, can develop at any time in childhood and is seen even before the first birthday. It is usually seronegative, i.e. IgM rheumatoid factor is not present, although a small proportion of patients (10 per cent) do have persistent IgM rheumatoid factor, they tend to be the older patients, aged ten and over (pp. 66 and 101). As yet the EULAR Classification has not suggested this further sub-grouping. The joint distribution as well as prognosis appears somewhat different. The two groups will therefore be discussed separately here.

Joint involvement in seronegative juvenile chronic arthritis

In a polyarthritic onset of juvenile chronic arthritis, or polyarthritis following a systemic onset of the illness, the most commonly involved joints initially are the knees (60 per cent), the carpi with the wrists (55 per cent) so that there is swelling right over the backs of the hands extending onto the metacarpi, and the ankles and tarsi (45 per cent) (Ansell, 1977). Hand involvement consists of a mixture of arthritis of proximal and distal interphalangeal joints

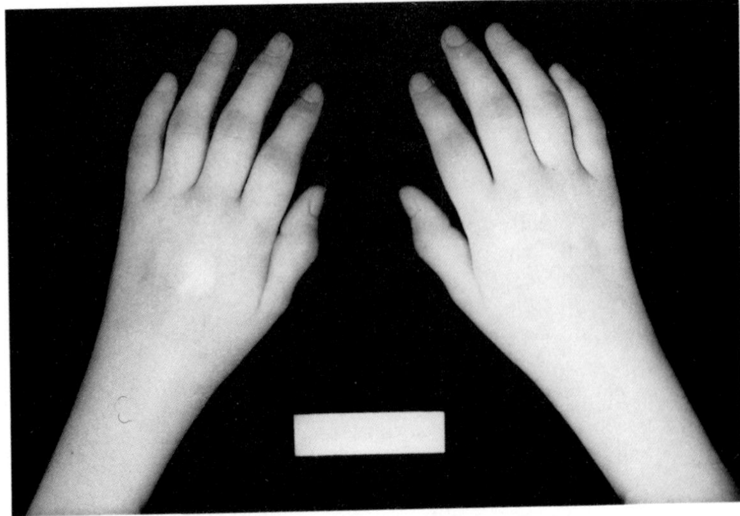

Figure 3.8. Juvenile chronic arthritis. Swelling of proximal and terminal interphalangeal joints which are already flexing because of flexor tendon involvement

(18 per cent) together with flexor tenosynovitis (*Figure 3.8*). Similarly, involvement of interphalangeal joints of the toes is not uncommon, while the first metatarsophalangeal joint is the only metatarsophalangeal joint involved at this stage. Tenosynovitis in toes is not unusual. Neck involvement is seen early in some 30 per cent, usually causing pain and loss of extension (*Figure 3.9*).

At times there may be a severe torticollis and this can be a presenting feature (*Figure 3.10*). It is rarely due to atlanto–axial subluxation but more commonly results from spasm due to unilateral involvement of the apophyseal joints or subluxation of C2 on C3.

Elbow involvement occurs early in a small proportion of children. Hip involvement is relatively uncommon in the first year of the disease as is shoulder involvement, both tending to occur late particularly in young children whose disease persists actively.

General features

There may be an occasional spike of fever or a low sustained fever, but the marked spiking fever of systemic illness is absent. Similarly, some degree of lymphadenopathy, not necessarily generalised, is not uncommon and occasionally splenomegaly is noted. There is thus a gradation between those with a systemic onset and those who have polyarthritis with some added features.

Investigations

Similarly, investigations tend to be intermediate. The ESR is raised but not usually above 60–70 mm/hour, the white cell count is somewhat raised at 12 000–15 000 predominantly polymorphonuclear leucocytosis, the haemoglobin is somewhat on the low side of normal. Platelets may be increased but not to the very high levels that are seen with a systemic onset. Similarly, modest rises

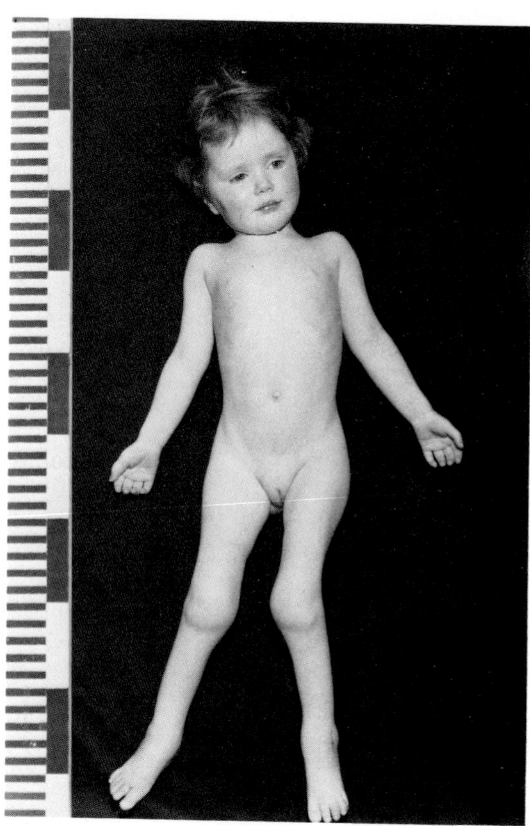

Figure 3.9. Juvenile chronic arthritis. Polyarthritic onset in a three year old with torticollis, elbow, hand, knee and ankle involvement

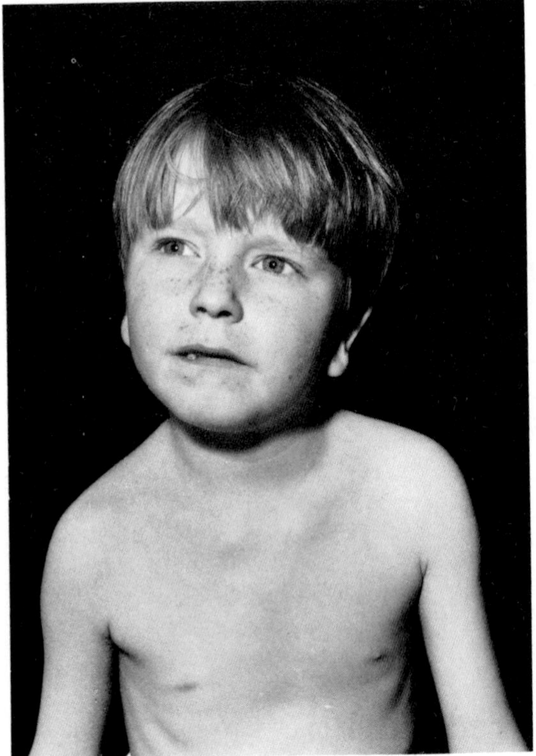

Figure 3.10. Juvenile chronic arthritis. Torticollis in a seven year old boy

of all immunoglobulins are not uncommon. Antinuclear antibodies are present in only a very small proportion of patients; other antibodies are absent.

With the exception of osteoporosis, radiological changes tend to be late (Ansell and Kent, 1977). Indeed, within the first year of disease the main purpose of the initial radiological assessment is to exclude other disorders such as leukaemia on the one hand or anomalies of epiphyseal development on the other.

Differential diagnosis

To some extent the age of presentation is helpful together, of course, with associated features. Thus the presence of bruising in a frightened baby who resists examination may make one suspect a battered child, a diagnosis which can usually be confirmed by the presence of fracture radiologically. Nowadays in Western countries scurvy is extremely uncommon in a baby; when it does occur it usually affects the hips and knees and it is associated with screaming on movement of the lower limbs but less of the upper limbs, at least initially. Another very rare cause of swollen joints with loss of movement in the first year of life is Farber's disease. This rare disease, which is associated with a deficiency in acid seramidase, tends to occur in the first few months of life and, in addition to the joint involvement, there are subcutaneous nodules and marked hoarseness of the voice (Toppet *et al.*, 1978).

The association of other disorders such as psoriasis may not be obvious initially. However, a family history and nail pitting in the patient (p. 71), may be helpful in distinguishing this sub-group. Similarly the synovitis associated with intestinal disorders such as ulcerative colitis and regional enteritis should be suspected in a child who is unduly anaemic, has a vague history of bowel dysfunction or has a family history of a relative suffering from some bowel disorder. Transient acute episodes of polyarthritis have been seen in children suffering from coeliac disease as well as from cystic fibrosis (Newman and Ansell, 1979). In many children, the post-dysenteric syndrome (p. 79) is associated with fever as well as arthritis, occasionally the presentation is as an arthritis, where sometimes there are other features suggestive of Reiter's syndrome such as conjunctivitis or urethritis (p. 78).

Other associations which are helpful in diagnosis include mouth ulcers as in Behcet's syndrome (p. 80), a history of repeated infections as in immunodeficiencies (p. 82), and rarely hypercholesterolaemia in the homozygous forms causes an episode of arthritis which is acute enough sometimes to mimic an attack of rheumatic fever (p. 81). Another problem is sarcoidosis where usually the presence of skin rash or bilateral lymphadenopathy will make further investigations for diagnosis essential. Occasionally bone tumours, usually secondary (pp. 236 and 260) or leukaemia (p. 230) can very closely simulate arthritis. Other oddities include Clutton's joints which have been seen in teenagers (Argen and Dixon, 1963) while the presence of finger clubbing and more generalised clubbing of digits should remind one of pseudohypertrophic osteoarthropathy (p. 258). Other problems in differential diagnosis include Thieman's disease (juvenile osteochondrodystrophy) which tends to occur in young people around the age of puberty (p. 265) and osteochondritis dissecans (p. 265) which when multiple, again simulates polyarthritic arthritis in the older child. Polychondritis may also be associated with features suggestive of arthritis (Blau, 1976).

IgM rheumatoid factor present

The main reason for separating out this sub-group is because of the difference in prognosis (p. 101). It is characterised by a female preponderance with an age of onset usually about ten years, although it has been seen in patients as young as five years. The presentation is with polyarthritis involving particularly the more distal joints of the limbs. The combination of soft tissue swelling of wrists and carpi with involvement of metacarpophalangeal joints,

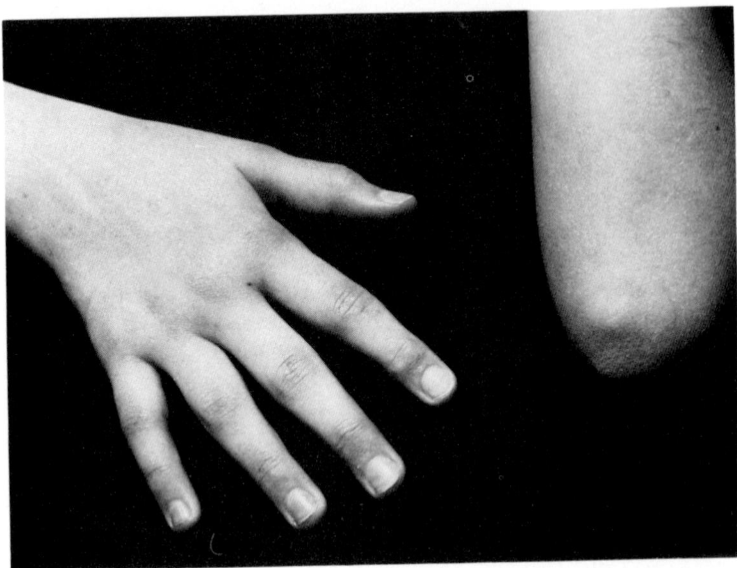

Figure 3.11. Juvenile chronic arthritis. IgM rheumatoid factor positive arthritis. Note involvement of the metacarpophalageal and proximal interphalangeal joints as well as the elbow nodule in a ten year old girl

proximal interphalangeal joints and metatarsophalangeal joints is closely associated with the persistent presence of IgM rheumatoid factor. In our computer study ulnar styloid lesions were also early – perhaps reflecting the age of the children. The large joints could also be involved early particularly knees and ankles, but usually in association with small joint involvement. Elbow nodules (*Figure 3.11*) with the histology characteristic of those seen in adult rheumatoid arthritis, can be seen.

That the age of onset is important is shown by the prospective study of Hanson *et al*. (1969) who noted that almost 80 per cent of those patients with positive rheumatoid factor tests had an onset between the ages of 12 and 16 years. Rheumatoid factor has been detected, using standard tests of latex, SCAT or commercial variants such as RAHA (p. 281), within six weeks of the first symptom and in the majority by three months. It is exceptionally rare for rheumatoid factor tests to become positive after more than one year of illness. These tests tend to remain positive unless long-term anti-rheumatic therapy has been given. Periostitis along

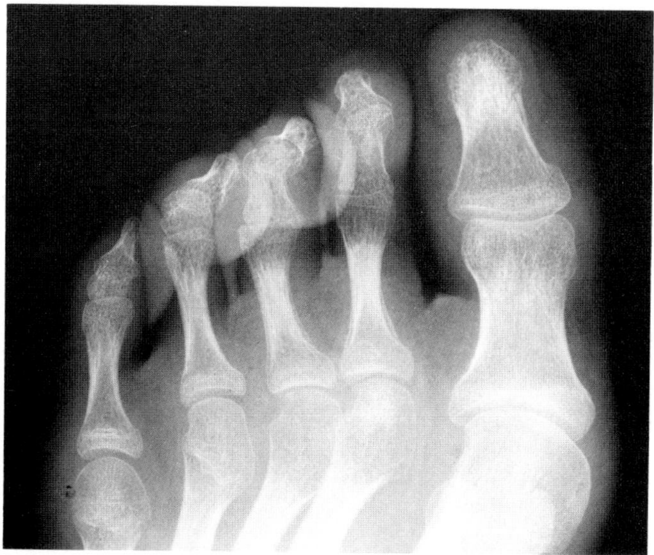

Figure 3.12. Juvenile chronic arthritis. IgM rheumatoid factor positive in a 14 year old girl. Note the periostitis, early erosion of the head of the metatarsal 2 and premature epiphyseal closure as compared to metatarsophalangeal 5

the shafts of metacarpals and metatarsals and bases of proximal phalanges extending into joints have been seen radiologically as early as six weeks, though more usually it occurs between three and 12 months (*Figure 3.12*). In all sites radiological change tends to be early (Ansell and Kent, 1977) but is particularly common in hands and feet.

Pauci-articular juvenile chronic arthritis (Still's, juvenile rheumatoid arthritis)

By pauci-articular juvenile chronic arthritis is meant arthritis of four or less joints in the first three months, and this is far the commonest mode of presentation of juvenile chronic arthritis. In

TABLE 3.6
Pauci-articular onset of juvenile chronic arthritis

Chronic iridocyclitis	Present or develops	Both sexes Young ANA +
Pauci-articular →	Polyarticular	Girls Any age ANA may be + Iridocyclitis
Persistent pauci-articular		HL-A D TMo
Monarticular		Girls 8 + ANA −
Juvenile ankylosing spondylitis		Boys 9 + HL-A B27 +

our experience it accounts for 65 per cent of cases seen within three months of onset. To date several sub-groups have been recognised (*Table 3.6*). The most commonly involved joints are the knee, ankle and elbow (*Figure 3.13*), while a single finger with a proximal interphalangeal joint swollen and flexor tenosynovitis or a toe similarly affected are also common. After this come the wrists and the neck.

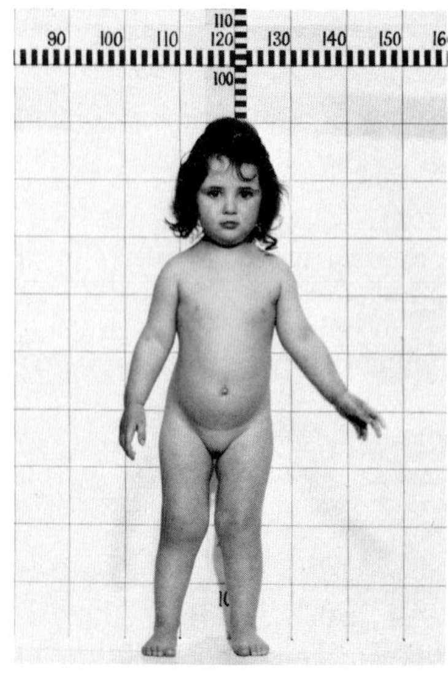

Figure 3.13. Juvenile chronic arthritis. Pauci-articular onset in a girl of three. Note swollen right knee and difficulty in extending right elbow

The most common sub-group is that of young children, i.e. between one and five years of age who either have chronic iridocyclitis at presentation or develop it in the course of the next year or so; both sexes are equally affected and they frequently carry anti-nuclear antibodies. There is a very close association between the presence of anti-nuclear antibodies in the serum and chronic iridocyclitis (p. 113). As yet, there is no way of distinguishing those children who present with two or three joints and then go on to polyarthritis; polyarthritis tends to be somewhat quiet and insidious with a gradual addition of one joint after another. Girls are more commonly affected than boys and the disease can occur at any age. Anti-nuclear antibodies may be present, particularly in those who commence young and there does appear to be an increased risk of iridocyclitis.

By contrast, those children who remain with just a few joints affected tend to carry tissue type HL-A D/TMo (Stastny and Fink, 1979). In our long-term follow-up there also seems to be a group of girls who commence with a swollen knee about the age of eight. They have a normal ESR, negative rheumatoid factor, negative anti-nuclear antibodies and the disease appears to be relatively benign affecting predominantly the knee (Ansell and Wood, 1976). It is within the pauci-articular group that radiological growth changes are noticeable early particularly in large joints such as the knee (*Figure 2.5*, p. 30) or elbows, (*Figure 2.1*, p. 21). An onset of pauci-articular arthritis in children aged nine or above, particularly boys, is very likely to be followed by the later development of sacro-iliac changes (*Figure 3.14*). A family history of ankylosing spondylitis or arthropathy associated with sacro-iliitis can be found in almost half the cases, after careful questioning. The most commonly affected joints in this sub-group are the hips (50 per cent) and knees (50 per cent) followed by the ankles (Ansell, 1980). These children carry HL-A B27. Juvenile ankylosing spondylitis (p. 77) may also develop in association with the intestinal diseases of ulcerative colitis and regional enteritis and give the same clinical picture as the lone disease. Suspicion should be aroused if the haemoglobin is somewhat low with an only slightly raised ESR or with only two or three joints involved, or there is fall off in growth.

Psoriatic arthritis (p. 71) too, not infrequently presents with a pauci-articular arthritis and again, it is the association of features such as nail pitting or a family history which will make one suspicious. Similarly, a previous history of an episode of diarrhoea will make one wonder about post-dysenteric arthritis. These children too, carry the tissue type HL-A B27.

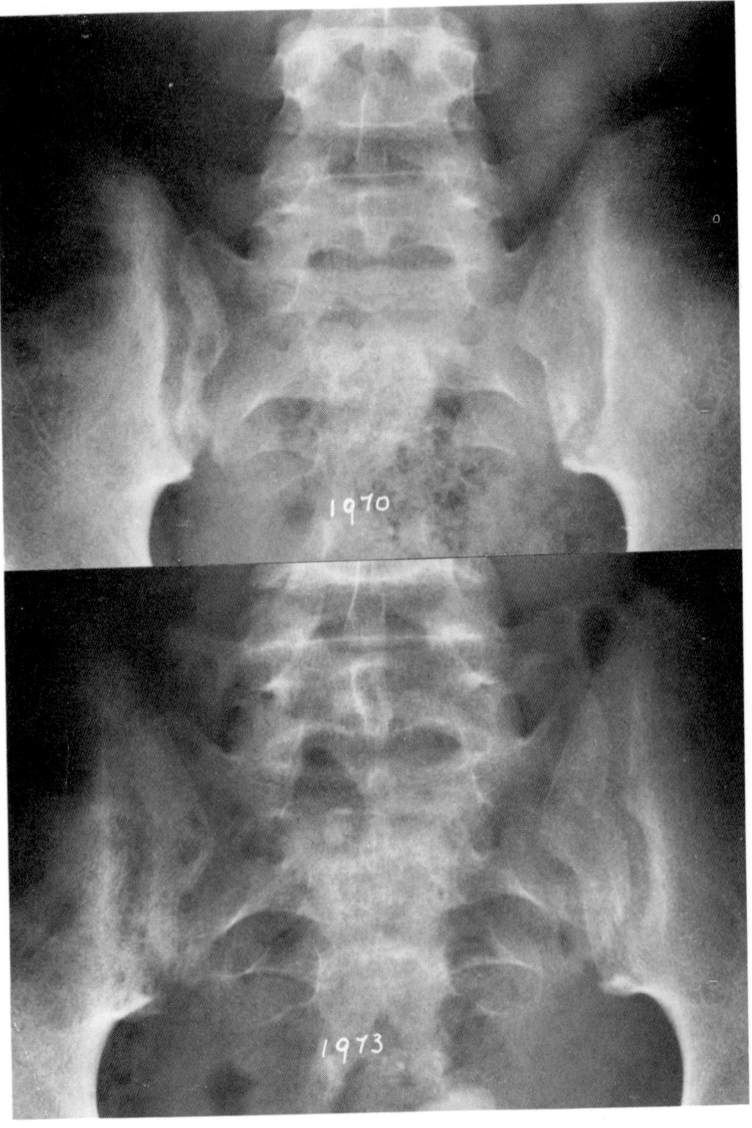

Figure 3.14. Juvenile chronic arthritis. Pauci-articular onset in a boy of nine. Note sacroiliac progression

The arthritis associated with immune deficiency (p. 821) also tends to have a pauci-articular onset, often involving the knees, but recurring frequently over a period of time. A history of recurrent infections should alert one to this possibility. Gout (p. 82) is uncommon in childhood except as a secondary phenomenon but will need to be suspected if acute episodes of arthritis occur in single joints. A form of rheumatism called palindromic rheumatism in which an acute episode of arthritis in one or two joints occurs and then regresses after a few days is occasionally seen in children, more commonly older ones, and in particular, those who ultimately develop IgM rheumatoid factor disease.

OTHER FORMS OF JUVENILE POLYARTHRITIS

Psoriatic arthritis

The onset of psoriasis is common between five and 15 years of age, 33 per cent of all cases starting by 15 years (Church, 1958). It is therefore somewhat surprising that there is relatively little information about psoriatic arthritis in childhood. Perhaps the wide pattern of disease that typifies this condition in the adult (Moll and Wright, 1973) and the lack of satisfactory definition in childhood are the main obstacles. We have therefore defined an inflammatory arthritis with an onset before 16 years, with psoriasis either preceding, coincident with or following the arthritis, and with no rheumatoid factor in the serum, as consistent with juvenile psoriatic arthritis (Lambert *et al.*, 1976). Our subsequent cases support the concepts given below.

Aetiology

Heredity probably plays a part in both uncomplicated and complicated psoriasis. It is not unusual to obtain a family history of psoriasis, psoriatic arthritis or spondylitis; it is very likely that the inherited aspect is multifactorial. This is supported by our studies on HL-A and B antigens, which show an increased incidence of HL-A B17 in psoriasis with peripheral arthritis and some increase in HL-A B27 in the spondylitis sub-group.

The peak age of onset is around ten years but both psoriasis and arthritis have been recorded as early as the first year of life. There is a marked female preponderance, conforming to the female dominance of childhood psoriasis. The psoriasis may ante-date the joint involvement, or the arthritis be followed by the psoriasis; relatively uncommonly the two occur simultaneously. There is probably a much wider group; Baker (1965) suggests that all adult patients with a strong family history of psoriasis, or with nail changes probably represent psoriatics. This would appear to be true in my juvenile cases as well. During the long-term follow-up

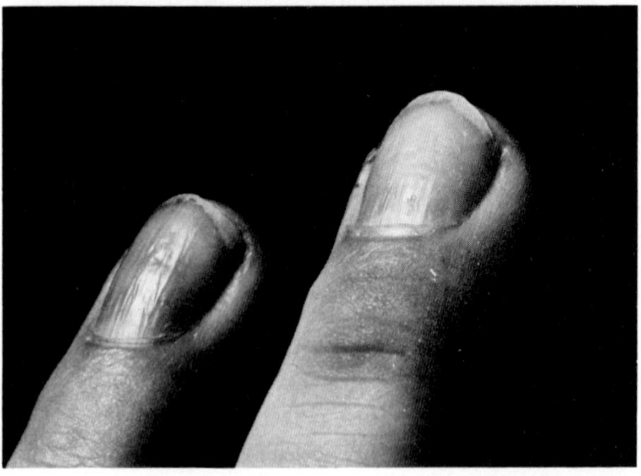

Figure 3.15. Psoriatic arthritis. Nail pits in an eight year old girl with asymmetric arthritis. Six years later she developed psoriasis

of children who have arthritis with nail pits (*Figure 3.15*) or sub-ungual atrophy, or with family history of psoriasis or psoriasis with arthritis, a number have ultimately developed psoriasis.

Manifestations

A monarticular onset is common but the pattern of joint involvement is wide-ranging; it is usually an asymmetical polyarthritis, often with intermittent episodes. One particularly common feature has been the involvement of metacarpophalangeal, proximal interphalangeal and terminal interphalangeal joints of a single digit often associated with severe flexor tendon involvement (*Figure 3.16*). There is a marked periosteal reaction along such a digit relatively early, and sometimes erosion of the joints (*Figure 3.17*). Tendon sheath involvement can be the major part of the disease with very little joint involvement, the flexor tendons of the hands being the most common site, followed by those around the ankles.

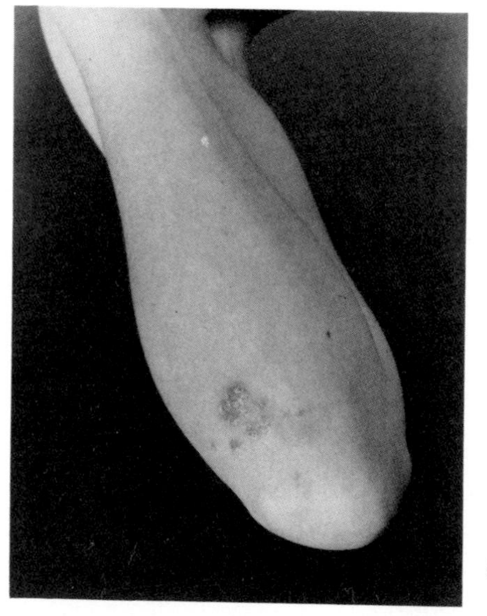

(a)

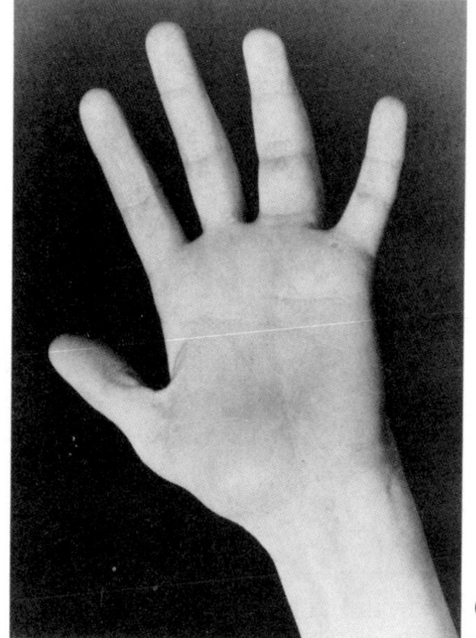

(b)

(c)

Figure 3.16. Psoriatic arthritis. (a) Psoriasis on elbow. (b) Flexor tendon synovitis of ring finger causing difficulty with flexion in a boy aged 12. (c) Periostitis in same patient as (b)

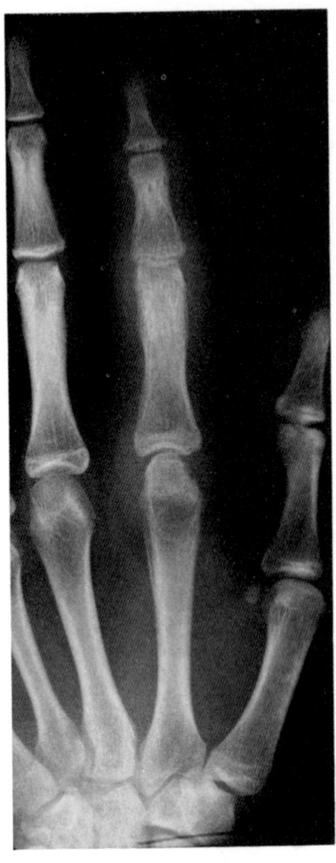

Figure 3.17. Extensive periostitis along the shafts of the metacarpus and proximal phalanx as a result of severe flexor tenosynovitis extending from the palm to its insertion. There is widening and shortening of the proximal and middle phalanx. In addition, synovitis of the metacarpophalangeal joint has led to the development of erosions

The major difference between juvenile chronic arthritis (Still's disease) and psoriatic arthritis the relative lack of systemic manifestations. Fever, rash and pericarditis are extremely rare, as is lymphadenopathy. The course is intermittent, with variable periods between exacerbations but it does continue into and through adult life. As in the adult form, very occasionally severe, destructive, asymmetrical disease occurs.

Indeed, there would appear to be two groups of patients, some who have the typical patterns of adult psoriatic arthritis as described by Moll and Wright (1973), and others in whom it is not possible to distinguish psoriatic arthritis from juvenile chronic arthritis (Still's disease). Thus, one of our patients had a family history of psoriasis and arthritis in the mother and psoriasis in the mother's mother; the patient herself had a pauci-articular onset of arthritis, she later developed psoriasis and also chronic iridocyclitis and carried anti-nuclear antibody in her blood. In general, anti-nuclear antibodies are found in the same proportion as in juvenile chronic arthritis and carry the same association with chronic iridocyclitis.

While agreeing with Calabro and Craig (1973) that the psoriatic arthritis has a somewhat later onset than juvenile chronic arthritis we would not agree that it is necessarily milder.

Arthritis with inflammatory bowel disease

Two major types of inflammatory bowel disease are generally recognised – ulcerative colitis and regional enteritis. The joint manifestations of the two disorders are indistinguishable. The incidence of arthritis in 136 children with inflammatory bowel disease in the USA was found to be 20 per cent (Lindsley and Schaller, 1974). There appeared to be little difference in the musculoskeletal complaints of children and adults with inflammatory bowel disease. The age of onset for children with inflammatory bowel disease is usually after the fourth year, with boys and girls equally affected. Onset of the arthritis usually follows bowel symptoms by intervals of months up to years but in some patients they develop at the same time, while occasionally the arthritis is the first manifestation.

In general, the episodes of arthritis occur when the underlying bowel disease is active. There is no demonstrable association between the severity of the underlying bowel disease and the arthritis. The most frequently involved joints are the knees, ankles, elbows and wrists but any joint can be affected. At times only a few joints are involved; the affected joints are swollen with varying degrees of pain, tenderness, warmth and loss of movement. These symptoms are indistinguishable clinically from those of arthritis due to other causes. Some patients will complain of arthralgia without any objective changes in the joints.

In general, the bouts of arthralgia or arthritis are brief, lasting a few weeks, and only rarely do they go on for months; but at least half such patients will have recurrent episodes. The prognosis for ultimate joint function is excellent.

Other manifestations

Recognised manifestations outside the alimentary tract include erythema nodosum, pyoderma gangrenosum and mucosal ulcers. These would appear to occur with increased frequency in patients who also have peripheral arthritis. Thus, Lindsley and Schaller (1974) found the prevalence of mucocutaneous lesions in children with inflammatory bowel disease considerably increased in those with arthritis. Fever can be a prominent finding in inflammatory bowel disease and may closely mimic the high spiking pattern of a systemic onset juvenile chronic arthritis. Weight loss is a well recognised concomitant of inflammatory bowel disease in children and, in addition, the children may suffer retardation of growth and severe anaemia. Thus, a child who presents with relatively few joints involved but has marked loss of weight with some growth retardation and a severe anaemia, particularly if there are mucocutaneous lesions as well, should suggest an associated bowel disorder (*Table 3.7*).

Spondylitis, which is indistinguishable from classic ankylosing spondylitis, is a well-recognised concomitant of inflammatory bowel disease in adults. Despite the lack of published reports of

TABLE 3.7
Complications of inflammatory bowel disease

Peripheral arthropathy
few joints
episodic
benign
Mucocutaneous lesions
erythema nodosum
pyoderma gangrenosum
mucosal ulceration
Gastro-intestinal symptoms
abdominal pain
diarrhoea
melaena
Fever
Anaemia

spondylitis and inflammatory bowel disease in children there is no doubt that it does occur. One of the main reasons for this is the fact that spondylitis in children often begins as a peripheral arthritis of large joints in the lower limbs, only considerably later do typical sacro-iliac changes (*Figure 3.14*) become obvious. There would appear to be no difference between uncomplicated ankylosing spondylitis and bowel disease. The incidence of HL-A B27 in our follow-up group is 90 per cent.

In our experience there is a high incidence (25 per cent) of acute iridocyclitis late in the spondylitic group so that this develops in the teenage period and in boys more often than girls. It is of some importance to try and distinguish the spondylitic peripheral arthropathy from that of the intestinal synovitis as the prognosis of the two conditions is entirely different. It is therefore occasionally justified to perform tissue typing. Mucocutaneous lesions do not occur with the spondylitic group.

Investigations

There are no specific laboratory findings in the blood, synovium or synovial fluid. The ESR is usually raised, there is usually anaemia which can be severe, the white blood cell count may be normal or elevated. Tests for rheumatoid factor and anti-nuclear antibodies are consistently negative. Low serum albumin will be found in patients with severe or protein-losing bowel disease. HL-A B27 is present in the majority of the spondylitics. Histologically the synovitis tends to be mild with polymorph infiltration but it is not possible to differentiate the lesion from other rheumatic disorders; in rare instances, granulomatous changes in the synovial tissue have been found in regional enteritis. The stools frequently contain occult blood.

Management

The management of this disorder is that of the underlying bowel disorder. Mild analgesia is usually all that is required; ibuprofen has proved very satisfactory as an analgesic anti-inflammatory agent in affected patients, and it has not caused further gastro-intestinal symptoms.

Reiter's syndrome

The most common cause of this syndrome in childhood is an infective diarrhoea although with sexual activity beginning earlier, one can expect to see more sexually acquired cases from the age of 13 or 14 years (Iveson *et al.*, 1975; Singson *et al.*, 1977). The dysenteric form can follow *Shigella* or *Salmonella* and probably other enteric infections. As it does not have to be associated with an epidemic, in all cases of acute arthritis it is wise to ask about preceding gastro-intestinal upsets. Boys are affected more commonly than girls.

The typical triad of urethritis, conjunctivitis and arthritis tend to develop within about ten days. Singson *et al.* (1977) suggest the range is usually three to 20 days after the initial incident. However, occcasionally an atypical arthritis in a teenager can be followed at a very much later date by other features suggestive of Reiter's syndrome. Irrespective of whether the illness follows diarrhoea or sexual intercourse, there is no consistent order in which symptoms develop. In small children it may indeed be difficult to observe a urethral discharge but a history of dysuria can often be obtained and,when the urine examined, pus found in it. Mucocutaneous lesions are not uncommon; these are usually mild and include erythematous ulceration of the hard palate, scattered pustules, inflammation of the glans penis and ulceration of the penis. Although Singson *et al.* (1977) report a child with a maculopapular rash, we have not seen the typical rash of Still's disease although the fever can mimic that of systemic disease. Acute iritis or keratitis is rare in these patients.

In addition to those manifesting all three features, children with polyarthritis may have either a history of diarrhoea or a definite other feature such as conjunctivitis. It could well be that this is more frequent than has previously been recognised and may account for some atypical juvenile arthritics. These children too carry the tissue type HL-A B27.

The arthritis varies from arthralgia, through a mild arthritis affecting two or three joints, to a severe widespread arthritis. The lower limb joints are usually involved first with the knee the most common site, followed by the ankle. Swelling of single toes and less commonly involvement of the upper limb joints have been noted, while in one of our post-dysenteric patients there was a marked flexor tenosynovitis. In young children the arthritis is very frequently symmetrical, the asymmetrical migratory involvement being more common in the teenager. Particularly in older boys, the arthritis can be very severe and persistent. Both typical Reiter's syndrome and post-dysenteric arthritis may go on to ankylosing spondylitis.

Basic laboratory tests are unhelpful in that the ESR is usually raised, there may be a mild polymorph leucocytosis, the haemoglobin is usually within the normal range as are the immunoglobulins. Rheumatoid factor and anti-nuclear factor are absent. In any patient with a history of preceding diarrhoea, stools should be cultured and blood obtained for routine antibody titres to *Salmonella* and *Shigella*, paratyphoid, etc. Most patients will carry HL-A B27.

Rarer causes

Serum sickness

The decline in the use of horse serum in therapeutics has caused a reduction in this type of illness but a similar reaction can be induced by drugs. Characteristically, some eight to 12 days after the injection or drug ingestion an urticarial rash develops which may cover the whole body. It is often associated with fever, rigors and occasionally pain and swelling develops in joints. Symptoms are seldom severe, antihistamines relieve the urticarial element of the skin rash and analgesics may be required. Only very rarely do corticosteroids have to be given. It is important to try and identify the allergen, often penicillin or Septrin, so as to warn the parents to avoid exposure in the future.

Behcet's syndrome

This syndrome is a triple symptom complex comprising recurrent oral and genital ulceration and relapsing iridocyclitis. In addition, a number of other features are seen with varying degrees of frequency, the basic lesion being a vasculitis. Skin lesions include erythema nodosum, small vasculitic lesions and thrombophlebitis, while arthritis and less commonly, involvement of the gastrointestinal tract, cardiovascular system and central nervous system can occur.

Behcet's syndrome affects males more frequently than females and is seen more commonly in patients from the Middle East and Japan than in British patients. It not uncommonly begins in childhood or adolescence, sometimes with just one feature. In our experience this feature has usually been oral ulceration while Mundy and Miller (1978) report its presentation with aphthous stomatitis. It is likely that incomplete forms of the syndrome exist in childhood, thus one young Turkish–Cypriot boy had recurrent oral ulceration and knee effusions beginning at the age of 11 but it was not until he was 15 that he started to get genital ulceration. Another nine year old boy who presented with abdominal symptoms and arthritis, some three years later developed iridocyclitis and later still, genital ulceration. Familial aggregation is not uncommon. Thus in an eight year old girl with recurrent mouth ulcers and arthritis, the father had had mouth ulcers all his life, while a paternal aunt had classic Behcet's syndrome.

Prognosis and, therefore, management depends on the manifestations. The recurrent ulceration usually requires only local treatment and the arthralgias mild analgesic anti-inflammatory agents. However, meningitic symptoms or pseudo-tumour cerebri will require high dose corticosteroids and bilateral iridocyclitis, cytotoxic drugs.

Familial Mediterranean fever

This disease is inherited as an autosomal recessive trait. It affects people from the Eastern Mediterranean, notably Sephardic Jews and occasionally Armenians and Arabs. It first appears in childhood or adolescence and recurs at irregular intervals throughout life. It is characterised by self-limiting episodes of fever with abdominal pain, due to a non-specific synovitis and sometimes an erysipelas-like erythema. Synovial episodes are cardinal features and occur in some 70 per cent of patients.

At times the joint episodes are the presenting features and indeed the only form of attack for a variable time. In the absence of a family history diagnosis may be very difficult until other features develop. The arthritis is usually polyarticular, can occur in isolation or with bouts of chest or abdominal pain (Heller *et al.*, 1966). The joints most commonly involved are the knees, ankles and hips. Occasionally episodes of synovitis are monarticular. The majority of such episodes are short-lived (three to seven days) but very occasionally joint destruction may develop in joints subjected to repeated attacks (Herness and Makin, 1975). In the hip, if the episode is prolonged, there appears to be a remarkable tendency to aseptic necrosis of the femoral head. It is suggested by Sneh *et al.* (1977) that this necrosis is not directly related to metabolic aberration underlying the disease but to attenuation of the arterial blood supply of the femoral head by synovial exudation. They therefore suggest that early aspiration of the exudate might alter this prognosis by preventing this complication. Lytic lesions are occasionally seen at other sites such as the knees, shoulder and metatarsophalangeal joints.

The development of secondary amyloidosis is of serious import, ultimately leading to death from renal failure; this can occur during childhood (Gafni *et al.*, 1968). Colchicine is considered to reduce both the attacks and the amyloidosis (Levy and Eliakim, 1977; Zemer *et al.*, 1974).

Familial hypercholesterolaemia (Type 2 hyperlipoproteinaemia)

Familial hypercholesterolaemia is a dominantly inherited condition, in which the majority of individuals are heterozygous for the abnormal gene. In the homozygous form, widespread xanthomata in skin and tendons develop in early childhood and ischaemic heart disease becomes clinically apparent during the first or second decade of life (Shapiro *et al.*, 1974). It is in this type that polyarthritis affecting the knees, ankles and hands can occur.

The onset is usually sudden and may be accompanied by fever and leucocytosis. The disease can mimic rheumatic fever because of the pre-existing ischaemic heart disease and if the xanthomata are mistaken for nodules. However, pre-existence and later yellow colour of the widespread skin and tendon xanthomata should help in diagnosis if the disease had not been already known or suspected, perhaps from a family history of early coronary disease. Confirmation of the diagnosis is made by the very high cholesterol level and type 2 pattern on lipoprotein electrophoresis.

The arthritis is self-limiting and in a few days requires only a simple analgesic for symptomatic relief.

Immunodeficiency

The arthritis seen in immunodeficiency tends to affect only a few joints with the knees the most common site; it is frequently episodic. Investigations for anti-nuclear antibodies and IgM rheumatoid factor are negative; x-rays are usually normal, minor growth anomalies can occur but bone erosion is extremely rare. It is generally considered more common in boys with sex-linked hypogammaglobulinaemia (Schaller, 1977) although Petty *et al.* (1977) noted chronic oligo-arthritis in 20 per cent of patients irrespective of whether the hypogammaglobulinaemia was familial or non-familial. It does not necessarily improve on adequate gammaglobulin therapy; indeed some of Petty's patients developed arthritis for the first time while on adequate therapy. This is in contrast to adults with acquired hypogammaglobulinaemia.

The disorder should be suspected in any child, but particularly in boys, with repeated episodes of oligo-arthritis, who have a past history of recurrent infections. Diagnosis is, of course, easy in those patients known to be immunodeficient!

Management is along the usual lines for chronic arthritis, i.e. maintenance of joints position and function by splints and physiotherapy. Simple analgesic anti-inflammatory drugs such as salicylates and ibuprofen are usually all that is required. It should also be realised that children with immunodeficiency are at greater risk of bacterial infection, which can affect more than one joint (p. 24).

Gout

A red-hot, swollen great toe mimicking sepsis will make one think of gout, but more than one joint can be affected and at any site. In childhood gouty arthritis is nearly always secondary to other disorders, such as neoplastic disease, particularly leukaemia: but it can also be seen in cyanotic congenital heart disease and in renal failure. It can also occur during the early treatment of leukaemia if the hyperuricaemia is not covered by allopurinol.

Primary gout is seen in the rare X-linked inborn error of purine metabolism associated with hypoxanthine phosphoribosyltransferase deficiency (Lesch–Nyhan syndrome); but it is not likely to present a problem in differential diagnosis because of the associated disturbances. These disturbances include mental retardation, chorea-athetosis, self-mutilation (especially of the lips and fingers) and high blood uric acid levels. Very occasionally in adolescence a partial defect of the enzyme will cause primary gout.

Sarcoidosis

Sarcoidosis is uncommon in childhood and, in particular, presentation as erythema nodosum with hilar lymphadenopathy is rare. It can present as fever, abdominal pain, enlargement of the liver with jaundice, a basal meningitis or arthritis. This is a chronic arthritis affecting particularly knees and ankles where there is gross boggy synovial proliferation with little pain, loss of movement or x-ray change (North *et al.*, 1970); histologically there are the typical granulomatous lesions. Other manifestations include chronic iridocyclitis, which is clinically indistinguishable from that of juvenile chronic arthritis, although anti-nuclear antibodies are absent from the serum. Localised cutaneous lesions are common, which again show granulomata histologically. Lymphadenopathy may be present. Constitutional symptoms are mild.

The increased prevalence seen among the adult black population in the USA is also noted in the childhood disease (Kendig and Brummer, 1976). One of our patients, a boy aged nine who presented with fever, arthralgia and iridocyclitis, was of Jamaican extraction; diagnosis was made on biopsy of an enlarged liver. Another young Kenyan Indian girl who presented with fever and a swollen knee had, in addition, infiltrative lung lesions. Indeed, to date, I have seen only one white child with polyarthritis due to sarcoidosis.

REFERENCES

Alarcon, G. S. and Townes, A. S. (1973). Arthritis in viral hepatitis; report of two cases and review of the literature. *Johns Hopkins Medical Journal,* **132**, 1

Ansell, B. M. (1977). Joint manifestations in children with juvenile chronic polyarthritis. *Arthritis and Rheumatism*, **20** (Suppl., 2), 204

Ansell, B. M. (1978). Chronic arthritis in childhood. *Annals of the Rheumatic Diseases*, **37**, 107

Ansell, B. M. (1980). Juvenile ankylosing spondylitis . In *Ankylosing Spondylitis.* Edited by J. Moll. London; Churchill Livingstone

Ansell, B. M. and Kent, P. A. (1977). Radiological changes in juvenile chronic polyarthritis. *Skeletal Radiology*, **1**, 129

Ansell, B. M. and Wood, P. H. N. (1976). Prognosis in juvenile chronic polyarthritis. *Clinics in Rheumatic Diseases*, **2**, 397

Argen, R. J. and Dixon, A. St. J. (1963). Clutton's joints with keratitis and periostitis; a case report with history of synovium. *Arthritis and Rheumatism*, **6**, 341

Baker, H. (1965). The relationship between psoriasis, psoriatic arthritis and rheumatoid arthritis. An epidemiological, clinical and serological study M.D. Thesis. University of Leeds

Bernstein, B., Takahashi, M. and Hanson, V. (1974). Cardiac involvement in juvenile rheumatoid arthritis. *Journal of Pediatrics*, **85**, 313

Blau, E. B. (1976). Relapsing polychondritis and retroperitoneal fibrosis in an 8-year-old boy. *American Journal of Diseases of Childhood*, **130**, 1149

Brewer, E. J., Bass, J., Baum, J., Cassidy, J. T., Fink, C., Jacobs, J., Hanson, V., Levinson, J. E., Schaller, J. and Stillman, J. S. (1977). Current proposed revision of JRA criteria. *Arthritis and Rheumatism*, **20** (Suppl., 2), 195

Calabro, J. J. and Garg, S. L. (1973). Psoriatic arthritis in children. *Arthritis and Rheumatism*, **16**, 117

Castleman, B., Scully, R. E. and McNeely, B. U. (1973). Rocky Mountain spotted fever. Case 26. *New England Journal of Medicine,* **288,** 1400

Church, R. (1958). The prospect of psoriasis. *British Journal of Dermatology*, **70**, 139

Emkey, R. D., Ragsdale, B. D., Ropes, M. W. and Miller, W. (1973). A case of lymphoproliferative disease presenting as juvenile rheumatoid arthritis – diagnosis by synovial fluid examination. *American Journal of Medicine*, **54**, 825

Frizzeria, G., Moran, E. M. and Rappaport, H. (1975). Angio-immunoblastic lymphadenopathy; diagnosis and clinical course. *American Journal of Medicine*, **59**, 803

Gafni, J., Ravid, M. and Sohan, E. (1968). Familial Mediterranean fever and amyloidosis. *Journal of Medical Science,* **4,** 995

Ginsburg, C. M., Henle, W., Henle, G. and Horwitz, C. A. (1977). Infectious mononucleosis in children; evaluation of Epstein-Barr virus-specific serological data. *Journal of the American Medical Association*, **237**, (8), 781

Gunawardena, D. A. Gunawardena, K. A., Ratnayaka, R. M. R. S. and Vasanthamathan, N. S. (1975). A clinical spectrum of Sweet's syndrome (acute febrile neutrophilic dermatosis) – a report of eighteen cases. *British Journal of Dermatology*, **92**, 363

Hanson, V., Drexler, E. and Kornreich, H. (1969). The relationship of rheumatoid factor to age of onset in juvenile rheumatoid arthritis. *Arthritis and Rheumatism*, **12**, 82

Heller, H., Gafni, J., Michaeli, D., Shahin, N., Sohar, E., Ehrlich, G., Karten, I. and Sokoloff, L. (1966). The arthritis of familial Mediterranean fever (FMF). *Arthritis and Rheumatism*, **9**, 1

Herness, D. and Makin, M. (1975). Articular damage in familial Mediterranean fever. *Journal of Bone and Joint Surgery*, **57A**, 265

Iveson, M., Nanda, B. S., Hancock, J. A. H., Pownall, P. J. and Wright, V. (1975). Reiter's disease in three boys. *Annals of the Rheumatic Diseases*, **34**, 364

Jones, M. C. (1970). Arthritis and arthralgia in infection with *Mycoplasma pneumoniae*. *Thorax*, **25**, 748

Kendig, E. L. and Brummer, D. L. (1976). The prognosis of sarcoidosis in children. *Chest*, **70**, 351

Kinsella, P., Ebringer, R., Hooker, J., Corbett, M., Cox, N. and Parry, C. B. W. (1978). Ankylosing spondylitis presenting at PUO. *British Medical Journal*, **2**, 19

Lambert, J. R., Ansell, B. M., Stephenson, E. and Wright, V. (1976). Psoriatic arthritis in childhood. *Clinics in Rheumatic Diseases*, **2**, 339

Larson, H. E., Nicholson, K. G., Loewi, G., Tyrrell, D. A. J. and Posner, J. (1977). Arthritis after meningococcal meningitis. *British Medical Journal*, **1**, 618

Levy, M. and Eliakim, M. (1977). Long-term colchicine prophylaxis in familial Mediterranean fever. *British Medical Journal*, **2**, 808

Lindsley, C. B. and Schaller, J. G. (1974). Arthritis associated with inflammatory bowel disease in children. *Journal of Pediatrics*, **84**, 16

Lister, P. D. and Hollingworth, P. (1980). Arthritis associated with leucocytoclastic angiitis. (In press)

McGill, R. C., Martin, A. M. and Edmonds, P. N. (1966). Rat-bite fever due to *Streptobacillus moniliformis. British Medical Journal*, **1**, 1213

Miller, J. J. and French, J. W. (1977). Myocarditis in juvenile rheumatoid arthritis. *American Journal of Diseases of Childhood*, **131**, 205

Moll, J. M. H. and Wright, V. (1973). Psoriatic arthritis. *Seminars in Arthritis and Rheumatism*, **3**, 55

Moran, H. M., Ansell, B. M., Mowbray, J. F., Levinsky, R. J. and Soothill, J. R. (1979). Antigen antibody complexes in the serum of patients with juvenile chronic arthritis. *Archives of Disease in Childhood*, **54**, 120

Mundy, T. M. and Miller, J. J. (1978). Behcet's disease presenting as chronic aphthous stomatitis in a child, *Pediatrics*, **62**, 205

Munoz, A. J. (1978). Gonococcal and meningococcal arthritis. *Clinics in Rheumatic Diseases*, **4**, 169

North, A. F., Fink, C. W., Gibson, W. M., Levinson, J. C., Schuchter, S. L., Howard, W. K., Johnson, N. H. and Harris, C. (1970). Sarcoid arthritis in childhood. *American Journal of Medicine*, **48**, 449

Newman, A. J. and Ansell, B. M. (1979). Episodic arthritis in children with cystic fibrosis. *Journal of Pediatrics*, **94**, 594

Petty, R. E., Cassidy, J. T. and Tubergen, D. G. (1977). Association of arthritis with hypogammaglobulinaemia. *Arthritis and Rheumatism*, **20**, (Suppl. 2), 441

Rahal, J. J., Millian, S. J. and Noviega, E. R. (1976). Coxsackie virus and adenovirus infection; association with acute febrile and juvenile rheumatoid arthritis. *Journal of the American Medical Association*, **235**, 2496

Rasmussen, J. E. (1976). Erythema multiforme in children; response to treatment with systemic corticosteroids. *British Journal of Dermatology*, **95**, 181

Reimann, H. R. (1948). Periodic disease; a probable syndrome including periodic fever, benign paroxysmal peritonitis, cyclic neutropenia and intermittent arthralgia. *Journal of the American Medical Association*, **136**, 239

Reimann, H. R., Coppola, E. D. and Villegas, G. R. (1970). Serum complement defects in periodic diseases. *Annals of Internal Medicine*, **73**, 737

Rossen, R. D., Brewer, E. J., Person, D. A., Templeton, J. W. and Lidsky, M. D. (1977). Circulating immune complexes and antinuclear antibodies in juvenile rheumatoid arthritis. *Arthritis and Rheumatism*, **20**, 1485

Schaller, J. G. (1977). Arthritis and immunodeficiency. *Arthritis and Rheumatism*, **20**, (Suppl. 2), 443

Schaller, J., Beckwith, B. and Wedgwood, R. J. (1970). Hepatic involvement in juvenile rheumatoid arthritis. *Journal of Pediatrics*, **77**, 203

Schaller, J. and Wedgwood, R. J. (1967). Classification of juvenile rheumatoid arthritis. *New England Journal of Medicine*, **277**, 1374

Schumacher, H. R. and Gall, E. P. (1974). Arthritis in acute hepatitis and chronic active hepatitis; pathology of the synovial membrane with evidence for the presence of Australia antigen in synovial membranes. *American Journal of Medicine*, **57**, 655

Shapiro, J. R., Fallat, R. W., Tsang, R. C. and Glueck, C. J. (1974). Achilles tendinitis and tenosynovitis; a diagnostic manifestation of familial type II hyperlipoproteinemia in children. *American Journal of Diseases of Childhood*, **128**, 486

Singson, B. H., Bernstein, B. H., Koster-King, K. G., Glovsky, M. M. and Hanson, V. (1977). Reiter's syndrome in childhood. *Arthritis and Rheumatism*, **20**, (Suppl. 2), 402

Sneh, E., Pras, M., Michaeli, D., Shahin, H. and Gafni, J. (1977). Protracted arthritis in familial Mediterranean fever. *Rheumatology and Rehabilitation*, **16**, 102

Sontheimer, R. D., Garibaldi, R. A. and Krueger, G. G. (1978). Stevens–Johnson syndrome associated with *Mycoplasma pneumoniae* infections. *Archives of Dermatology*, **114**, 241

Stastny, P. and Fink, C. W. (1979). Different HLA-D associations in adult and juvenile rheumatoid arthritis. *Journal of Clinical Investigation*, **63**, 124

Steere, A. C., Malawista, S. E., Hardin, J. A., Ruddy, S., Askenase, P. W. and Andiman, W. A. (1977). Erythema chronicum migrans and Lyme arthritis. *Annals of Internal Medicine*, **86**, 685

Trentham, D. E., Masi, A. T. and Bale, G. F. (1976). Arthritis with an inflammatory dermatosis ressembling Sweet's syndrome; a report of a unique case and review of the literature on arthritis associated with inflammatory dermatoses. *American Journal of Medicine*, **61**, 424

Toppet, M., Vamos-Hurwitz, E. Jonniaux, G., Cremer, N., Tondeur, M. and Pelc, S. (1978). Farber's disease as a ceramidosis: clinical, radiological and biochemical aspects. *Acta Paediatrica Scandinavica*, **67**, 113

Utsinger, P. D. (1977). Immunologic study of arthritis associated with adenovirus infection. *Arthritis and Rheumatism*, **20**, 138

Van H. Souter, S. and Utsinger, P. D. (1978). Viral arthritis. *Clinics in Rheumatic Diseases*, **4**, 225

Windom, R. E. Sanford, J. P. and Ziff, M. (1961). Acne conglobata and arthritis. *Arthritis and Rheumatism*, **4**, 632

Whittle, H. C., Abdullahi, M. T., Fakunle, F. A., Greenwood, B. M., Bryceson, A. D. M., Parry, E. H. O. and Turk, J. L., (1973). Allergic complications of meningococcal disease I – Clinical aspects. *British Medical Journal*, **2**, 733

Zemer, D., Revach, M., Pras, M., Modan, B., Schor, S., Sohar, E. and Gafni, J., (1974). A controlled trial of Colchicine in preventing attacks of familial Mediterranean fever. *New England Journal of Medicine*, **291**, 932

CHAPTER 4

Juvenile Chronic Arthritis

The cause or causes of the different patterns of juvenile chronic arthritis remain to be elucidated. Except for post-dysenteric arthritis, including Reiter's syndrome, the initial triggering mechanism is unknown. Despite the suggestion of Rahal *et al.* (1976) that it is caused by adenoviral infection there have been no other reports of early viral isolation. The increased incidence of rubella titres noted by Ogra *et al.* (1975) may merely reflect an increased immune responsiveness, because when, in children under the age of five, with an onset of disease, the sera was examined, there was no increase in the expected incidence of rubella titres (Schnitzer *et al.*, 1977).

Certainly a large number of non-specific immunologic changes have been described. These changes include antiglobulin activity which is increased whatever technique is used, but IgG antiglobulins can be present in normal children! As yet, it has not been possible to demonstrate a significant difference in function of those antiglobulins found in juvenile chronic arthritis which would lead us to assume they have a pathogenic role. Similarly, the role of immune complexes which can be detected either by the $C1_q$ or Levinsky technique (p. 54) is not certain; neither is the role of thymus-dependent lymphocytes (T lymphocytes) in initiating or maintaining this illness (Miller, 1979).

Genetic aspects are also difficult to unravel, partly, at least, because of the heterogeneity of the groups that have been studied. Certainly in juvenile ankylosing spondylitis and occasionally in postdysenteric arthritis more than one sibling can be affected, and a family history of spondylitis is not uncommon in such patients.

Similarly, in psoriatic arthritis, a family history of similar illness is noted in about a quarter, and more than one sibling has been affected in some instances.

The overall prognosis as regards life is good, the two main causes of death being infection early and amyloidosis later. The course tends to be unpredictable and relapses can occur after prlonged remission: the vast majority of children do go into remission, but with varying degrees of residual deformity. In management, patience and a good relationship with the family are essential.

PROGNOSIS

Prognosis suggests the ability to predict outcome. Its accuracy is influenced by a number of factors which include the reason for referral (there are no population statistics available for juvenile chronic arthritis) and the homogeneity of the group under study, as well as the duration of disease at the time of referral. Thus, in the initial Taplow series those children seen within one year of onset (mean 5.7 months) fared considerably better than those seen later in the course (mean duration at inclusion in the study 4.7 years) when comparing function at the 15-year follow-up. Sixty per cent of the early referrals had no limitation of activity compared with 25 per cent of the late ones (Ansell and Wood, 1976). In looking at reports it is important to know their source, e.g. orthopaedic hospital, national referral centre or local hospital but with a special interest, etc., as well as the duration of illness. In the Taplow and other series not only the age at onset but also the mode of onset were associated with differences in outcome (Calabro, 1977). The following remarks are based on the Taplow and other retrospective studies with respect to the different syndromes that can be identified. Prospective studies, using the sub-grouping described in Chapter 3 (p. 48) are in progress in a number of countries in Europe, including the UK, as well as in the USA. It is hoped that these studies will shed more light on the value of current laboratory practice and the clinical state initially in allowing prediction of outcome.

Systemic illness

Systemic illness accounts for a fifth of patients in our present prognosis studies (*Table 4.1*). As already indicated on p. 50, systemic illness affects young children. At presentation only a few

TABLE 4.1
Mode of onset – cases seen by three months after onset, 1970–73, Taplow

	Number	%
Systemic	30	20.4
Polyarticular	20	13.6
Pauci-articular	95	64.6
Other	2	1.4
	—	—
	147	100

will have any evidence of arthritis but our recent prospective study has shown that by three months arthritis had developed in just over half. The younger the child at onset the more difficult it is to prevent the development of contractures and deformities. This may well account for the rather poor functional outcome in those who have an onset before the first birthday. Looking at the five-year state of our present study group, 14 of the 30 had had one episode of systemic illness and were in complete remission with minimal residua at this follow-up. Those children who were in remission by five years have tended to be markedly improved with loss of most of the systemic features and only a relatively mild arthritis by the one-year follow-up. This is also true of our previous studies (*Figure 4.1*). Of the remainder, three had had a remitting and relapsing course with periods of more than six months completely free of symptoms; relapses were usually associated with intercurrent infections, particularly of the throat. The other 13 showed varying degrees of systemic illness still present, but active arthritis was the main feature.

Exacerbation of systemic disease can also be associated with all previously described features (p. 50); thus recurrent pericarditis may occur and a case of cardiac tamponade has been recorded (Scharf *et al.*, 1976). Similarly myocarditis is occasionally seen but usually only when pericarditis is already present. Pneumonitis or pleuritis may accompany carditis; rarely it occurs alone.

The liver in children with systemic illness and, to a lesser extent, in the polyarthritic group appears particularly vulnerable; this vulnerability may be part of the disease but the liver is also intolerant to viral, chemical or other insults.

Cerebral manifestations are not uncommon (Jan *et al.*, 1972), again particularly in the sub-group with systemic illness (Calabro, 1976). These manifestations consist of drowsiness, meningismus

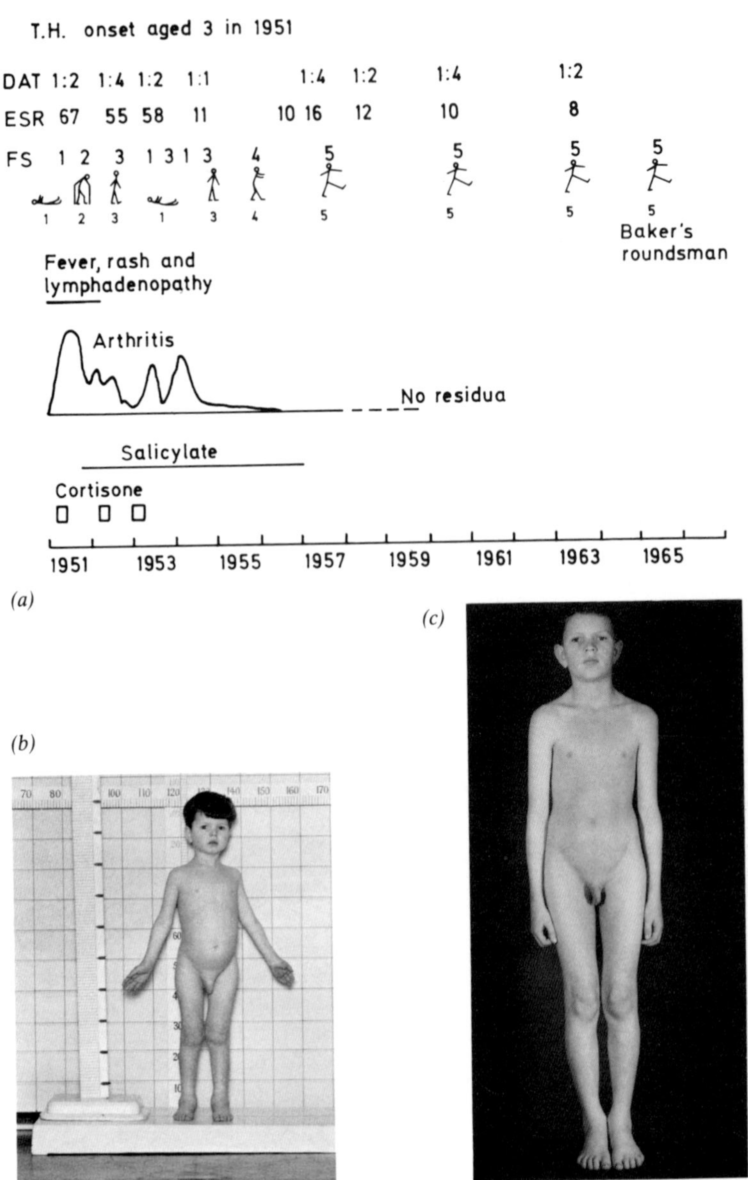

Figure 4.1. Systemic juvenile chronic arthritis. (a) Chart showing course with recovery at five years. (b) State one year from onset. Note swelling of the knees and ankles. (c) State nine years from onset, asymptomatic and with no residua

and seizures. The EEG may show transient very specific focal or diffuse abnormalities. The picture is further confused by the development of pseudo-tumour cerebri on reduction of cortico-steroids and, even more rarely, fat embolus after collapse of vertebrae or joint surgery.

In the Taplow series predictive factors are still being examined but we would concur with Endresen *et al.* (1977) that high platelet levels within the first few months of illness suggest a prolonged and difficult outcome as do high IgA levels.

In this small group seen within three months of onset and followed for five years, there were no deaths; in previous studies of 161 cases seen within one year of onset and followed for 15 years, eight of the 14 deaths had occurred in the systemic group (*Table 4.2*) (Ansell, 1978). The causes of death were equally divided between infection early in the course of the disease and amyloidosis late. In those patients with a systemic onset where active disease persists, there appears to be a very much greater risk of amyloidosis developing than in any of the other sub-groups (Ansell and Wood, 1976).

TABLE 4.2
Cause of death prior to 15-year follow-up among 161 patients seen within one year of onset by 1962

	Infection	*Amyloidosis*	*Other*	
Juvenile chronic arthritis				
Systemic onset	3	3	2	Cardiac failure – congenital; Renal failure
Polyarthritic onset	1	0	1	Aplastic anaemia
Pauci-articular onset	0	0	0	
Sero-positive juvenile rheumatoid arthritis	1	0	2	Fat embolus; Cardiac failure
Juvenile ankylosing spondylitis	0	0	0	
Psoriatic arthritis	0	0	1	Carcinoma colon

Polyarthritis

Whether the onset is polyarthritic or the polyarthritis follows systemic illness there appears to be little diffference in manifestations clinically or radiologically. When polyarthritis follows a pauci-articular onset, asymmetry is not uncommon, so that particularly in the early stages, there may be growth anomalies both clinically and radiologically. There is an impression that while the majority of children with polyarthritis show prolific synovitis, a few, in our experience about 10 per cent, show little palpable synovial thickening but gradually contract up in a manner which later leads to marked loss of function.

Girls are more commonly affected by polyarthritis than boys. There appears to be a bimodal distribution with a peak age of one to three, when the polyarthritis often follows systemic illness, in which boys and girls are equally affected, and a second group eight to ten when girls are more affected.

The knees, wrists and carpi, ankles and tarsi are involved symmetrically, as already described (p. 61). This is usually followed by symmetrical inflammation of the smaller more distal joints, particularly the proximal interphalangeal joints which tend to flex (*Figure 4.2*); though the metacarpophalangeal joints are frequently splinted by flexor tendon involvement, they are less severely involved primarily. In the presence of severe hindfoot involvement, metatarsophalangeal joints are not uncommonly affected later, while as in the hand, soft tissue swelling of interphalangeal joints may occur early. Particularly in those children where the illness starts before the age of five and persists actively for more than one year, hip involvement is common. Usually this slowly progresses and is the ultimate cause of functional disability. Some restoration of the hip joint is, however, possible (Bernstein *et al.*, 1977).

In general, sub-cutaneous nodules are rare in seronegative juvenile chronic arthritis, but when they do occur it is in the polyarthritic group. The nodules tend to develop in the usual sites such as at elbows, heels, occiput and over vertebrae as well as in the flexor tendons of the hands and feet; in the absence of IgM rheumatoid factor histologically, they resemble those of rheumatic fever more than those of adult rheumatoid arthritis.

Overall growth is probably less retarded in children with a polyarticular onset than in those with a systemic onset (Bernstein *et al.*, 1977). Growth rate improves as the disease goes into remission or is controlled by drug therapy, e.g. penicillamine (Ansell and Simpson, 1977).

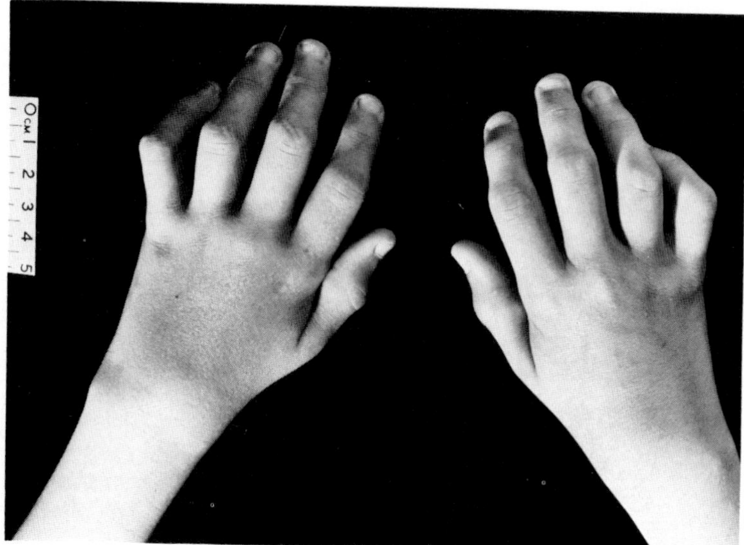

Figure 4.2. Juvenile chronic arthritis. Polyarticular onset aged four, five years previously. Note the marked flexion contractures at the proximal interphalangeal joints with metacarpophalangeal joints minimally affected. Wrist involvement is also obvious

While children with polyarticular disease may have mild fever and some lymphadenopathy it is relatively rare to find a rash. It is uncommon for them to go into a systemic phase of illness, unless the polyarthritis has followed systemic illness, in which case intercurrent infections may be associated with exacerbations of systemic illness. As in systemic illness, thrombocytosis and very high immunoglobulin levels probably portend a poor prognosis.

Although significant renal involvement is not a feature, urinary sediment abnormalities are not uncommon in juvenile chronic arthritis. There would appear to be an increased incidence of urinary tract infections when those children are compared with school populations. In a specific study Anttila and Laaksonen (1969) found up to a quarter of all children had haematuria or pyuria, with proteinuria less frequently. A number of these children had renal biopsies in which mild abnormalities were noted but the significance of these is not known; except when amyloidosis is present, renal function is rarely impaired. The evaluation of the kidney during gold and penicillamine therapy, however, becomes more difficult. Analgesic nephropathy, including renal papillary necrosis, has been seen, although the overall incidence is difficult to determine.

Early radiological changes are minimal (Ansell and Kent, 1977). They are predominantly juxta-articular osteoporosis and soft tissue swelling (*Figure 4.3*); later periosteal new bone formation adjacent to involved joints may be seen particularly along the phalanges, as a result of flexor tenosynovitis. Radiological asymmetrical growth anomalies are rare unless the onset is pauci-articular, but overall failure of development is not uncommon in protracted disease.

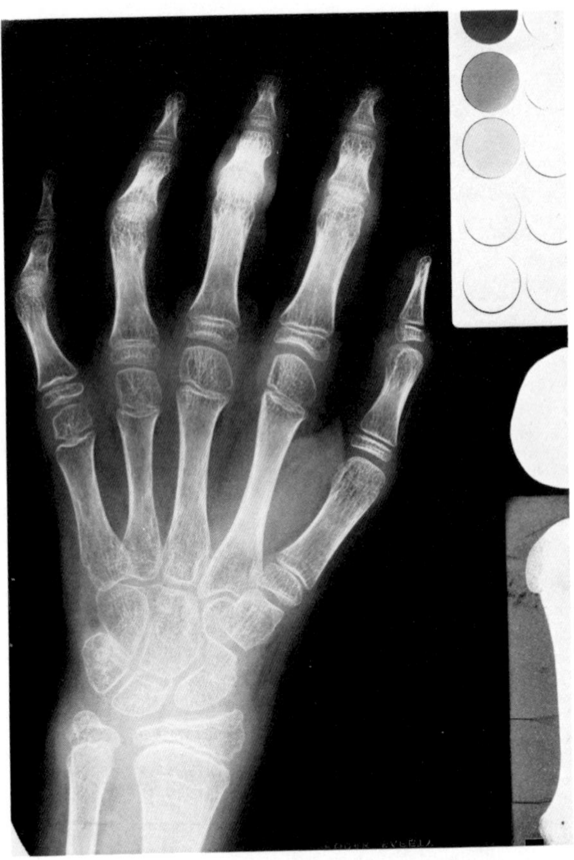

Figure 4.3. Radiological state five years after onset. Note the general porosis of bone, the normal metacarpophalangeal joints and flexed proximal interphalangeal joints without erosive change

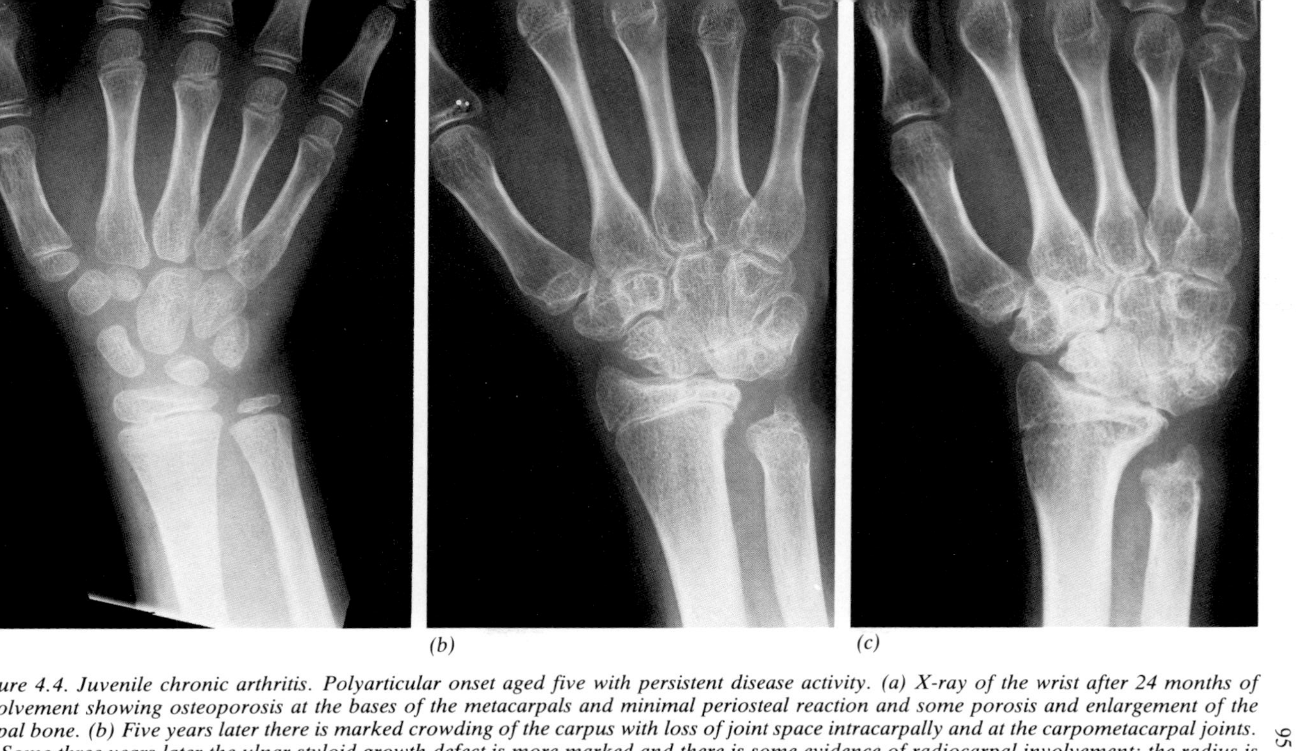

(a) (b) (c)

Figure 4.4. Juvenile chronic arthritis. Polyarticular onset aged five with persistent disease activity. (a) X-ray of the wrist after 24 months of involvement showing osteoporosis at the bases of the metacarpals and minimal periosteal reaction and some porosis and enlargement of the carpal bone. (b) Five years later there is marked crowding of the carpus with loss of joint space intracarpally and at the carpometacarpal joints. (c) Some three years later the ulnar styloid growth defect is more marked and there is some evidence of radiocarpal involvement; the radius is tending to move away from the carpus

Persistent disease activity is associated after several years with progressive bony change (*Figure 4.4a, b,* and *c*). This is most commonly seen in the hands (*Figure 4.5*), knees (*Figure 4.6*) and tarsus (*Figure 4.7*). Cervical spine involvement is associated with radiological changes in 30–40 per cent of the whole group by five years. The most common manifestation is fusion of the apophyseal joint starting at C2/3 (*Figure 4.8*). With prolonged activity,

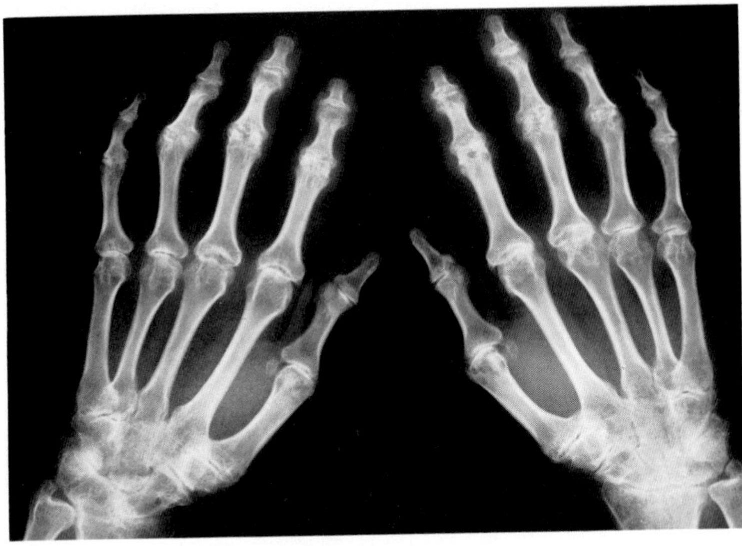

Figure 4.5. Juvenile chronic arthritis. Systemic onset aged nine followed by severe arthritis affecting all joints. Disease is now inactive but note the narrowing of the radiocarpal joints, the partial bony fusion of the carpus, the loss of joint space at metacarpo and interphalangeal joints with bony proliferation at terminal interphalangeal joints. Despite radiological appearances, the hands function adequately for daily life

particularly in the absence of adequate measures to maintain mobility, failure of development of vertebrae and widespread apophyseal joint fusion occurs (*Figure 4.9*). This is frequently associated with failure of development of the lower jaw (*Figure 4.10*) irrespective of whether or not there is temperomandibular involvement.

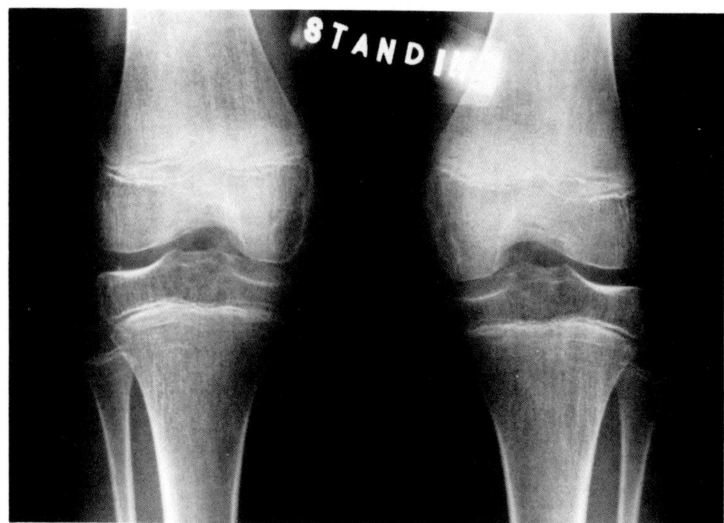

Figure 4.6. Polyarticular juvenile chronic arthritis. Knee involvement of five years' duration. Note the remodelling of the femoral epiphysis with apparent increase in size of the medial condyle, widening of the intercondylar notch, some narrowing of the medial joint space and modelling of the tibia below the enlarged femoral condyle

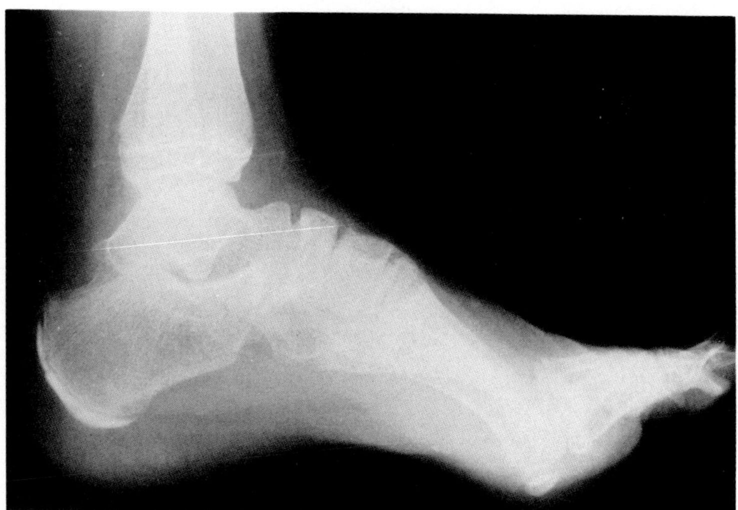

Figure 4.7. Juvenile chronic arthritis. Polyarticular onset in patient aged five, of five years' duration. Note the bony enlargement of the navicula which tends, together with narrowing of joint spaces and irregularity of tarsal bones, to be the earliest radiological finding in the tarsus

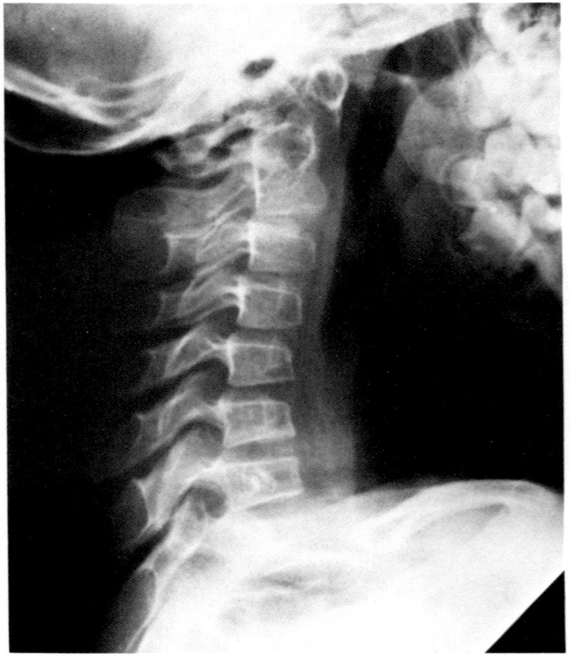

Figure 4.8. Juvenile chronic arthritis. Polyarthritic. Cervical spine showing apophyseal and disc changes at the C2/3 level. Note the small vertebra with step-like pattern

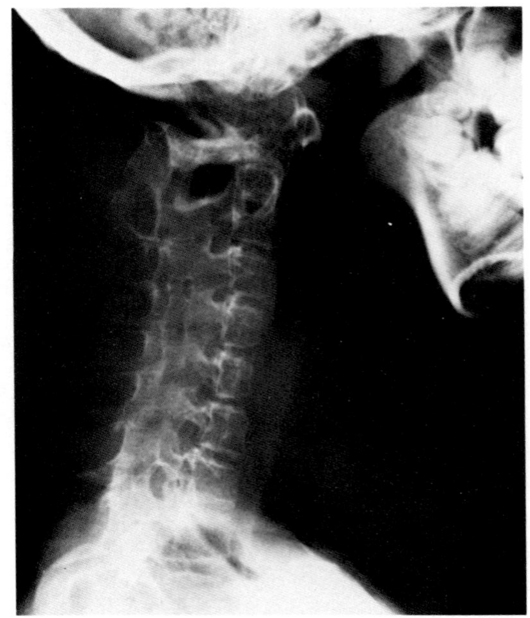

Figure 4.9. Juvenile chronic arthritis. Polyarthritic onset in patient aged two, with neck involvement from the onset. Now aged 12 with persistent activity and widespread deformity. Note the small but elongated vertebrae and bony fusion of all the apophyseal joints as well as the small chin

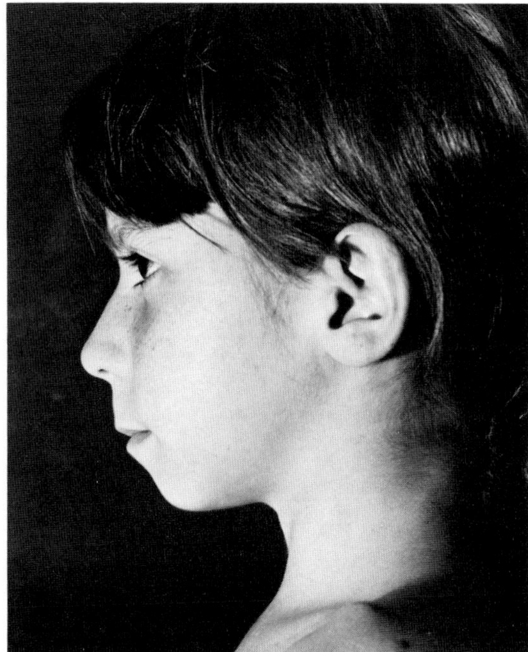

Figure 4.10. Juvenile chronic arthritis. Polyarthritic onset, patient now has limited neck movement and withdrawn chin

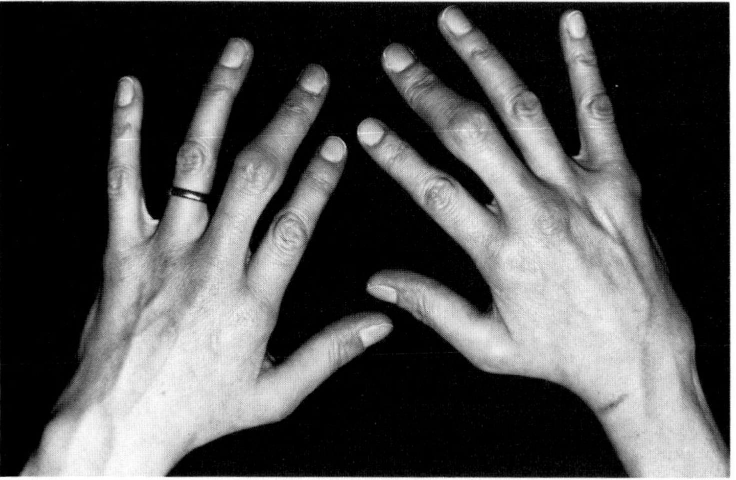

Figure 4.11. Juvenile chronic arthritis. Polyarthritic onset in patient aged seven. Now 35 years later bony enlargement of ulnar styloid and a number of proximal interphalangeal joints with flexion deformities of the third; hands function well

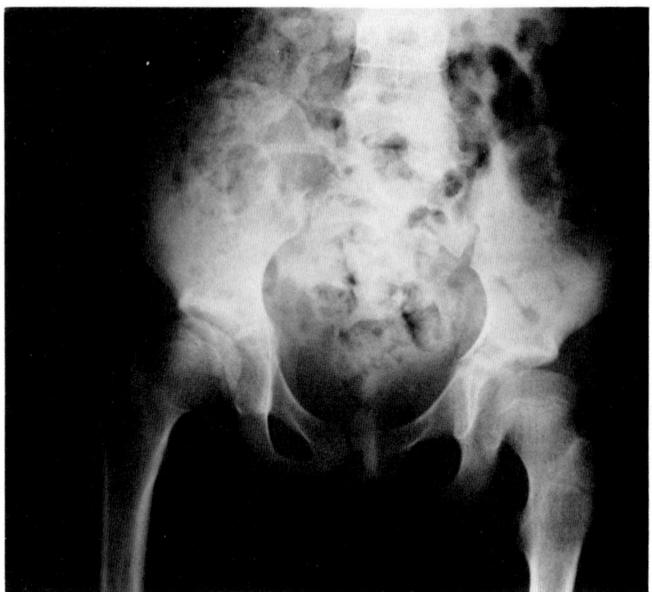

(a)

Figure 4.12. Juvenile chronic arthritis. Hip involvement. (a) Systemic onset in a girl of one year. Now six years later, the disease is inactive and she is asymptomatic but with coxa magna on the right with relatively poorly developed acetabulum and the straight femoral neck and narrowing of the joint space on the left. These are the only residua

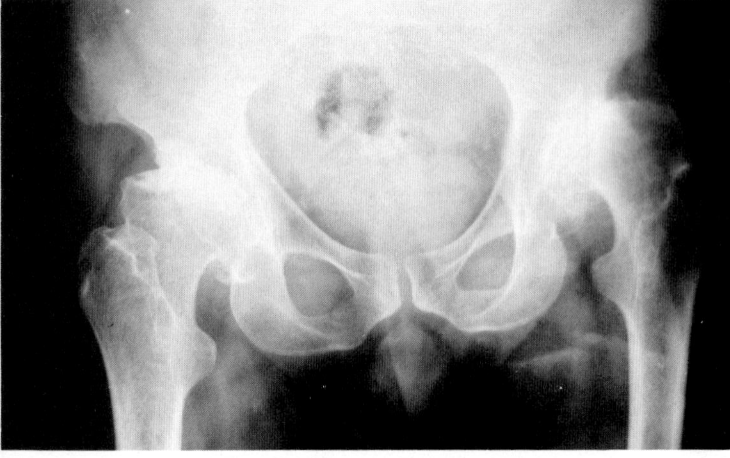

(b)

Figure 4.12(b). State of the hips of a man now aged 48 who had systemic juvenile chronic arthritis aged two and had an active disease for approximately eight years. All his life he has had what he described as 'a nautical gait', but in the last one or two years has had progressive pain and loss of movement at the hips

In our most recent study of early cases (p. 89) only three of the 20 with a polyarthritic onset had had one episode and were in remission at five years. In general, although many cases do have a monocyclic course with a good functional outcome, this tends to be prolonged over several years. The proportion which have an unremitting course with poor functional outcome is not yet known. Various series, not sub-divided into seropositive and seronegative, have suggested something like 30 per cent will still be active at approximately 15 years after onset but that this is not necessarily associated with marked disability. Thus (*Figure 4.11*) this patient had juvenile chronic arthritis some 35 years ago but has led a normal life. Long continued persistent activity is associated with the later involvement of elbows, hips and shoulders. When there is prolific synovitis Baker's cysts can develop at knees, shoulders and elbows. Radiological changes other than those associated with growth occur late in large joints (*Figure 4.12a* and *b*).

It is important, from time to time, to assess various features which include soft tissue swelling, effusion and pain on movement of joints, the functional capacity of the patient and the presence or absence of radiological changes, so that should deterioration be occurring appropriate medical and/or surgical management can be introduced. In those patients with persistently active disease over a prolonged period there is a risk of amyloidosis, but less than if the onset has been systemic.

IgM rheumatoid factor

IgM rheumatoid factor was present in 14 per cent of 162 early cases seen before 1962 and followed to the present time (*see Table 4.2*). This high incidence may reflect the number of adolescents seen.

In the Taplow series, sero-positivity is closely correlated with the presence of nodules. In a cross-sectional review of 110 patients with disease commencing under the age of 14 Cassidy and Valkenberg (1976) also noted a significant correlation between serological reactions, age of onset, the presence of nodules and bone erosions. As already indicated (p. 66) this usually commences in children aged ten or more; the early radiological changes demonstrated in *Figure 3.12* on p. 67 tend to progress rapidly so that, even with slow-acting drugs, five years from onset serious radiological damage can have occurred (*Figure 4.13*).

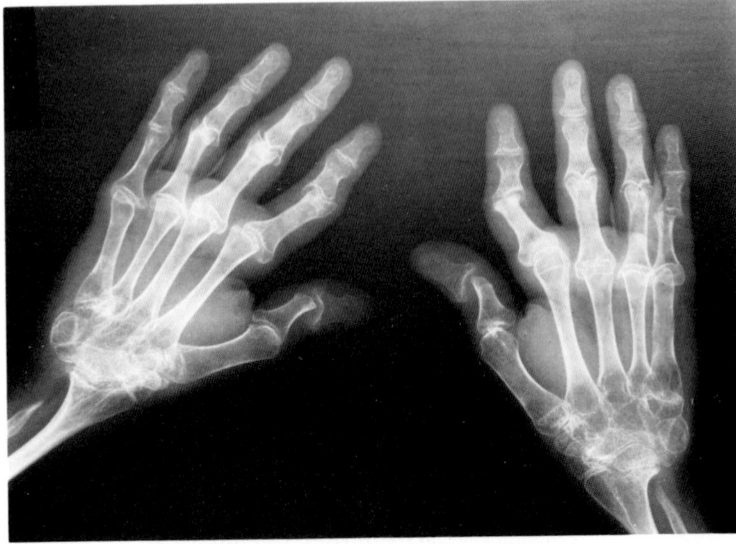

Figure 4.13. Seropositive juvenile chronic arthritis. Hand x-ray of a 17 year old girl five years after onset showing widespread destructive changes; the ulnar styloid processes have been removed. She had received myocrisin for two years early in the disease but this had to be discontinued because of leucopenia

Complications of adult sero-positive rheumatoid arthritis were also observed in this sub-group. These complications included the relatively mild one of carpal tunnel syndrome requiring decompression, the more sinister atlanto-axial subluxation (*Figure 4.14*), as well as rupture of extensor tendons. Other joint problems include a high incidence of hip involvement with a marked tendency to the development of protrusio acetabulae; destructive changes in the hip can be seen as early as seven months from onset.

In addition to the early destruction of joints, the disease tends to stay active so that patients seen in the late 1940s and early 1950s are still attending for control of active disease with progressive damage. At the 15-year follow-up of those cases seen within one year of onset, one-third had severe limitation of functional capacity and the majority were still active. It is accepted that, in considering the findings in this follow-up survey, therapy with gold and other slow-acting drugs was introduced somewhat later than would now be considered desirable (Ansell, 1978).

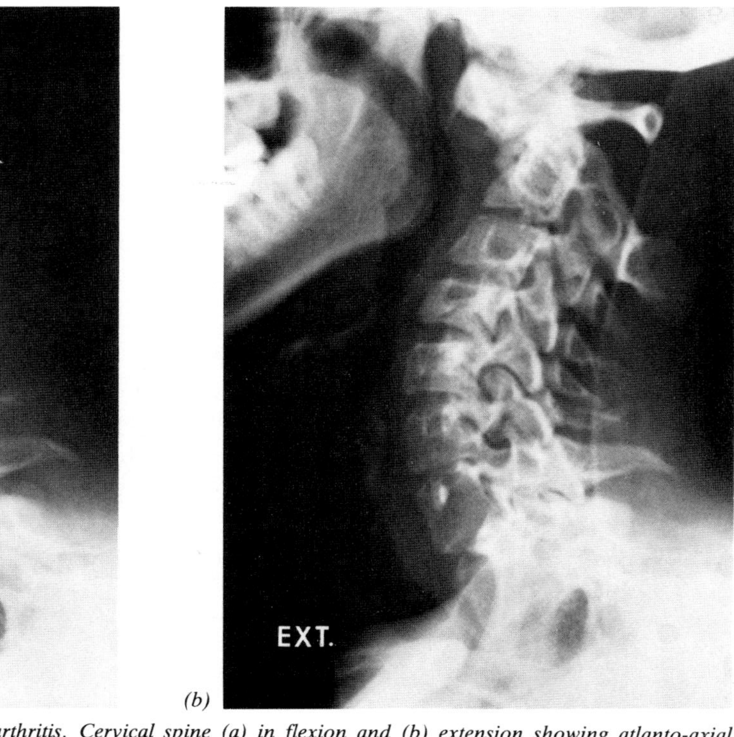

Figure 4.14. Seropositive juvenile chronic arthritis. Cervical spine (a) in flexion and (b) extension showing atlanto-axial subluxation causing neurological symptoms and signs in a 17 year old girl who had arthritis for ten years. Initially well-controlled on gold but deteriorated while on low dose maintenance therapy

Pauci-articular disease

As already indicated (p. 68 *Table 3.6*) pauci-articular disease probably represents a number of entities. Of those children who present with a single affected joint, i.e. monarticular disease, the majority will develop a pauci-articular pattern, frequently within weeks to months and usually within one year. However, in these patients the disease is usually limited to a few joints. It is within the pauci-articular group that radiological changes in the form of growth anomalies are seen relatively early (*Figure 2.5*, p. 30) and ultimately more destructive changes may be present. The presence of antinuclear antibodies with pauci-articular onset in a young age, i.e. under five years, suggests that the child is at risk from chronic iridocyclitis (p. 113). In general, in this sub-group joints can be controlled easily and the eye involvement remains a serious problem (*Figure 4.15a, b*); this warrants meticulous monitoring for many years.

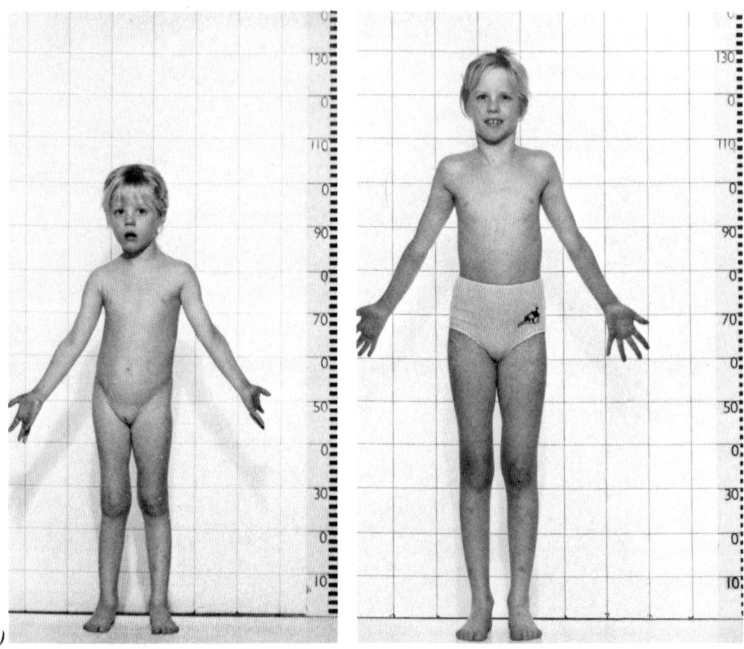

Figure 4.15. Juvenile chronic arthritis. Pauci-articular arthritis. (a) A girl of three and a half presenting with stiff neck and swollen knee of four months' duration and found to have chronic iridocyclitis. (b) Four years later she is growing straight with minimal joint residua but still requires constant local therapy for her chronic iridocyclitis

Those children who have negative antinuclear antibody appear to be at less risk of iridocyclitis, but are not completely free from this problem. There does, however, appear to be a group with a good prognosis which is associated with the carriage of HLAD, TMo (p. 69). As yet, there are no identifying features for those children who insidiously develop polyarthritis after starting with pauci-articular disease; some will have antinuclear antibodies and iridocyclitis, but not the majority. Such cases as do become polyarthritic tend to have raised immunoglobulins and higher ESRs initially but these are, of course, non-specific. Attention should therefore be paid to monitoring the number of joints involved at each visit. In addition, there is a small group who,

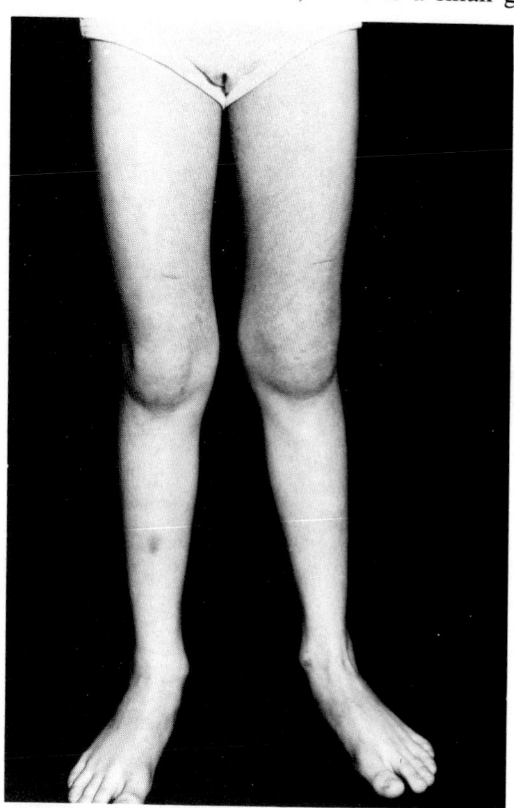

Figure 4.16. Juvenile chronic arthritis. Pauci-articular disease. Onset aged five with swelling of the left knee. Now, three years later, has a slight flexion contracture and valgus deformity at the left knee with a secondary valgus deformity at the foot

while still maintaining only two or three active joints at any one time, may get a total of seven or eight joints involved. They carry as good a prognosis with regards to joint function as the persistent pauci-articular group. However, in such patients meticulous care is required if local deformities are to be avoided (*Figure 4.16*) (*Figure 4.17*).

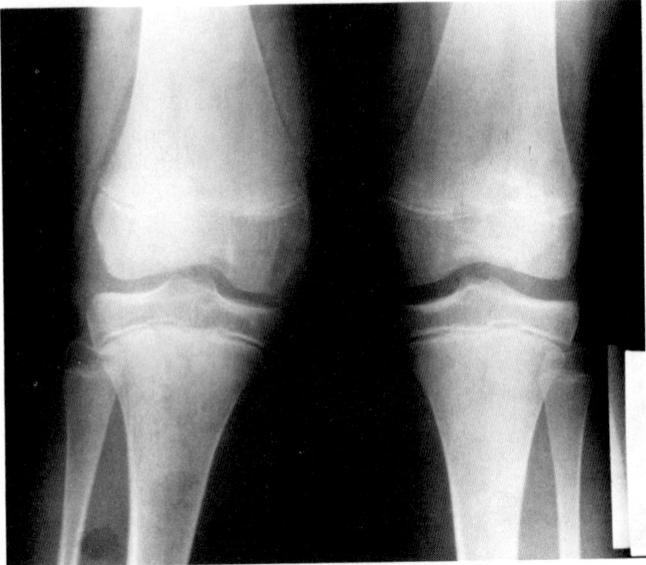

Figure 4.17. Juvenile chronic arthritis. Persistent monarticular arthritis of the right knee in a girl with onset aged seven; note the overgrowth of the metaphysis and epiphyses on the affected side together with marked valgus deformity at the five-year follow-up

In general, the clinical course is characterised by exacerbations and remissions but without much functional impairment. In this sub-group it is extremely rare to get amyloidosis. In our recent five-year follow-up study 36 of 95 patients had gone into complete remission by five years; a number were having repeated episodes; and ten, i.e. a ninth, had become polyarticular. Other series suggest that ultimately a quarter may go on to develop polyarthritis.

Pauci-articular onset of juvenile ankylosing spondylitis

This is the only form with a male predominance and in the follow-up of pre-1962 cases it accounted for 17 per cent of the total (*Table 4.3*). While the age of onset is usually in children above

TABLE 4.3
Patterns of disease according to 15-year follow-up (161 early cases seen within one year of onset prior to 1962)

Juvenile chronic arthritis	65%
Juvenile ankylosing spondylitis	17%
Juvenile rheumatoid arthritis	14%
Psoriatic arthritis	4%

nine years, it can start throughout the teens and very occasionally it is seen in children as young as three or four years. The family history of ankylosing spondylitis or arthropathy associated with sacroiliitis will not be obtained unless careful investigations, with detailed questioning, and often contact with other hospitals, is made.

The most commonly affected joints are the hips, knees and ankles, often asymmetrically. There is relative sparing of the upper limbs except for the elbows. Very occasionally there are constitutional symptoms such as fever and weight loss (p. 53). The peripheral arthritis may remit completely (*Figure 4.18a, b, c* and *d*) and then recur several years later or there may be just a progressive increase in the number of lower limb joints affected. There may be involvement at associated sites, giving symptoms such as heel pain due to plantar fasciitis (*Figure 4.19*) or bursitis of the tendo-achilles. Asymmetrical residual limitation and deformity of toes is seen in a quarter of the cases, while loss of movement at subtalar joints is also common. Knees and ankles tend to remit completely.

At presentation sacro-iliac films rarely show any abnormality but by about five years, in the majority, minor sacro-iliac changes have developed (*Figure 4.20*). Limitation of movement of the back may take many years longer to occur (*Figure 4.21*). Very uncommonly, atlanto-axial subluxation may be the presenting feature of this sub-group (Ansell, 1980); it occurs either with no other arthritis, or relatively mild involvement of peripheral joint or spine, and sometimes absent or only minimal sacro-iliac changes. By the 15-year follow-up acute iridocyclitis affecting one or both eyes has occurred in a quarter. Much less frequent problems include the development of lone aortic incompetence (in two of 70 patients), amyloidosis and bowel disorders. Over a third of patients have serious hip involvement (*Figure 4.22a, b* and *c*) and this is reflected in the functional status (*Table 4.4*) at the 15-year follow-up.

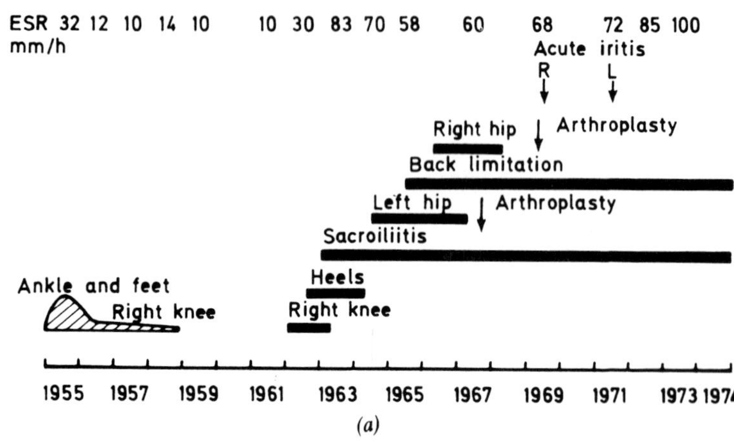

(a)

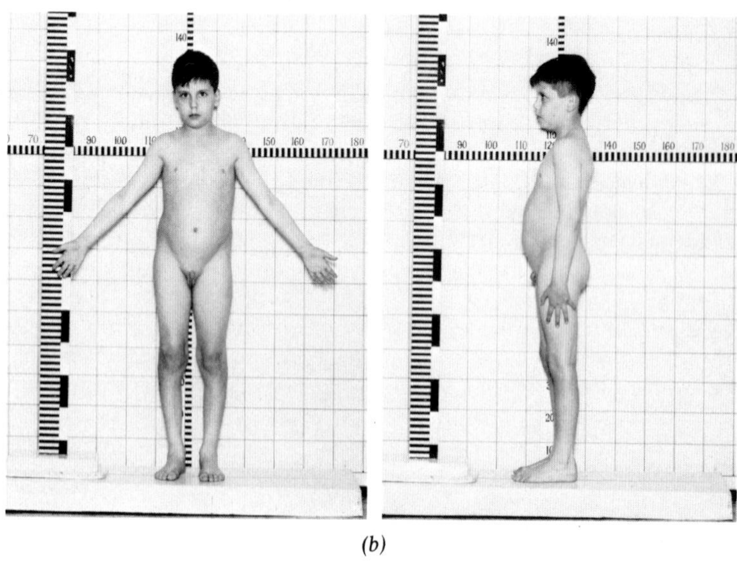

(b)

Figure 4.18. Juvenile ankylosing spondylitis. (a) Chart of course of a boy who presented at nine with a lower limb peripheral arthropathy; after a period of remission he developed new joint and back involvement followed by acute iridocyclitis. Amyloidosis was diagnosed on rectal biopsy 20 years from onset. (b) PA and lateral of RR aged nine

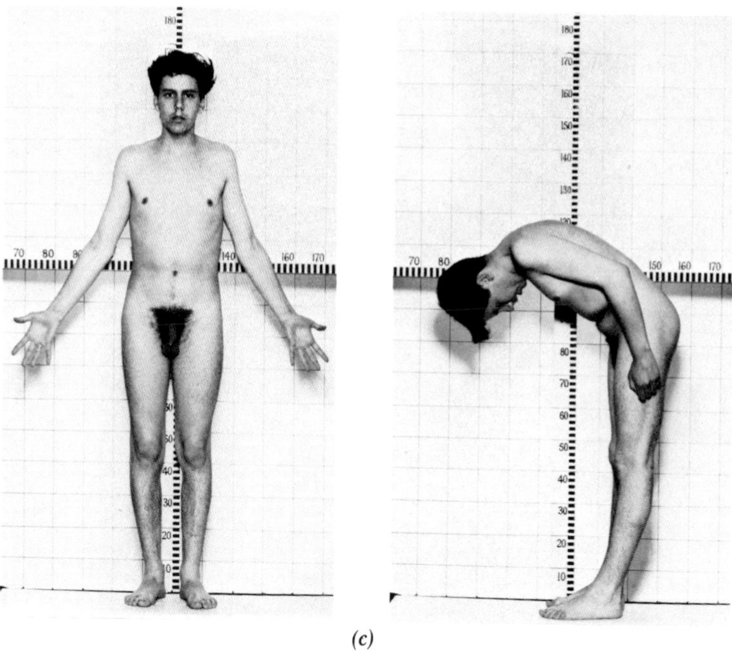

(c)

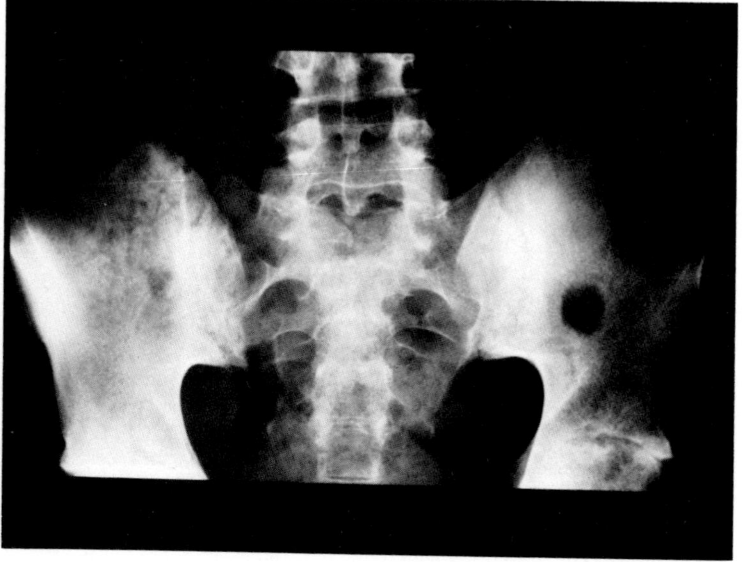

Figure 4.18(c). PA and lateral of RR aged 20. (d) Sacroiliac joints aged 21

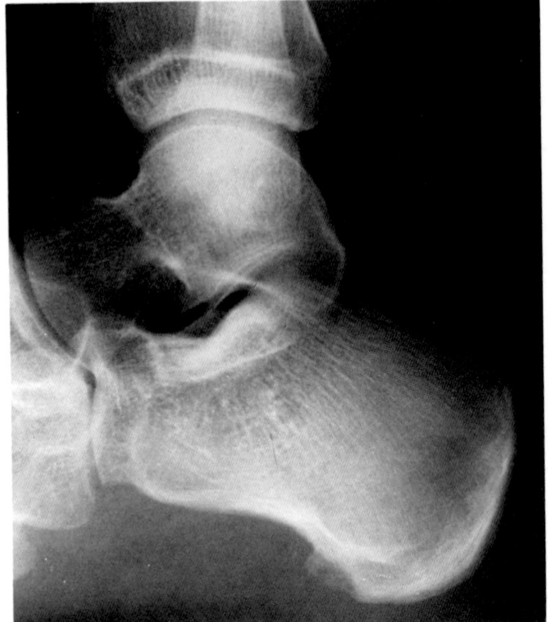

Figure 4.19. Juvenile ankylosing spondylitis. Heel spur secondary to plantar fasciitis

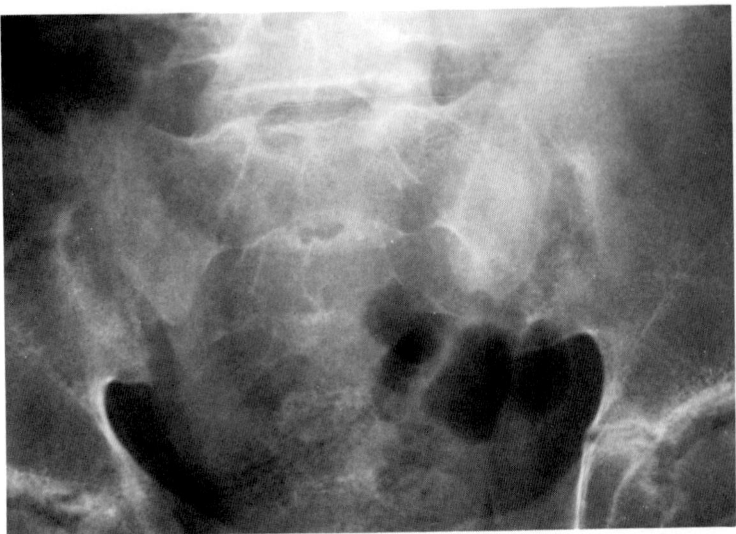

Figure 4.20. Juvenile ankylosing spondylitis. Early sacro-iliac changes in a boy who presented with atlanto-axial subluxation and a swollen knee

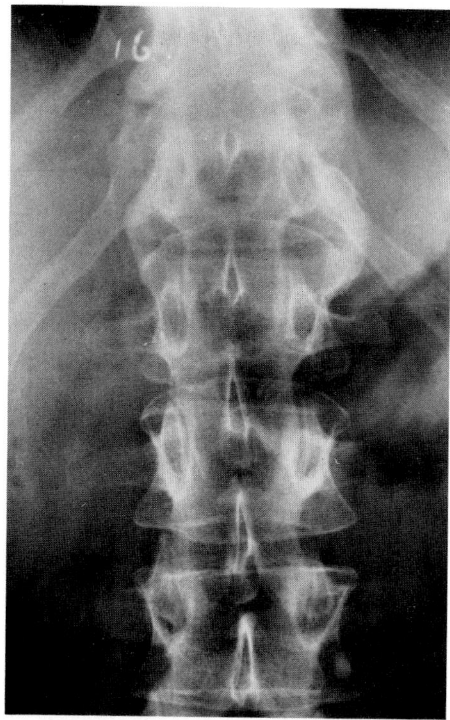

Figure 4.21. Juvenile ankylosing spondylitis. Classic bony bridging 14 years after presentation with pain in the metatarsophalangeal joints of one foot and the heel of the other

It has been suggested that the apparent excess of HL-A B27 in juvenile chronic arthritis may be due to these patients with pauci-articular onset not having been recognised. Certainly, by the time sacro-iliitis or ankylosing spondylitis has developed (Edmonds *et al.*, 1974; Ansell, 1978) there is a 90 per cent chance

TABLE 4.4
Functional status in juvenile ankylosing spondylitis 15 years from onset

NORMAL	60%
Slight limitation	28%
Severe limitation	12%

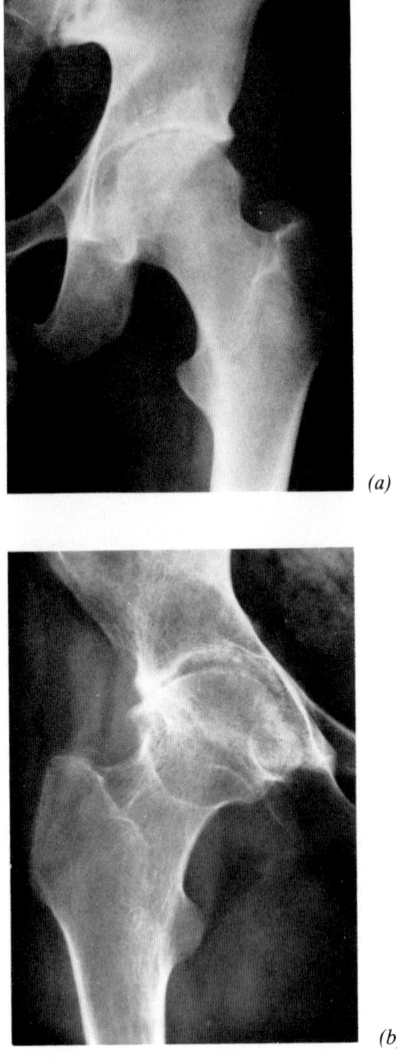

Figure 4.22. Juvenile ankylosing spondylitis. Hip changes of three types in adolescence. (a) Loss of joint space with narrowing and early erosion indistinguishable from seropositive juvenile rheumatoid arthritis. This type is associated with severe pain and loss of function. (b) Change in shape of the femoral head with widening, osteophyte formation and early 'ruff'. The joint space is well-maintained as is function, although there may be some loss of movement and discomfort on prolonged use

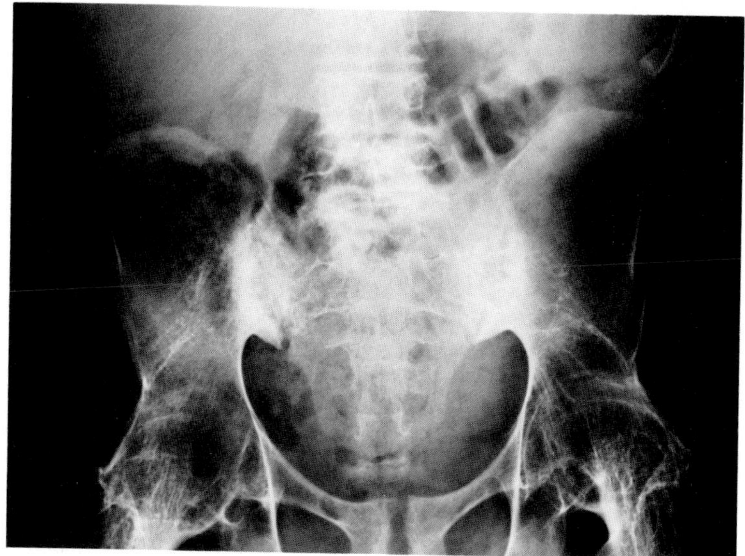

Figure 4.22. (c) Bony fusion after a period of immobilisation in a 14 year old patient

of carrying HL-A B27. Follow-up of those early cases reported by us in 1975 (Hall *et al.*, 1975), when it was noted that 25 per cent of early cases showed HL-A B27, shows that by the five-year follow-up the majority had developed sacro-iliac changes.

SPECIAL PROBLEMS

Eye complications

Chronic iridocyclitis

Chronic iridocyclitis affects young children, the mean age of onset in our series being 3.9 years. In two-thirds, both eyes are affected; the second eye becoming inflamed within a few months, or not at all. There is no relationship to the activity of the arthritis. It usually follows the onset of pauci-articular arthritis by a few months or even years; we have seen it as late as 18 years after the onset of arthritis in a single joint. The sera of affected children do *not* contain IgM rheumatoid factor but nearly 90 per cent are positive for antinuclear antibodies (Schaller *et al.*, 1974). Indeed the involvement of a few joints and a strongly positive antinuclear antibody suggest that the child is at real risk of developing iridocyclitis.

Chronic iridocyclitis can also precede the arthritis. In such cases, one or two joints are affected slightly, often only transiently, in the first few years but occasionally there is a more definitive arthritis. We have seen one patient with bilateral chronic iridocyclitis and a positive antinuclear antibody test who did not develop arthritis until 12½ years later. In such cases the iridocyclitis is the main problem in the disease.

The condition is not seen during the systemic phase of the illness but can develop later in a few cases, particularly if one or two joints are troublesome and the child develops antinuclear antibodies. Similarly, it occasionally develops in patients with chronic polyarthritis. The overall incidence in our series is 10 per cent but in the pauci-articular group it is much higher.

Symptoms and signs are minimal so a routine regular eye examination is essential in every child with juvenile chronic arthritis. In the presence of inflammation, examination with a slit lamp microscope reveals cells in the aqueous and keratic precipitates on the corneal endothelium. Posterior synechiae form in the majority (*Plate 4*) and exudate frequently coats the anterior lens and trabecular meshwork. The inflammation tends to drag on relentlessly for years with the formation of band keratopathy, complicated cataracts and secondary glaucoma. Band keratopathy appears at an early stage in eyes that are otherwise unscathed and with potentially good function. Initially, the sub-epithelial opacities are paralimbal at 3 o'clock or 9 o'clock or both; they may remain localised, but frequently extend centripetally to coalesce just below the centre of the pupil. Very occasionally, the eyes become hypotonic and phthisical due to the destruction of the secretory ciliary epithelium.

Management

Because the eye involvement is insidious it is essential that slit lamp microscope examination, to look for cells in the aqueous and keratic precipitates on the corneal endothelium, is carried out at regular intervals in those children at risk, i.e. pauci-articular arthritis with a positive antinuclear antibody test. This examination should be carried out not less frequently than four-monthly; in children with systemic illness, yearly assessment is all that is necessary, as it is in the children with polyarticular onset of arthritis who have negative antinuclear antibodies. Early detection and prompt treatment, with the use of local potent corticosteroids drops (dexamethasone) and mydriatics, are essential; slit lamp monitoring must continue after the institution of therapy, the frequency dependent on the severity of the inflammation and the ease with which it is controlled. The condition may drag on for years, during which time it needs adequate control.

Treatment of band keratopathy

Calcium salts are readily extracted from the cornea by chelation. The corneal epithelium overlying the opacity is removed by curettage and a 0.01M solution of sodium versonate is applied to the cornea. The corneal epithelium regenerates in a few days; the transparency of the cornea is invariably improved by this simple manoeuvre, and recurrence is rare even if inflammation persists (Smiley and Kanski, 1978).

Cataract

Cataract is the commonest cause of blindness in patients with chronic iridocyclitis; approximately one-third of eyes show some degree of complicated cataract, and this may be present at detection of iridocyclitis or develop over a few years. The development is insidious and may be difficult to observe through a small pupil which is resistant to dilatation because of posterior synechiae; in addition the anterior lens surface is frequently coated by iris pigment and exudate, and the cornea clouded by band keratopathy and keratic precipitates. These pathological changes allied to continuing inflammation combine to make removal of the cataract technically difficult and hazardous. In the past, conventional techniques of cataract surgery gave poor results. The recent introduction of more sophisticated instrumentation has enabled a less traumatic and safer operation to be performed at an earlier stage, with good visual results (Smiley and Kanski, 1978). Cataract secondary to corticosteroid therapy is discussed on p. 134.

Glaucoma

Hypertensive uveitis, which may occur as a result of acute iridocyclitis or during an exacerbation of chronic iridocyclitis, is due to the increased resistance to outflow of aqueous humour through the trabecular meshwork which is narrowed by inflammatory oedema. Obstructive glaucoma occurs as a result of mechanical interference with the circulation of aqueous humour at the pupil or in the angle. Every effort should be made to control intra-ocular pressure medically by the use of systemic Diamox and Timolol drops. When cataract and glaucoma occur together and the intra-ocular pressure is only moderately raised, the cataract surgery should be undertaken first, both for practical and psychological reasons; if this does not reduce the intra-ocular pressure then cyclocryotherapy is indicated (Smiley and Kanski, 1978).

Amyloidosis

The incidence of amyloidosis appears to vary. Thus, in our own 15-year follow-up series it is 7.4 per cent, which is similar to findings in other parts of Europe where the hospital acts as a national referral centre, whereas in Australia and North America this complication seems rare, possibly because the patient population is not comparable.

In general, amyloidosis appears to develop after many years of activity, thus we have seen it as late as 28 years from onset in one patient but more usually after five to ten years of unremitting activity, particularly with a systemic onset and relapsing systemic disease. As yet, we have no other correlations; the most sensitive index appears to be the development of proteinuria which is either intermittent or persistent, even though mild. Any rise in blood pressure, particularly if there has been an occasional trace of protein in the urine, should also be viewed with suspicion. In the year or so before the diagnosis of amyloidosis, CRP levels and IgG levels appear to be higher than in patients who do not show this complication. If the child with juvenile chronic arthritis goes into remission or can be satisfactorily controlled with therapy, it would appear that the patient's life expectancy can be considerably improved (Schnitzer and Ansell, 1977).

Mortality

There is an increased mortality in juvenile chronic arthritis which is probably related to infection within the first five years of onset and in later cases to amyloidosis (Baum and Gutowska, 1977). In addition there are occasional lethal complications of therapy, which include adrenal failure and blood dyscrasia (*see Table 4.2*).

MANAGEMENT

Principles

Juvenile chronic arthritis is a chronic disease which may persist actively for many years. The aim is to achieve a state whereby the child lives at home under adequate supervision and treatment, and attends school regularly. Every effort is required to prevent contractures and growth deformities from developing and, at the same time, to promote the proper growth of body, mind and spirit. To achieve this vigilance must be maintained throughout the whole period of activity of the disease process.

In assessments both initially and subsequently it is essential to take into account not only the pattern of disease present, but also the family background. The intelligence, willingness and ability of the parents to cooperate is extremely important, as the outlook in any individual case depends to a considerable extent on the persistent courage and capacity of the parents to help their child through what is often a long and difficult time. Drug treatment is only one of many measures in the management of this disorder; adequate splinting, exercises, rest of joints in good position; social measures and occasionally, surgery, but above all, the maintenance of psychological support is of paramount importance (Ansell, 1975; Bywaters, 1976).

Rest

While the disease is active the child will require an adequate period of rest each night, as well as a rest period during the day. Weight bearing should be restricted only if there is severe pain in the hips or knees or when flexion deformities of these joints require correction. It is important to emphasise that irreversible damage can result from prolonged bed-rest. Muscles and bones waste, joints ankylose, contractures develop, renal calculae and bed-sores can occur, and above all, time is lost, perhaps the most valuable commodity of childhood.

During periods of systemic illness bed-rest will be required; at such times every effort is needed to maintain functionally good posture by appropriate splints and movement of all joints by adequate physiotherapy. Thus, unless severe systemic illness, severe pain in the hips or knees, or gross contractures are present, every effort should be made to get the child up and walking for a period each day.

Maintenance of posture

This requires prevention of deformities. In the acute phase wrist and knee deformities can largely be prevented by the proper use of rest splints. If there is severe ankle involvement a foot piece can be incorporated at 90 degrees to maintain the ankle in a good position. Any involvement of these joints requires the use of rest splints. Work splints are rarely required in the acute phase but may occasionally be needed for a painful knee or wrist. If there is

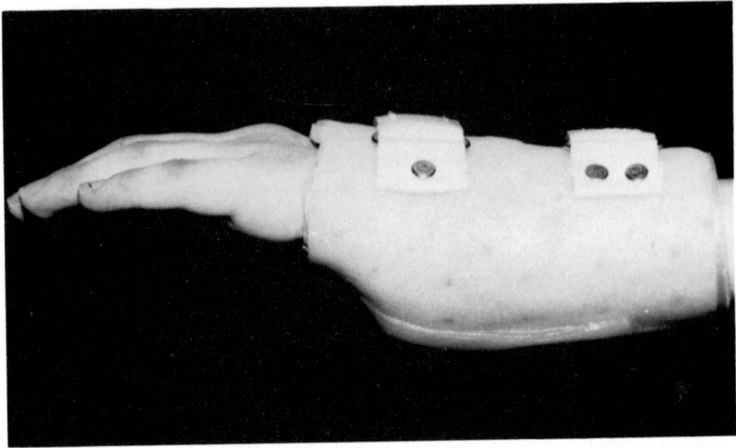

Figure 4.23. Juvenile chronic arthritis. Work wrist splint in vitrathene which allows full use of fingers

severe pain it is better to wear a splint and maintain the wrist in good position while using the hand, as in writing (*Figure 4.23*), otherwise deformity will develop.

If flexion contractures of knees or wrists are already present when the child is first seen, correction by serial splinting with plaster of Paris should be undertaken at the earliest opportunity (*Figure 4.24a, b*). After extra analgesia a hot damp pack is applied to the affected joint and maximum extension subsequently obtained. A cylindrical plaster is placed on the joint in this

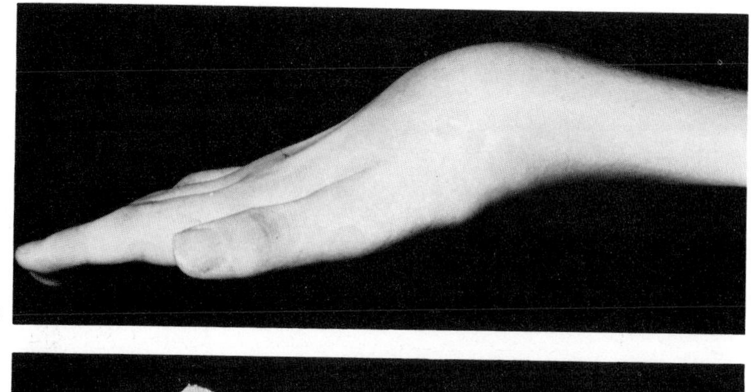

(a)

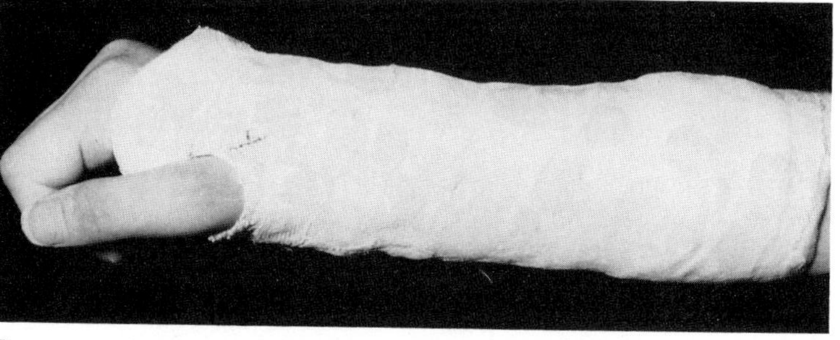

(b)

Figure 4.24. Juvenile chronic arthritis. (a) Dropped wrist after only nine months of illness. (b) Correction with plaster of Paris serial splint

position and left *in situ* for 48 hours. It is then removed and the patient given physiotherapy.

At Taplow, we tend to use weekdays for active physiotherapy and the weekends for serial splinting. In between periods of active physiotherapy a divided plaster continues to be worn. After one or two weeks a further serial splint is applied. In this way, gradual correction of deformities of wrists, and often knees, can be achieved. However, if three such splints do not give marked improvement, a surgical opinion should be obtained. Once satisfactory correction has occurred, the child should use a light splint until the muscles have been satisfactorily re-developed. This is particularly important in the knee (*Figure 4.25*).

After knee correction, weight bearing is gradually achieved with the help of either a frame, if the child has been immobile for some time, or a stick or crutches. Knee contractures are frequently consequent on hip flexion and when both are present they require correction at the same time.

To prevent and correct hip flexion, prone lying is of great value; this can be done during the daily rest period and for a short period

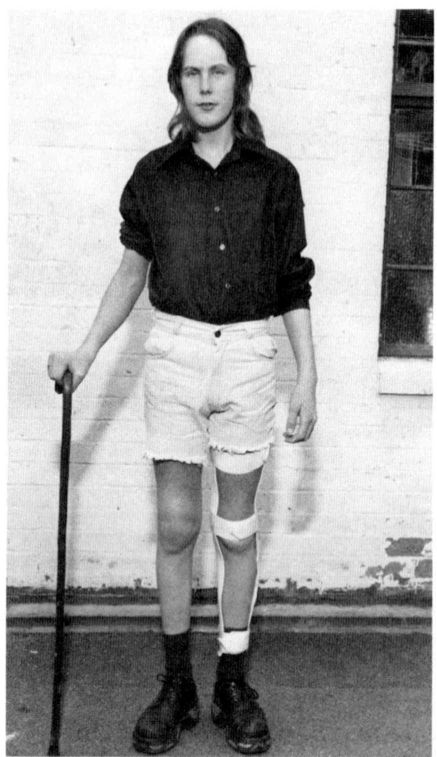

Figure 4.25. Juvenile chronic arthritis. Work splint for knee

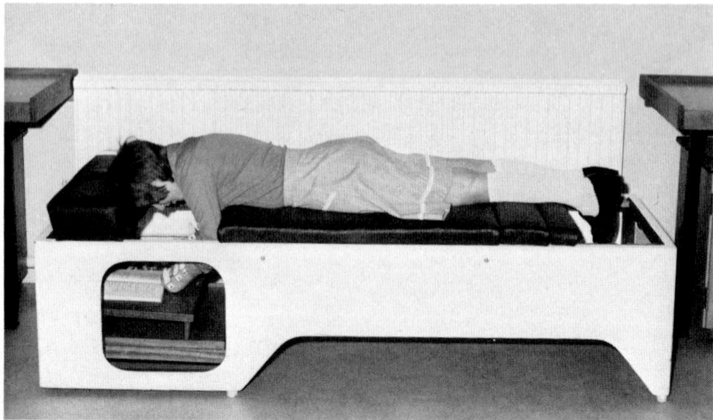

Figure 4.26. Juvenile chronic arthritis. Prone-lying bed which maintains extension of spine, hips and knees while allowing reading and writing

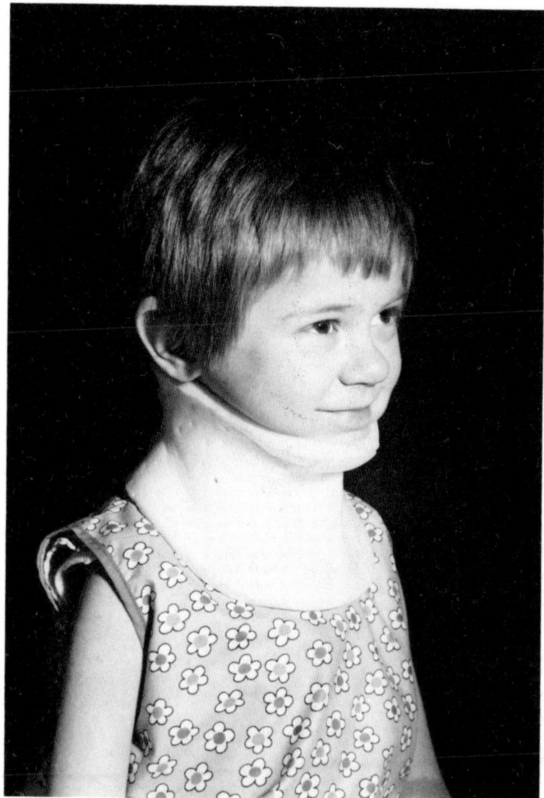

Figure 4.27. Juvenile chronic arthritis. Neck collar to maintain extension

when the child goes to bed at night. It can also be maintained while watching television and can even be done in a special school using an appropriate prone-lying bed (*Figure 4.26*). Acute spasm around the hip is best treated by continuous traction. Any tendency to flexion contracture due to active involvement of the hip requires skin traction at night which may need to be continued for several months. Traction used in this way is also a very valuale way of overcoming flexion contractures at the knees, thus allowing both deformities to be corrected at the same time. It does, however, require an old-fashioned type of bed or a special board at the end of a divan bed over which the traction can be used (Allin and Lawton, 1977).

In view of the tendency to bony fusion of apophyseal joints, neck involvement requires special mention. As one cannot prevent this once severe apophyseal involvement has occurred, the best possible position should be obtained by use of a collar which can be in plastic or plastazote. It is particularly important that this is worn when the patient is sitting at a table or desk doing tasks which involve the head leaning forwards (*Figure 4.27*). Torticollis occasionally occurs and this may respond to splinting although traction or manipulation is occasionally necessary. Again, this requires appropriate orthopaedic cooperation.

In the feet varus or valgus deformities occur due to involvement of the ankle and tarsus. Adequate shoes are required to give good support, and to these can be added insoles (*Figure 4.28*) which

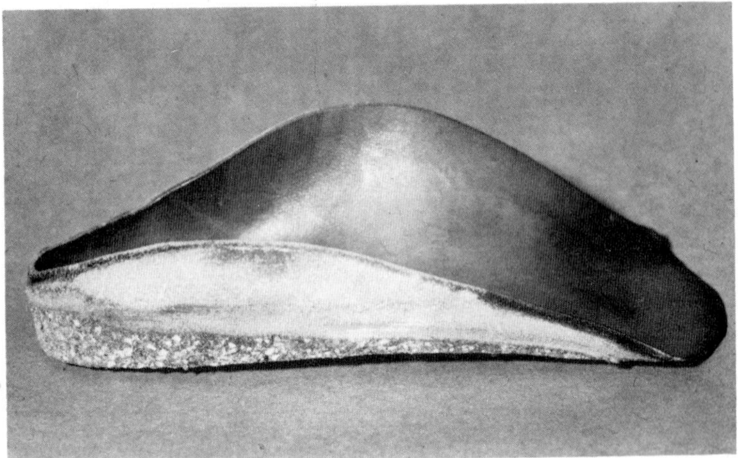

Figure 4.28. Juvenile chronic arthritis. Moulded leather on cork insole to maintain subtalar and mid-tarsal in a neutral position

maintain the child's foot in a good position. If the deformity has already occurred it may be necessary to correct this by means of serial plasters. Correction in this way should be followed by either a T-strap and irons (*Figure 4.29*) or a cosmetic caliper for several months. Occasionally, if an insole is not holding the foot in a good position, a cosmetic caliper may be the support of choice. This last is particularly valuable if there is also severe pain in the ankle.

Physiotherapy

Exercise is the most valuable form of physiotherapy. In the acute stage of the illness and particularly when the child is seriously ill with systemic illness, exercises need to be assisted. As soon as possible, however, these should be followed by active exercises. Later in the course of the disease resisted exercises may be undertaken to build up muscles. As soon as the general condition permits, exercises in the hydrotherapy pool should be started (*Figure 4.30*); there, walking can be instituted even when weight bearing on dry land is impossible because of acute spasm of the hip joint or flexion contractures of the knee, hip or both.

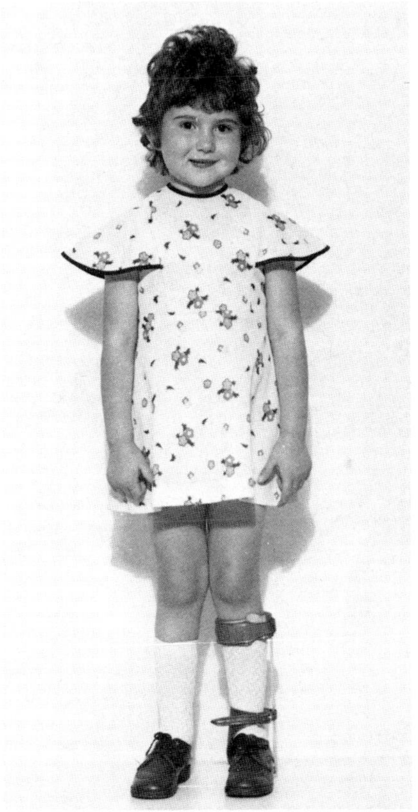

Figure 4.29. Juvenile chronic arthritis. T-strap and iron to hold hind foot in a neutral position

Once flexion contractures of hips or knees have been corrected, mobilisation with the use of walking aids and splints will be required and this will need constant encouragement by the physiotherapist. The walking frame will be followed by crutches and then, depending on the child's state, the question of whether to allow the child to walk without aids or with a stick or even a

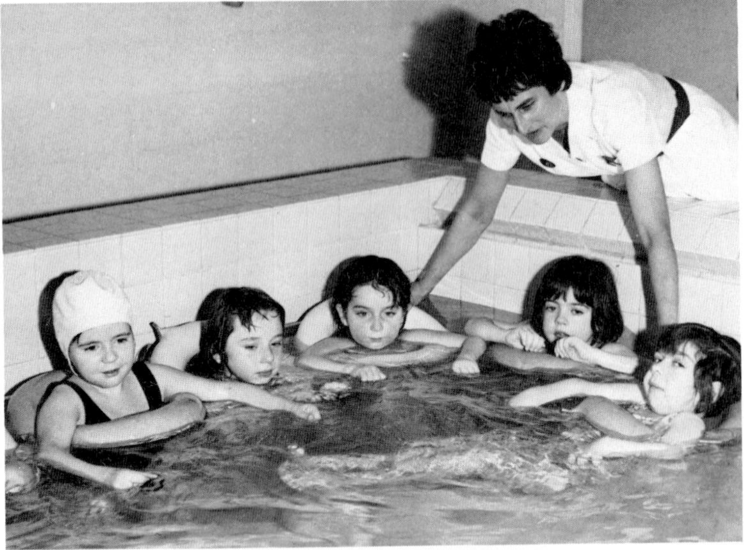

Figure 4.30. Juvenile chronic arthritis. Exercises in the hydrotherapy pool

crutch will have to be considered. Persistent hip involvement may mean restricted weight bearing by the use of a crutch or stick, but this always has to be individualised to each child's need and when these aids are used the child must learn to walk properly with them.

Once discharged from hospital, the exercise programme cannot stop; it must go on at home daily under parental supervision. To this end it will be necessary for the parents to be taught the exercises and this usually requires several sessions. The majority of parents are able to supervise their child successfully, but repeated visits, e.g. once or twice weekly to the hospital at first, with longer intervals later, to reinforce their supervision may be required. Certainly at each follow-up it is essential that the physiotherapist checks whether the exercise programme is satisfactory and, when necessary, adjusts it. As an exercise programme will need to be maintained throughout the period of disease activity this must become as much a part of the child's daily life as washing, dressing, eating and so on.

In general, during the whole of the period of disease activity sports which will strain joints or cause considerable body contact (e.g. rugby football and soccer) are best avoided. Regular swimming, however, is encouraged from an early age as this will aid muscle development and allow the child with painful joints to enjoy one sport at which he can excel. If hip involvement is present, riding astride a horse is best avoided as this can cause extremely painful spasm in the hips after the ride is over.

Drug therapy

The basic rule is to administer those agents for which the demonstrated value is greater than the threat of serious toxicity. In selecting the type of drug one is influenced by the pattern of disease process present, serious disease complications and the possible side effects of the drugs used. Many children with chronic polyarthritis do not complain of pain, though protective muscle spasm is present around involved joints; in such circumstances an analgesic anti-inflammatory agent should be used. In serious systemic illness one uses high dose aspirin immediately, followed, if necessary, by other potent analgesic anti-inflammatory drugs such as indomethacin. If these fail, the early use of corticosteroids or corticotrophin may be considered. Conversely, with a single joint, particularly if there is little pain or spasm, one may give simple analgesics on a self-demand regime. As the prognosis of sero-positive juvenile rheumatoid arthritis, in respect of continuing activity and joint destruction, is more serious than sero-negative disease, the advisability of introducing anti-rheumatic drugs (such as gold or penicillamine) early needs to be considered. The pauci-articular arthritis of juvenile ankylosing spondylitis appears to respond better to indomethacin or naproxen than to aspirin.

Analgesic anti-inflammatory agents (*Table 4.5*)

Aspirin

Aspirin is still the most valuable drug in the management of this illness. It can relieve fever and joint pain, and children tolerate it well. There are many preparations available. While older children can swallow tablets, soluble preparations, which include palaprin, are better for young patients. Provided the timing and dosage is appropriate to the medication used, round-the-clock suppression of disease activity can be achieved.

The dosage should be in the order of 80 mg aspirin/kg bodyweight daily (although Mäkelä, 1979 suggests 2 g/m^2). In children with serious systemic illness it may be necessary to

TABLE 4.5
Non-steroid anit-inflammatory drugs

Approved name	*Proprietory name*	
	UK	*USA*
Flufenamic acid	Meralen	Not available
Ibuprofen	Brufen	Motrin
Indomethacin	Indocid	Indocin
	Imbrilon	
Mefenamic acid	Ponstan	Ponstel
Naproxen	Naprosyn	Naprosyn
Oxyphenbutazone	Tanderil	Tandearil
		Oxalid
Phenylbutazone	Butazolidin	Azolid
	Butazone	
	Ethibute	
	Flexazone	
	Oppazone	
	Tetnor	
Piroxicam	Feldene	Feldene
Tolmetin	Tolectin	Tolectin

increase the dosage to 100 or 120 mg/kg bodyweight daily for short periods to bring the disease under control. In such circumstances the child should be observed closely for evidence of salicylism; over-breathing, vomiting or drowsiness are the usual signs. If any one of these signs occurs, or if the dosage is continued for more than a week, the blood salicylate level should be measured. In general, it is desirable to try to maintain the serum salicylate level near 2 mmol/l mid-way between doses. When this is done it is unlikely that serious hepatotoxicity will occur, as in our experience high transaminase levels are only recorded when blood levels are particularly high. Indeed, despite the worry about rises in transaminase levels, serious liver impairment has not been recorded in children (Athreya *et al.*, 1975; Bernstein *et al.*, 1977). The dosage of salicylate may need to be modified from time to time to maintain control of the disease activity as well as to take account of increases in the size of the child!

Benorylate, at 200 mg/kg daily, given in a twice-daily dosage, usually maintains an ambulant child in a satisfactory state. As the paracetamol level appears to parallel the salicylate level, monitoring of the latter is all that is necessary. This medication has been particularly useful in providing twice-daily dosage for children at school.

Indomethacin

The initial report of sudden death occurring in two children receiving indomethacin (Jacobs, 1967) was extremely disturbing. However, these children had received multiple drugs and it was difficult to be certain that indomethacin was the actual cause of their demise. Our studies have shown 2.5 mg/kg to be as effective as 80 mg/kg of aspirin in controlling joint symptoms, and of value in suppressing fever. It also seems that it is possible to add in for patients who have failed to respond adequately to aspirin (*Figure 4.31*). For children who are particularly slow or appear to their parents to be stiff in the mornings, the use of 1–1.5 mg/kg as a night dose has been found to be extremely valuable in relieving morning stiffness. Indeed, indomethacin at night, often using the

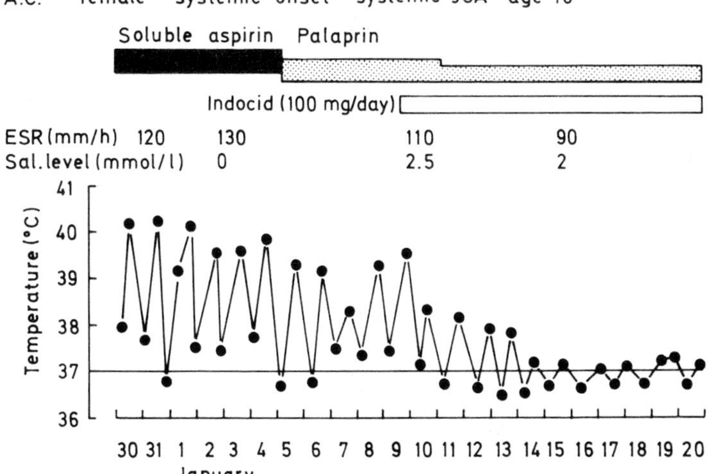

Figure 4.31. Systemic juvenile chronic arthritis. Failure to control fever on soluble aspirin which gave poor salicylate levels. Palaprin of some value, Indocid added with considerable benefit

suspension preparation, and full salicylate dosage by day, is a satisfactory combination. Other studies (Bhettay and Thompson, 1978) confirm its value. Side effects are similar to those seen in adults, although complaints of dizziness and headaches are relatively rare. Particularly in young children, recurrent vomiting and loss of appetite have proved to be more troublesome than headaches. The more usual gastro-intestinal complaints of adults, including haematemasis, have been seen but usually in referred cases on a much higher dosage than suggested here.

Ibuprofen

Initial studies with this drug were on the basis of 20 mg/kg bodyweight, when it compared favourably with aspirin at 80 mg/kg bodyweight in the control of joint symptoms. Ibuprofen has proved particularly useful in children in whom aspirin is not tolerated, either because of gastro-intestinal disturbances or deafness. The only side effects encountered have been very occasional minimal dyspepsia, or rashes. Because of this it has become customary in recent years to increase the dose if control of symptoms is inadequate; dosages of 60 mg/kg have, on occasions, been given, when they appear also to have some effect on the fever.

Naproxen

In a double-blind study, naproxen at 10 mg/kg (in two divided doses) compared favourably with aspirin at 80 mg/kg bodyweight (in four divided doses) in controlling pain and stiffness of joints as well as in maintaining function. However, at this dosage naproxen did not appear to control fever (Ansell *et al.*, 1979; Mäkelä, 1977). This drug also appears to be extremely well tolerated in children and has been welcomed by parents frightened of aspirin.

More recent studies suggest that a dosage of 15 mg/kg, given in two divided doses, produces very little in the way of side effects. The only side effect noted by us has been mild dyspepsia.

Tolmetin

A comparative study has shown that 15–30 mg/kg bodyweight daily in divided doses has compared favourably with 80–100 mg/kg daily of aspirin in the control of joint symptoms over a three-month comparative period (Levinson *et al.*, 1977). This appears to be another effective, non-steroidal, analgesic anti-inflammatory drug for children who find aspirin difficult to tolerate. It too has little effect on fever at this dosage.

Fenamates

Mefenamic acid in a dosage of 20 mg/kg bodyweight daily in divided doses proved a useful adjunct for acute episodes. As it has been suggested that the drugs used should be limited to seven days at any one time because of the possibility of side effects, such as haemolytic anaemia, it is not of value as long-term therapy in children. However, mefenamic acid can be added to salicylate therapy to cover a short period of more intense pain. Although flufenamic acid has been reasonably effective as an analgesic anti-inflammatory agent, the high incidence of diarrhoea and rashes during prolonged therapy prohibit its use.

Fenclofenac (Flenac)

This relatively recently introduced drug has just begun to be used in juveniles. A pilot study has shown it to be well tolerated with the only side effect a rash. The dosage used has been 20 mg/kg bodyweight. It is possible that this drug may exert some effect on the underlying mechanisms because its use there does appear to be a slow but steady decrease in immunoglobulins over a six-month period.

Phenylbutazone and oxyphenbutazone

In children below the age of seven years side effects are relatively common with these two drugs. These side effects have included fever, rash, hepatitis and pancytopaenia. With the large number of other, much safer analgesic anti-inflammatory agents available, it is rarely necessary to use these drugs. Just occasionally, with juvenile ankylosing spondylitis, presenting as a pauci-articular arthritis, in older boys who cannot be controlled by aspirin, naproxen or indomethacin, one may have to turn to phenylbutazone (Butazolidin). The dosage of these drugs needs to be tailored to bodyweight; it is suggested that something in the region of 5 mg/kg bodyweight daily of phenylbutazone is the maximum dose that should be employed.

Steroid therapy

Steroid therapy will need to be considered in serious systemic illness, or with severe joint involvement, particularly when associated with deterioration of general health and failure to respond to a basic regime (splints, modified rest, and analgesic anti-inflammatory drugs) and very, very, occasionally in severe bilateral chronic iridocyclitis. As children rapidly develop hyper-cortisonism with suppression of the hypothalamic pituitary adrenal axis, the use of daily corticosteroids in divided doses is undesir-able; once suppressed the child is at risk for any stressful event, so that a minor episode of diarrhoea and vomiting or other intercurrent infection can precipitate coma. In addition, the majority of children so treated fail to grow and this can be complicated by severe osteoporosis with crush fractures of vertebrae (*Figure 4.32*).

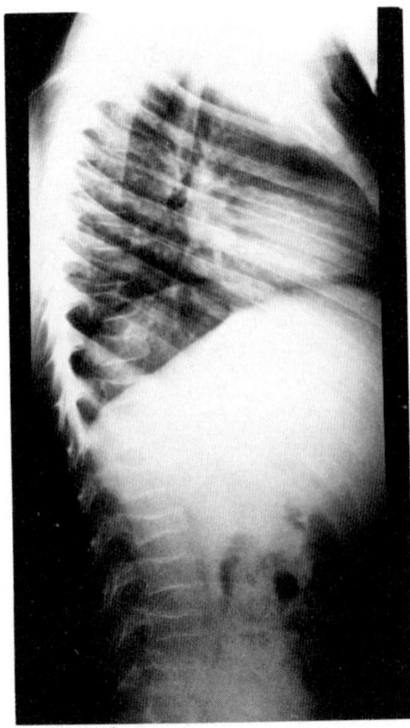

Figure 4.32. Juvenile chronic arthritis. Multiple crush fractures of vertebra after 5–10 mg of prednisone daily over two years

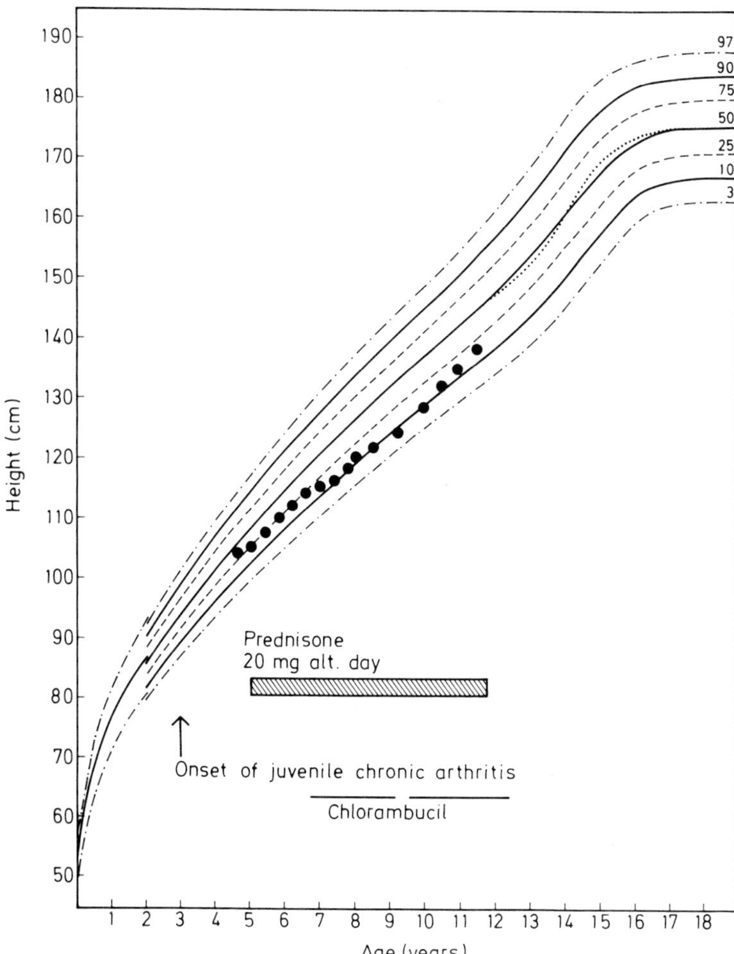

Figure 4.33. Juvenile chronic arthritis. Maintenance of growth, albeit not at the correct percentile on alternate-day corticosteroid in severe systemic disease in a boy aged three at onset

Thus, for the child with severe systemic illness continuing despite the use of aspirin, ibuprofen in high dosage and indomethacin, corticosteroids (e.g. prednisone) may need to be given, preferably as a single morning dose. If at all possible, one should try to use different dosages on two alternate days. Even if a child is extremely ill it is better to start with a 40 mg dose alternating with a 10 mg dose of prednisone, in the realisation that there will be some escape on the 10 mg day, rather than to maintain the child on 40 mg daily. Once acute manifestations subside the dose can be reduced on the high dose day to approximately 20 mg and then on the low dose day to approximately 2 mg; in this way some maintenance of hypothalamic pituitary adrenal reserve is usually achieved and growth continues, albeit not at the expected rate (*Figure 4.33*). This does not mean that one is able completely to control all manifestations, and indeed this is probably not desirable as it tends to lead to a false sense of security. However, one aims to maintain children in such a state that they are not unduly distressed on both alternate days by their illness. On the low dose day it will usually be necessary to supplement the corticosteroid with one of the analgesic anti-inflammatory drugs already described. If one attempts to use

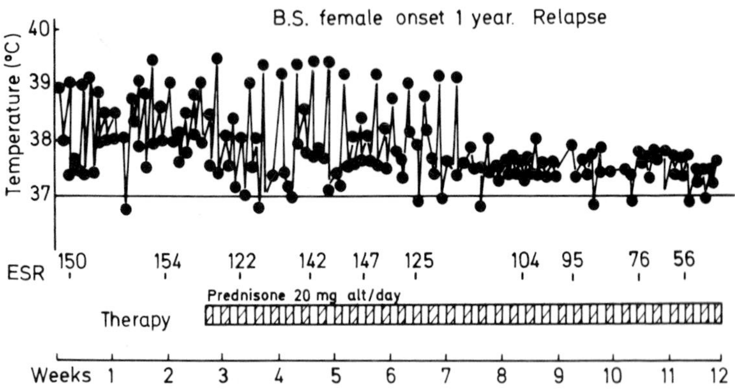

Figure 4.34. Juvenile chronic arthritis. Alternate-day corticosteroid therapy will control systemic illness. It takes considerably longer (see text)

alternate-day corticosteroid therapy it will often take some six to eight weeks for systemic disease to come under control (*Figure 4.34*). This is the ideal way though unfortunately it is not always a practical proposition.

Corticotrophin (ACTH) is also useful for systemic manifestations. Should it need to be continued for a prolonged period of time, and provided the interval between injections is suitably spaced for the preparation employed, suppression of the hypothalamic pituitary adrenal axis does not occur and growth usually continues. In practice, therefore, one tends to use ACTH suspended in gelatin given initially daily, and subsequently on alternate days, thus allowing recovery of the axis between injections.

For those patients whose indications for corticosteroids are a serious joint problem and deterioration in general health, there is little to choose between alternate-day corticosteroid, e.g. prednisone given at a dosage of 10–20 mg/single dose every 48 hours and a small dose of corticotrophin, e.g. acthar gel 20 units given every 48 hours. More prolonged preparations of corticotrophin, such as Tetracosactrin, need very careful handling if hypercortisonism is to be avoided, with a weekly dose not exceeding 0.5 mg. Again the dose given here will not completely control all manifestations but should allow the child to cope with physiotherapy, remobilisation and, probably, school. There will be stiffness on the afternoon of the off day and in the morning when the child is due for a dose of steroid. This can usually be overcome by the suitably timed use of an analgesic anti-inflammatory agent such as indomethacin or a propionic acid derivative. There is no place for combining corticotrophin with oral corticosteroids.

Once a child has been put on daily divided corticosteroid therapy, with its concurrent dangers, it is extremely difficult to return to a daily, let alone alternate-day regime. Attempts to do this are associated with acute exacerbations of arthritis and often systemic features, while the child may have symptoms of hypoadrenalism on the day off the steroid. Because of this, if a child needs to be converted from a daily divided dose to alternate-day therapy it is usually necessary to bring the patient into hospital. One then starts by changing to a single morning dose. Once the child has acclimatised to this morning dose, and it may take several weeks, then one can start to reduce the dose on the alternate day. This can be done gradually or suddenly; if the latter, one increases the usual daily dose to twice its amount on one day and gives 2 mg as a single morning dose on the alternate day. This 2 mg of prednisone needs to be continued until there is evidence that the resting cortisol levels have returned to normal; it is then possible to discontinue the 2 mg dose gradually without the child becoming generally unwell and apathetic on the off day. After even two to three months of daily divided dose it will take anything up to six to 12 months to transfer the child to a single dose of corticosteroid on alternate days. It is, however, extremely important that this be done if recovery of the hypothalamic pituitary adrenal axis is to occur and if growth is to be resumed (*Figure 4.35*) and osteoporosis improved (Ansell and Bywaters, 1974).

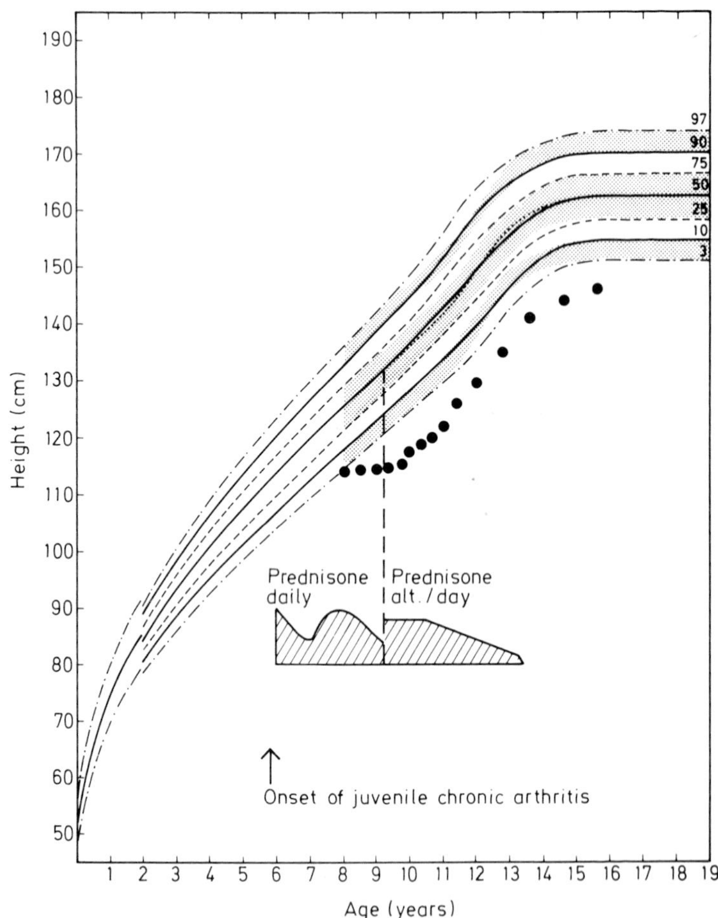

Figure 4.35. Juvenile chronic arthritis. Resumption of growth some nine months after conversion to alternate-day prednisone. (By courtesy W. B. Saunders Company Ltd)

Cataract may develop as the result of long-term administration of systemic corticosteroid, and very occasionally following the prolonged use of topical corticosteroids. With systemic administration the lens opacities are always bilateral. In the early stage these opacities have a characteristic appearance on slit lamp microscopy showing as discrete grey subcapsular dots near the posterior pole coalescing into a plaque which gradually extends axially and peripherally (Smiley and Kanski, 1978). The lenticular tolerance to corticosteroids shows a high individual variation. Previous work at Taplow (Furst *et al.*, 1966) suggested an incidence of some 11 per cent developing on an average daily dose equivalent to 10 mg of prednisone administered over four years; however opacities have been seen with as little as the equivalent to 7 mg of prednisone daily for 15 months and 10 mg of prednisone on alternate days for three years. As the pupil is mobile and easy to dilate, the removal of a steroid cataract is usually straightforward.

Slow-acting drugs

Antimalarials, gold and penicillamine

The indications for these agents are (a) severe, persistent activity with functional or radiological deterioration despite good basic management over several months, or (b) to control disease activity in a child already corticosteroid dependent, and so to allow reduction in dosage. It is rarely necessary to consider such drugs in sero-negative chronic arthritis of childhood of less than two years' duration, but if activity continues for more than three or four years they will need to be considered seriously. In those cases in which IgM rheumatoid factor is present they should be considered early, preferably as soon as erosions have been seen to develop. It is important that full supportive therapy continues. These drugs do not become effective for a minimum of 12 weeks, and unless side effects occur they should be continued for a minimum of six months in the first instance.

Chloroquine and hydroxychloroquine

Although these agents have been used extensively in Scandinavia there have been relatively few formal studies on their place in chronic polyarthritis in childhood. In general, we have tended to use them when we have not felt the disease is quite severe enough to warrant gold or penicillamine, when gold or penicillamine are contra-indicated (either because of difficulties in regular blood control or refusal by parents) or when side effects have occurred with these drugs. Because of the risk of eye complications chloroquine and hydroxychloroquine should only be used when eye monitoring is available; but this should present no problem because eyes should be always closely monitored in juvenile chronic arthritis.

The dosage is tailored to the patient's weight; it is suggested that 4 mg/kg daily of chloroquine phosphate and between 5 and

7 mg/kg daily of hydroxychloroquine (Laaksonan *et al.*, 1974) will not be associated with the development of serious side effects. Corneal deposition is reversible, because on stopping treatment with chloroquine or hydroxychloroquine the depositions are absorbed. The real problem is that of macular degeneration; this has only been recorded on high dosage continuous therapy but not in children.

At the end of six months, if there has been no effect at all, it is desirable to reconsider whether other drugs should be employed. If there has been a considerable improvement the child should be reduced to an alternate-day regime, and an attempt be made to wean him off anti-malarials gradually so that no more than a maximum of two years is given in any one course. In addition to the possibility of eye complications, bleaching of the hair is occasionally encountered; as yet neuromuscular problems have not been recorded in juvenile chronic polyarthritis.

Gold

Myocrisin does not appear to be more toxic in children than in adults. The dosage can be either 1 mg/kg bodyweight given weekly, or it can be standardised at 10 mg weekly for children with a bodyweight of up to 19 kg; it rises to 20 mg weekly for those weighing between 20 and 30 kg, increasing proportionately to the adult dosage of 50 mg weekly for larger children. Injections should be given weekly for a minimum period of six months unless the side effects of proteinuria, rash or blood dyscrasias occur; it is only after six months that it is possible to appreciate whether one is affecting the underlying disease process. It is therefore desirable to have a full appraisal at this time. If there has been no clinical or haematological effect, as judged by a reduction in the number of joints showing soft tissue swelling, a falling ESR and a rising haemoglobin, it may be worth considering changing to another drug. If there is some benefit, therapy should be continued weekly for a further six months unless untoward effects occur. If there is marked benefit, therapy can be reduced to fortnightly, or even monthly doses, depending on the state of remission of the disease.

At the end of the second six month period, the whole situation needs review. If satisfactory improvement has occurred, maintenance therapy monthly, later reducing to two-monthly, should usually be continued for several years, the reason being that there is a significant relapse rate after one six month course of gold

C.B. 69562 Onset age 13 in 1962

DAT 1:2 1:1 1:2 1:1 1:1 1:1

Hb(g) 8.5 14 9.5 12 14 14 13.5

ESR 90 10 20 62 60 18 15 15 6 20 14

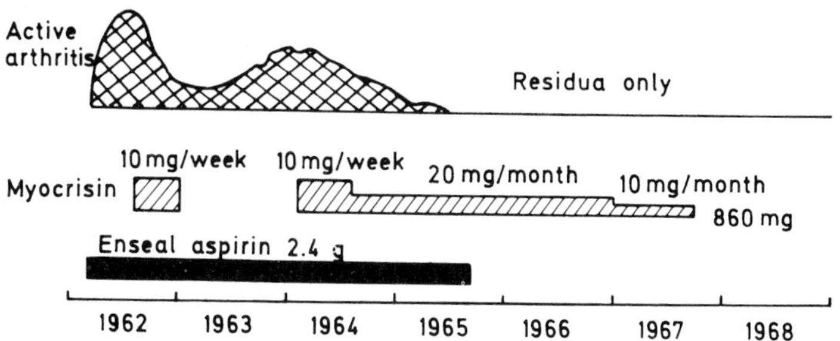

Figure 4.36. Juvenile chronic arthritis. Myocrisin therapy. Note the relapse after discontinuation at six months and the improved state on using maintenance therapy. (By courtesy W. B. Saunders Company Ltd)

(*Figure 4.36*). The development of persistent proteinuria during gold therapy should lead to investigation for amyloidosis, a much more common cause of persistent proteinuria in juveniles than is gold nephropathy, although the latter has been seen on occasions.

In our experience, some 60 per cent of children with severe progressive disease can be expected to improve on gold therapy (*Figure 4.37*).

Penicillamine

Penicillamine has been used in children only in the last five years. The optimum dosage is still not certain. At Taplow the idea is to use slowly increasing dosages beginning with 50 mg daily in children weighing less than 20 kg, and 100 mg daily in those over 20 kg increasing to a maximum of 20 mg/kg. At Taplow we have aimed to maintain this for up to two years unless the disease goes into remission, in which case we reduce to a maintenance dosage of 125 or 250 mg daily (*Figure 4.38*). Comparative studies with gold suggest that both drugs are equally effective. While penicillamine poses rather more problems in management, perhaps because of our lack of expertise, it is generally preferred by patient and parents. This is probably because it is given by mouth rather

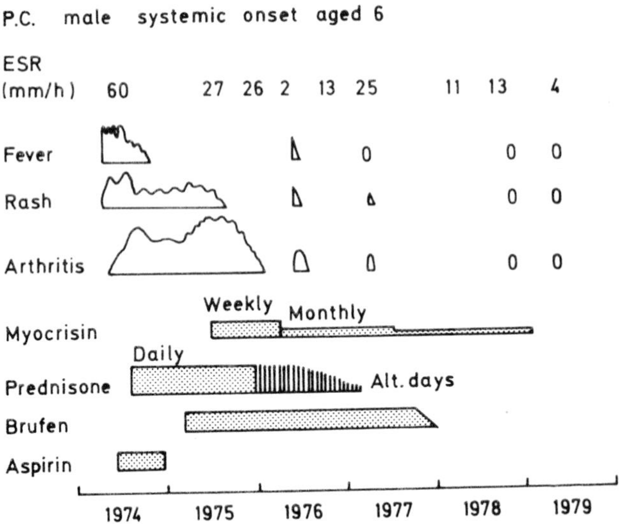

Figure 4.37. Juvenile chronic arthritis. Myocrisin to control disease activity and allow withdrawal of the prednisone (see text)

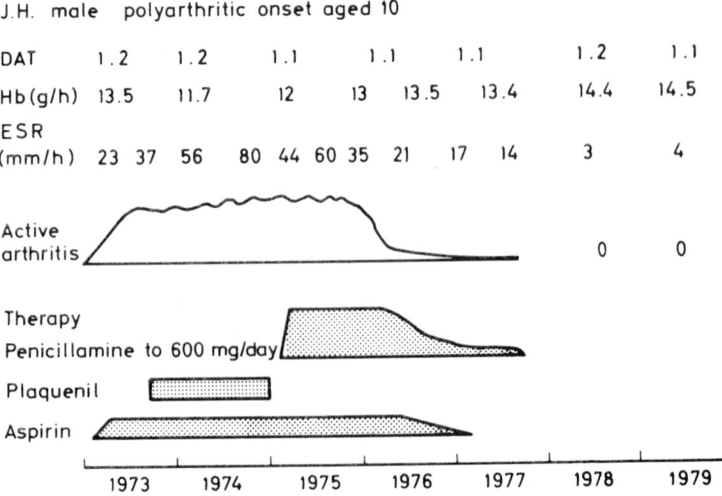

Figure 4.38. Juvenile chronic arthritis. Penicillamine therapy which was associated with the decline in disease activity; note the gradual withdrawal of the drug

than by injection, and because we have been able to carry out monthly monitoring rather more quickly than with gold injections. Side effects are very similar to gold; it is of interest that children have not complained of any disturbance of taste although anorexia is occasionally noticed. Rash, transient leucopenia and thrombocytopenia do not necessarily require therapy to be stopped but only some modification of dosage. Proteinuria may occur, particularly after some months of satisfactory maintenance therapy and has occasionally been the result of amyloidosis; investigation as to the cause of the proteinuria must be instituted. To date we have not seen any of the more serious complications of penicillamine therapy, such as myasthenia, which are common in the adult, but one child did develop pleurisy and a rise in antibodies to DNA, which settled after discontinuing penicillamine.

Immunosuppressive therapy

Because of the possible mutagenic and oncogenic effects of these types of drugs, they need to be used with extreme caution. They should certainly not be introduced as a routine in the management of active sero-negative chronic arthritis of childhood. They will, however, need to be considered if amyloidosis, the one potentially fatal complication of juvenile chronic polyarthritis, is present or very serious side effects have occurred with other forms of therapy.

Azathioprine in a daily dosage of 2.5 mg/kg bodyweight is of use, but blood monitoring is essential as there is a definite risk of suppression of the bone marrow (Kolle, 1969; Dale 1972). Azathioprine is less likely to have serious mutagenic effects than are alkylating agents. Azathioprine is recommended for those cases in which immunosuppressive therapy is indicated because of serious side effects from corticosteroids, gold or penicillamine in the presence of severe active disease. Although there has been one encouraging report on the use of cyclophosphamide (Skoglund *et al.*, 1971), another does not support it (Walters, 1972). One cannot recommend cyclophosphamide therapy, because of the possibility of permanent damage to the bladder and genital organs, and hair loss can be very distressing.

In our hands, the alkylating agent chlorambucil has been particularly potent in controlling disease activity in those cases complicated by amyloidosis, and it has been found to be acceptable to the patients (Schnitzer and Ansell, 1977). From the haematological point of view it has been difficult to monitor, and viral infections, particularly herpes zoster and chickenpox, have been troublesome, often requiring cessation of therapy and the administration of prophylactic gammaglobulin. The dosage employed was 0.15 mg/kg bodyweight initially, but this has always had to be adjusted as a result of regular blood monitoring, with the aim of controlling disease activity while maintaining the white blood count at about 3000/mm^3 and the platelets above 120 000/mm^3.

Combined therapies

A small proportion of children with juvenile chronic arthritis have a prolonged period of severe activity. In such circumstances it may be necessary to use a number of medications combined to control the disease process. To avoid side effects from daily divided dosage of corticosteroids the patients should receive an alternate-day regime and non-steroidal analgesic anti-inflammatory drugs. When long-acting drugs are added to try to withdraw corticosteroids gradually, full supportive therapy with non-steroidal anti-inflammatory agents should continue once the disease activity comes under control. It must be appreciated that it can take months or years for improvement to show. The same is also true for the occasional case when it is desirable to use an immunosuppressive agent. Only when these drugs become effective is it reasonable to attempt to withdraw, first, corticosteroids and then, considerably later, analgesic anti-inflammatory drugs and finally all anti-rheumatic therapy.

Management of certain sub-groups

The general principles of management are similar to those of juvenile chronic arthritis as a whole, notably the maintenance of good joint position and function by appropriate splinting and physiotherapy. However, a few specific points needs to be re-emphasised.

Seropositive juvenile rheumatoid arthritis

In view of the prognosis of this disease, both as regards persistent activity and the rate of erosive changes, slow-acting anti-rheumatic drugs are introduced early; thus, if erosions are present at any site

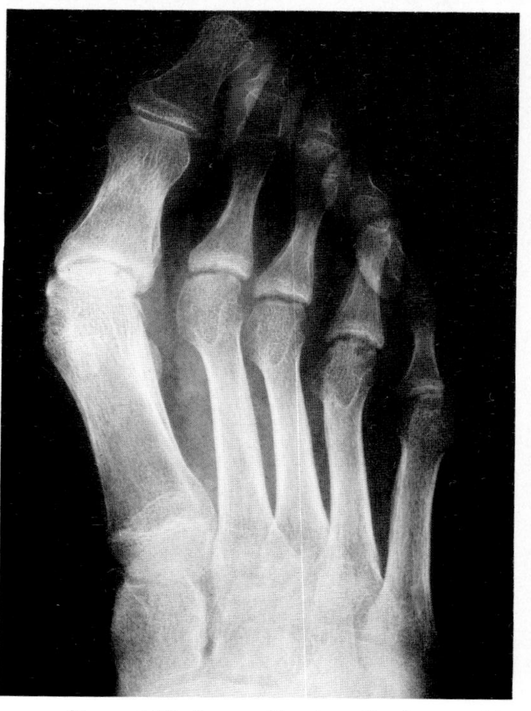

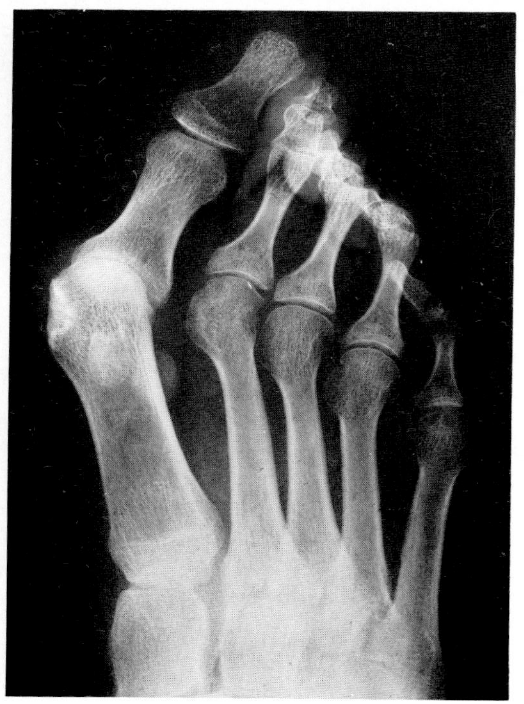

Figure 4.39. Seropositive juvenile rheumatoid arthritis. Healing of erosions after five years of maintenance therapy with gold

these drugs must be considered. Should there be only hand and foot involvement with minor changes it is justifiable to use an anti-malarial drug initially. However, if more joints become involved, so that by the end of six months there are more active joints or increasing erosions, it would be wise to consider gold or penicillamine. There is as yet, no good evidence that either of these two drugs is superior to the other. Both appear to cause a reduction of soft tissue swelling and nodule formation and also be associated with healing of erosions (*Figure 4.39*). It is important, however, that maintenance therapy should be adequate, otherwise minor activity can continue causing further damage. In only approximately half the patients is the disease well controlled, and it is particularly important in these to ensure adequate maintenance therapy. As patients approach adolescence the incidence of side effects appears to rise, particularly with penicillamine. These side effects include loss of taste and immune complex nephritis, which has been seen with both gold and penicillamine. For such patients treatment with azathioprine needs to be considered early before irreparable damage has occurred.

The high incidence of hip involvement, often associated with severe destructive changes in the knees, means that total replacement arthroplasty is required relatively frequently. Similarly, hand surgery to relieve carpal tunnel symptoms, repair ruptured tendons and realign tendons is also required. Thus, although some 11 per cent of all patients admitted to the special unit for juvenile rheumatism at Taplow have undergone surgery, almost half of this has been performed in the seropositive group which constitutes barely a tenth of all admissions.

Juvenile ankylosing spondylitis

Schaller (1977) has suggested that patients with peripheral arthropathy associated with ankylosing spondylitis do not necessarily do well on salicylates and this has also been the Taplow experience; also gold or penicillamine are not helpful. It is therefore usual to try to control the inflammatory arthritis with either naproxen in high dosage (a minimum of 15 mg/kg bodyweight daily) or indomethacin in full dosage. It is particularly important that these patients should not be encouraged to rest affected joints as the joints tend to stiffen easily. A notable exception is the patient with hip disease when, in the presence of acute spasm, it may be necessary to advise rest with traction. But he should also have hydrotherapy at least once daily. Valium or a similar preparation will often help relax both muscles of the hip and the general tension in the patient!

Early recognition is also helpful in anticipating and preventing subsequent back and neck deformities. Rehabilitation may occasionally need to be considered in hip disease, particularly unilateral, while hip arthroplasty particularly for the type of lesion in *Figure 4.22a* gives good results. The other types (*Figure 4.22b* and *4.22c*) have relatively poor movement post-operatively but even a small range of flexion is helpful to the patient.

Psoriatic arthritis

The majority of patients will require only analgesic anti-inflammatory drugs. Local steroid injections into tendon sheath effusions may be essential to reduce inflammation and maintain function. If this is not successful or recurrence is rapid surgical decompression, particularly where there is loss of function, may be required (p. 144). Occasionally, when episodes of severe acute arthritis occur, it may be necessary to consider alternate-day corticosteroids for a relatively short period of time to bring the child into remission. For those few patients who develop a progressive arthritis, gold has presented no special skin or other problems despite the presence of psoriasis; while in the few cases which pursue a rapidly destructive course cytotoxic therapy may be considered. In our experience, azathioprine is very useful in this small sub-group, while methotrexate has also been recommended (Biorksten and Back, 1975).

SURGERY

Apart from diagnostic biopsy in monarticular disease (p. 22) there is no indication for surgery early in the disease. Guidance will, however, be required from orthopaedic colleagues as to the best methods of splinting, the type of materials available, and the appropriate use of appliances on severely affected joints. The management of fractures frequently calls for a combined consultation as fractures require treatment with the minimum of immobilisation of nearby involved joints, so that ultimately function will be maintained.

Local corticosteroid injections

For severe flexor tendon synovitis in the hands, local injections of hydrocortisone appear to provide a useful means of regaining function (Macauley *et al.*, in preparation). As the patients requiring these injections are often young, and need multiple injections because of the widespread nature of the synovitis, it is our custom for them to be performed under general anaesthesia by the hand surgeon. In this way the risk of not getting into the tendon sheath (because of a frightened child moving) is avoided. For a single flexor tendon in older children, the injection can frequently be done under local anaesthesia. Very occasionally a single flexor tendon, particularly if there is a nodule present causing triggering, may require surgical decompression. Whether there has been local therapy with corticosteroids, or surgery as soon as feasible, an active physiotherapeutic regime is required if movements are to be improved.

Other sites where local corticosteroids may be useful are the knee, the elbow and the shoulder. In general one is wary of putting either hydrocortisone or the longer-acting corticosteroids into joints in children because of the possibility of causing damage to the articular cartilage, but in the presence of progressive deformity and prolific synovitis with only minimal radiological damage, it is fully justified to consider one injection of a long-acting corticosteroid such as triamcinolone hexacetonide. The accepted dosage is 20 mg for an elbow and 40 mg for a knee. In the majority of cases this is followed by amelioration of symptoms. If this does not occur the injection should not be repeated, instead a surgical opinion should be obtained. Should the improvement last for some months followed by a relapse, it is reasonable to consider a further local steroid injection after approximately six months. This mode of treatment is of particular value in children with pauci-articular arthritis, especially when growth problems are occurring. In Scandinavia, osmic acid intra-articularly is widely used in the knee as a means of controlling synovitis; this is usually combined with hydrocortisone as it causes a temporary exacerbation of synovitis with severe pain. It would appear to have a limited place in the management of severe persistent knee synovitis (Martio *et al.*, 1972).

Synovectomy

Synovectomy is considered occasionally. It is particularly useful in patients with few joints involved and when overgrowth of the epiphyses or metaphyses is occurring. The most common sites are the knee and elbow. As radiological change, apart from growth anomalies, is very much later in children than in adults, persistent involvement for more than a year or so does not contra-indicate surgery (Arden and Ansell, 1978). There is no place for synovectomy if the overall disease activity has not been controlled, so that there are many joints still active. In general, operation is deferred until children are old enough to cooperate in an active physiotherapeutic regime. Remobilisation is certainly much more difficult than in adults and many more knees have needed manipulation after synovectomy.

Correction of deformity

When conservative measures fail to correct flexion deformities of hips and knees, particularly in the young child, soft tissue releases should be considered (Granberry, 1977). These are particularly valuable when there are severe flexion contractures of the hip, but surgery needs to be followed by prolonged traction and intensive physiotherapy to maintain and improve the gain achieved at operation. In the knees, flexion contractures without hip involvement have also responded extremely well. When hip and knee flexion contractures are present together, both will need to be corrected at the same time or one very shortly after the other if satisfactory alignment is to be achieved.

For the child who still has severe flexion contractures of the knees with the epiphyses only moderately damaged, the question of femoral osteotomy for correction will need to be considered. There is likely to be slight loss of movement, so that most patients loss 5–10 degrees of movement but the new position of the leg compensates very satisfactorily for this. If severe valgus deformities of the knees are present at the age of ten or 11, and growth is being maintained, stapling of the femoral and tibial epiphyses on the medial side of the knee may be undertaken. The rate at which correction occurs will depend on the rate of growth of the child; it is therefore important to check the rate of growth from an appropriate chart before surgery. If growth is rapid post-operative observations should be frequent, e.g. two to three monthly, to make sure over-correction into a varus position does not occur. Once satisfactory correction has been achieved the staples should be removed. Older patients may require a tibial osteotomy to achieve a satisfactory correction. In teenage patients, valgus deformities of the great toe may be corrected by a Mitchell's osteotomy. Severe established deformities in adolescence require more intensive orthopaedic measures. These will vary from osteotomies at different sites, fusion of carpus or tarsus in good position, lengthening of tendo Achillis or extensor tendons of the fingers, to reconstructive surgery and even arthrodesis.

Arthroplasty

Total replacement arthroplasty of the hip is a practical procedure, although at times specially made small prostheses will be required (Arden and Ansell, 1978) while some surgeons favour cup arthroplasty (Lang and Klassen,1977). It is possible in years to come that the double surfacing procedure of Wagner may be better for young patients.

As yet, knee arthroplasty is not entirely satisfactory, but new prostheses which involve taking less bone away are being developed. It is hoped that improved arthroplasty of the knee will soon be a readily available procedure for severely damaged knees. To date at Taplow, particularly in younger patients, we have tended to try to hold the knees with osteotomies, either a single one or the double osteotomy of Benjamin, which will give them a good position (even with limited movement) until such time as more suitable replacement therapy becomes available. There is still the occasional need for arthrodesis of a knee. Arthroplasty at other joints is currently being investigated; to date our group has attempted shoulder arthroplasty and elbow arthroplasty with reasonable success.

Special problems

Juvenile rheumatoid arthritis

The complications of juvenile rheumatoid arthritis resemble those of the adult disease. Thus rupture of the extensor tendons at the wrist, and less commonly flexor tendons particularly of the thumb, occurs and this has to be repaired in the usual way. In addition, atlanto-axial subluxation (*Figure 4.14*,p. 103) is not uncommon in severe seropositive juvenile rheumatoid arthritis. While a number of patients stabilise with six months in a collar this condition will, from time to time, require surgical treatment. Hip involvement is common; this accounts for a large number of the hip arthroplasties done on young people. As the patients frequently have a combined hip and knee problem, and erosions develop rapidly, they also account for the greatest number of patients with four joint replacements in the lower limbs. In the feet Fowler's procedures, i.e. excision of damaged metatarsal heads and bases of phalanges, are helpful but tend to make the foot small, while formal fusion of subtalar joints is another useful operation.

Juvenile ankylosing spondylitis

The high incidence of hip involvement in young people with ankylosing spondylitis often leads to serious problems because, with a stiff back and stiff painful hips, the maintenance of mobility is very difficult. Total replacement arthroplasty has been undertaken in a number of these patients. Although the range of movement achieved is not as great as in the other types of juvenile arthritis, even 60 degrees of flexion allows normal sitting and entry into a motor car with a moderate degree of ease. There is, of course, a risk of re-ossification around the new arthroplasty so whenever possible a prosthesis with a particularly long neck is used. To date, all our cases of atlanto-axial subluxation have stabilised and fused with collars alone.

Anaesthesia

Anaesthesia may be difficult because of micrognathia, poor bite due to temporomandibular joint involvement and rigidity of the cervical spine. It is therefore important, however minor the surgical procedure, that the anaesthetist understands the problems that may present and is capable of dealing with them (D'Arcy *et al.*, 1976).

SOCIAL ASPECTS

Most children with arthritis are only away from normal activities for a short time: for others there will be some permanent restrictions. These restrictions will vary from being unable to join in physical education and sports at a normal school to difficulty in managing to move about, write or dress in comfort. Children or young persons who have to grow up within the limitations of a crippling disease will be deprived of experiences that are essential to normal development. If children have to be in hospital for several long periods they will lack a normal home life with opportunities to mix in their own community. In addition they will often be unable to take part in many of the activities of healthy children. It is very important that parents, and indeed everybody around, including doctors, physiotherapists, school teachers, friends, etc., should appreciate the need to compensate for these deprivations so as to give such children as full a life as possible. It is a great blow to children to realise that they have a condition which separates them from some of the activities of friends. This is particularly noticeable in children aged from eight or nine upwards. At times they may become moody or depressed or may tend to go back to the ways of a younger child.

When children reach adolescence or are adolescent when arthritis is diagnosed they are confronted not only with adjusting to the disease and its treatment regime, but are also concerned with how it will affect the future both socially and vocationally.

Social activities and opportunities to go out and about are just as important for children with arthritis as for their brothers and sisters. Similarly, such children should be allowed to help choose clothes for themselves, and presents for the other members of the family and friends, and should be encouraged or enticed into appropriate hobbies. Children need to be helped to undertake the normal tasks, e.g. dressing at the appropriate age, even if they take a long while. In just the same way they will need to learn to cross the street, to eat in a restaurant, etc.

Should their illness not start until early teens, or should the arthritis in childhood have been so severe that they are left with problems of mobility, they should still have the chance to take part in activities of their age group, either through a youth club and, for those few who are severely handicapped, through 'PHAB' (Physically handicapped able-bodied) clubs or through their school friends. Teenagers require encouragement to use their initiative in creating activities and interests. Financial independence is important to young people – it is often a bitter blow to a teenager that she is unable to do a Saturday job and earn extra pocket money. At the age of 16 a handicapped teenager can apply in his own right to the Department of Health and Social Security for an allowance.

REFERENCES

Allin, R. E. and Lawton, D. S. (1977). *The management of juvenile chronic polyarthritis*. The Association of Paediatric Chartered Physiotherapists

Ansell, B. M. (1975). Treatment of juvenile chronic polyarthritis. *Clinics in Rheumatic Diseases*, **1**, 443

Ansell, B. M. (1977). Joint manifestations in children with juvenile chronic polyarthritis. *Arthritis and Rheumatism*, **20**, Suppl. 2, 204

Ansell, B. M. (1978). Juvenile chronic polyarthritis. In *Drug Treatment of the Rheumatic Diseases*. Edited by F. Dudley Hart. Adis Press

Ansell, B. M. (1980). Juvenile ankylosing spondylitis. In *Ankylosing Spondylitis*. Edited by J. Doll. Edinburgh; Churchill Livingstone

Ansell, B. M. and Bywaters, E. G. L. (1974). Alternate-day corticosteroid therapy in juvenile chronic arthritis. *Journal of Rheumatology*, **1**, 176

Ansell, B. M., Hanna, B., Moran, H., Hall, M. A. and Engler, C. (1979). Naproxen in juvenile chronic polyarthritis. *European Journal of Rheumatology and Inflammation*, **2**, 79

Ansell, B. M. and Kent, P. A. (1977). Radiological changes in juvenile chronic polyarthritis. *Skeletal Radiology*, **1**, 129

Ansell, B. M. and Simpson, C. (1977). The effect of penicillamine on growth as height in juvenile chronic polyarthritis. *Proceedings of the Royal Society of Medicine*. **70**, Suppl. 3, 123

Ansell, B. M. and Wood, P. H. N. (1976). Prognosis in juvenile chronic polyarthritis. *Clinics in Rheumatic Diseases*, **2**, 397

Anttila, R. and Laaksonen, A. L. (1969). Renal disease in juvenile rheumatoid arthritis. *Acta Rheumatologica Scandinavia*, **15**, 99

Arden, G. P. and Ansell, B. M. (1978). *Surgical management of juvenile chronic polyarthritis*. London; Academic Press

Athreya, B. H., Moser, G., Cecil, H. S. and Myers, A. R. (1975). Aspirin-induced hepatotoxicity in juvenile rheumatoid arthritis – a prospective study. *Arthritis and Rheumatism*. **18**, 347

Baum, J. and Gutowska, G. (1977). Death in juvenile rheumatoid arthritis. *Arthritis and Rheumatism*, **20**, Suppl. 2, 253

Bernstein, B. H., Forrester, D., Singsen, B., Koster-King, K., Kornreich, H. and Hanson, V. (1977). Hip joint restoration in juvenile rheumatoid arthritis. *Arthritis and Rheumatism*, **20**, 1099

Bernstein, B. H., Singsen, B. H., Koster-King, K. and Hanson, V. (1977). Aspirin induced hepatotoxicity and its effect on juvenile rheumatoid arthritis. *American Journal of Diseases of Children*, **33**, 659

Bernstein, B. H., Stobie, D., Singsen, B. H., Koster-King, K., Kornreich, H. K. and Hanson, V. (1977). Growth retardation in juvenile rheumatoid arthritis (JRA). *Arthritis and Rheumatism*, **20**, Suppl. 2, 212

Bhettay, E. and Thomson, A. J. (1978). Double-blind study of ketoprofen and indomethacin in juvenile chronic arthritis. *South African Medical Journal*, **54**, 276

Bioeksten, B. and Back, O. (1975). Methotrexate and prednisolone prescribed for a child with psoriatic arthritis. *Acta Paediatrica Scandinavia*, **64**, 664

Bywaters, E. G. L. (1976). The management of juvenile chronic polyarthritis. *Bulletin of Rheumatic Diseases*, **27**, 882

Calabro, J. J. (1977). Other extra-articular manifestations of juvenile rheumatoid arthritis. *Arthritis and Rheumatism*, **20**, Suppl. 2, 237

Calabro, J. J., Holgerson, W. B., Sonpal, G. M. and Khoury, M. I. (1976). Juvenile rheumatoid arthritis; a general review and report on 100 patients observed for 15 years. *Seminars in Arthritis and Rheumatism*, **5**, 257

Cassidy, J. T. and Valkenberg, H. A. (1976). A five year prospective study of rheumatoid factor tests in juvenile rheumatoid arthritis. *Arthritis and Rheumatism*, **10**, 83

Dale, I. (1972). The treatment of juvenile rheumatoid arthritis with azathoprine. *Scandinavian Journal of Rheumatology*, **1**, 125

D'Arcy, D. J., Fell, R. H., Ansell, B. M. and Arden, G. P. (1976). Ketamine and juvenile chronic polyarthritis (Still's disease). *Anaesthesia*, **31**, 624

Edmonds, J., Metzger, A., Terasaki, P., Bluestone, R., Ansell, B. and Bywaters, E. G. L. (1974). HL-A antigen W27 in juvenile chronic polyarthritis. *Annals of the Rheumatic Diseases*, **33**, 576

Endresen, G. K. H., Høyeraal, H. M. and Kåss, E. (1977). Platelet count and disease activity in juvenile rheumatoid arthritis. *Scandinavian Journal of Rheumatology*, **6**, 237

Fürst, C., Smiley, W. K. and Ansell, B. M. (1966). Steroid cataract. *Annals of the Rheumatic Diseases*, **25**, 364

Granberry, G. M. (1977). Soft tissue release in children with juvenile rheumatoid arthritis. *Arthritis and Rheumatism*, **20**, (2), 565

Hall, M. A., Ansell, B. M., James, D. C. O. and Zylinski, P. (1975). HL-A Antigens in juvenile chronic polyarthritis (Still's disease). *Annals of Rheumatic Diseases,* **34,** 36

Hanson, V., Drexler, E. and Kornreich, H. (1969). Relationship of rheumatoid factor to age of onset in juvenile arthritis. *Arthritis and Rheumatism*, **12**, 82

Jacobs, J. C. (1967). Sudden death in arthritis children receiving large doses of indomethacin. *Journal of the American Medical Association*, **199**, 932

Jan, J. E., Hill, R. H. and Low, M. D. (1972). Cerebral complications in juvenile rheumatoid arthritis. *Canadian Medical Association Journal*, **107**, 623

Kölle, G. (1969). Knochenmarksschadigung bei immunsuppressiver Therapie der juvenilen rheumatoiden Arthritis und des Still-Syndroms mit Azathioprin. *Deutsche medizinische Wochenschrift*, **94**, 2268

Laaksonen, A. L., Koskiahde, V. and Juva, K. (1974). Dosage of antimalarial drugs for children with juvenile rheumatoid arthritis and systemic lupus erythematosus. A clinical study with determination of serum concentration of chloroquine and hydroxychloroquine. *Scandinavian Journal of Rheumatology*, **3**, 103

Lang, A. G. and Klassen, R. A. (1977). Cup arthroplasties in teenagers and children. *Journal of Bone and Joint Surgery*, **59A**, 444

Levinson, J. E., Baum, J., Brewer, E. J., Fink, C., Hanson, V. and Schaller, J. (1977). Comparison of tolmetin sodium and aspirin in the treatment of juvenile rheumatoid arthritis. *Journal of Paediatrics*, **91**, 799

Macauley, D., Evans, D. and Ansell, B. M. (In preparation). Local steroid injections in flexor tenosynovitis in juvenile chronic arthritis. *IXth European Congress of Rheumatology*, Wiesbaden, Abstract No. 896

Mäkelä, A. L. (1977). Naproxen in the treatment of juvenile rheumatoid arthritis; metabolism, safety and efficacy. *Scandinavian Journal of Rheumatology*, **6**, 193

Mäkelä, A. L. (1979). Dosage of salicylates for children with juvenile rheumatoid arthritis; a prospective clinical trial with three different preparations of acetylsalicylic acid. *Acta Paediatrica Scandinavia*, **68**, 423

Martio, J., Isomaki, H., Heikkola, T. and Laine, V. (1972). The effect of intro-articular osmic acid in juvenile rheumatoid arthritis. *Scandinavian Journal of Rheumatology*, **1**, 5

Miller, J. J. III (1979). *Juvenile rheumatoid arthritis*. PSG Publishing Company

Ogra, P. L., Chiba, Y., Ogra, S. S., Dzierba, J. L. and Herd, S. S. (1975). Rubella-virus infection in juvenile rheumatoid arthritis. *Lancet*, **1**, 1157

Rahal, J. J., Millian, J. S. and Noriega, E. R. (1976). Coxsackie virus and adenovirus infection; association with acute febrile and juvenile rheumatoid arthritis. *Journal of the American Medical Association*, **235**, 2496

Schaller, J. G. (1977). Ankylosing spondylitis of childhood. *Arthritis and Rheumatism*, **20**, (2), 398

Schaller, J. G., Johnson, G. D., Holborow, E. J., Ansell, B. M. and Smiley, W. R. (1974). The association of antinuclear antibodies with the chronic iridocyclitis of juvenile rheumatoid arthritis (Still's disease). *Arthritis and Rheumatism*, **17**, 409

Scharf, J., Levy, J., Benderly, A. and Nahir, M. (1976). Pericardial tamponade in juvenile rheumatoid arthritis. *Arthritis and Rheumatism*, **19**, 760

Schnitzer, T. J. and Ansell, B. M. (1977). Amyloidosis in juvenile chronic polyarthritis. *Arthritis and Rheumatism*, **20**, Suppl. 2, 245

Schnitzer, T. J., Ansell, B. M., Hawkins, G. T. and Marshall, W. C. (1977). Significance of rubella virus infection in juvenile chronic polyarthritis. *Annals of the Rheumatic Diseases*, **36**, 468

Skoglund, R. R., Schanberger, J. E. and Kaplan, J. M. (1971). Cyclophosphamide therapy for severe juvenile rheumatoid arthritis. *American Journal of Diseases of children*, **121**, 531

Smiley, W. K. and Kanski, J. J. (1978). *Surgical management of juvenile chronic polyarthritis*. Edited Arden, G. P. and Ansell, B. M., p. 235. London; Academic Press: New York; Grune & Stratton

Walters, D. (1972). Poor response in two cases of juvenile rheumatoid arthritis to treatment with cyclophosphamide. *Medical Journal of Australia*, **2**, 1070

CHAPTER 5

Rheumatic Fever – A Changing Scene

In the late 1940s florid rheumatic fever was common in many parts of the world. In Britain, the Juvenile Rheumatism Unit at the Canadian Red Cross Memorial Hospital, Taplow, was opened in 1947, and its 100 beds were constantly full of children with either first attacks or with recurrences of rheumatic fever or chorea, which were usually associated with serious carditis. However, by the mid-1950s rheumatic fever was in decline (*Figure 5.1*). Not

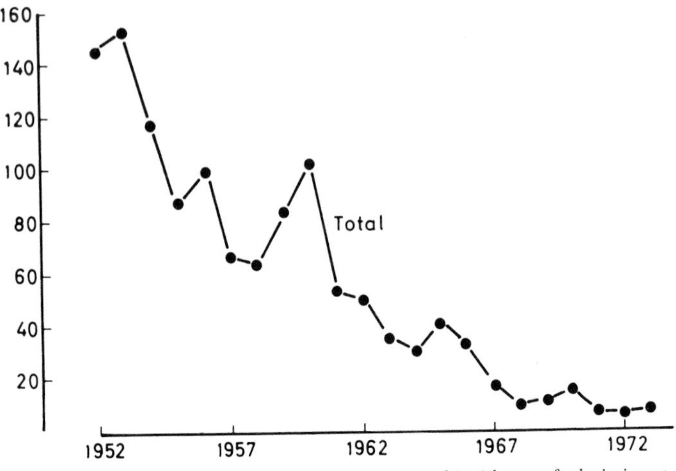

Figure 5.1. Rheumatic fever. Decline in the annual incidence of admissions to the Rheumatism Unit at Taplow

only has there been a decline in incidence but the severity of the disease has also decreased (Markovitz, 1977) (*Figure 5.2*). Today it is rare, so that in 1978 a solitary case of non-carditic rheumatic fever was admitted to Taplow! In developing countries, however, one still sees serious rheumatic fever; and on visiting them one notes rheumatic pancarditis, which was so common in the early 1950s in Britain. This is unlikely to be due to a racial susceptibility but is probably due to crowded living conditions with large families

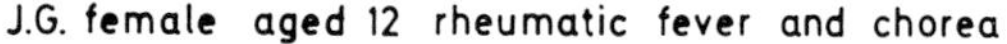

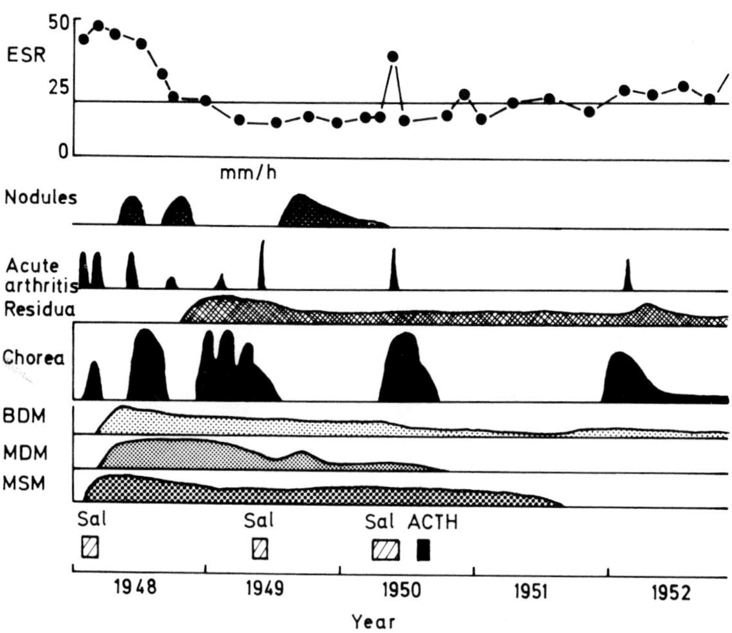

Figure 5.2. Rheumatic fever. Chart showing the pattern of illness 30 years ago with repeated episodes of arthritis, chorea, carditis and residual joint changes

and low incomes. Thus, 'tropical' rheumatic fever probably relates to poverty, overcrowding, poor housing and relatively inadequate health services. A recent prospective study of rheumatic fever and rheumatic heart disease in India (Sanyal, 1974) showed first attacks resembling those previously seen in developed countries, but also showed frequent recurrences.

As pointed out by Strasser (1978), it is difficult to determine the extent of rheumatic fever and rheumatic heart disease in the world today, partly because rheumatic fever is infrequently a notifiable disease, and partly because there are scarcely any mortality statistics for either rheumatic fever or rheumatic heart disease available from developing countries. In reviewing the whole problem he reminds us that, despite the marked decline in rheumatic fever in most developed societies today, there are in these societies still, small groups of high risk population who exist at a much lower socio-economic status.

In Britain acute rheumatic fever attacks occur in schoolchildren, with boys and girls equally affected, the age of onset having risen from seven or eight to early teens. Chorea tends to affect adolescent girls. In developing countries the age of onset tends to be younger. The clinical onset is some two to three weeks after a sore throat caused by a Group A haemolytic streptococcus. This infection may have been quite mild, so that the story has frequently to be sought, while in some 10 per cent of patients no definite story of sore throat can be obtained. Anti-streptolysin O-titres will rise in about 80 per cent of patients. Stollerman (1975) suggests that if one looks for other evidence of previous streptococcal infection, notably anti-hyaluronidase and anti-streptokinase antibodies, the proportion of positives will rise to near 98 per cent. However, these are not standard tests in laboratories today in this country.

AETIOLOGICAL FACTORS

A Group A haemolytic streptococcal infection always precedes an attack of rheumatic fever. There is no evidence that it is immediately responsible for the manifestations or, indeed, that haemolytic streptococci are present in any of the lesions: various suggestions have been made as to its role and the mechanisms involved but as yet the evidence is inconclusive, although immunologically mediated damage seems the most likely (Bywaters, 1978). It is generally agreed that in the rheumatic fever group as a whole, antibody titres are higher and last longer than in uncomplicated streptococcal infections; but the immunological activity of rheumatic fever subjects to non-streptococcal antigens does not differ from healthy controls. The presence of antibodies reacting both to streptococci and myocardial sarcolemma is, however, strong evidence that the streptococcus is concerned in the development of heart damage, although these antibodies themselves do not appear to be the active agents as they can be found in non-rheumatic patients after cardiac surgery and in other diseases. It is probable that the infrequency of rheumatic fever after streptococcal infection is associated with human individual peculiarity which could be genetic. A little support is given to this concept by the studies of Caughey *et al.*, (1975) who suggest that HLA B17 occurs with undue frequency in patients with rheumatic fever.

CLINICAL FEATURES

Acute rheumatic fever is characterised by a fever which is usually sustained (*see Figure 3.2*, p. 51) and a large joint polyarthritis with red hot, acutely tender joints, often a single joint at a time. The first joint involved may well mimic a septic arthritis but the involvement of further joints and the flitting character, i.e. one joint regressing after two to three days and another becoming affected, are characteristic. The child appears ill and sweating. At

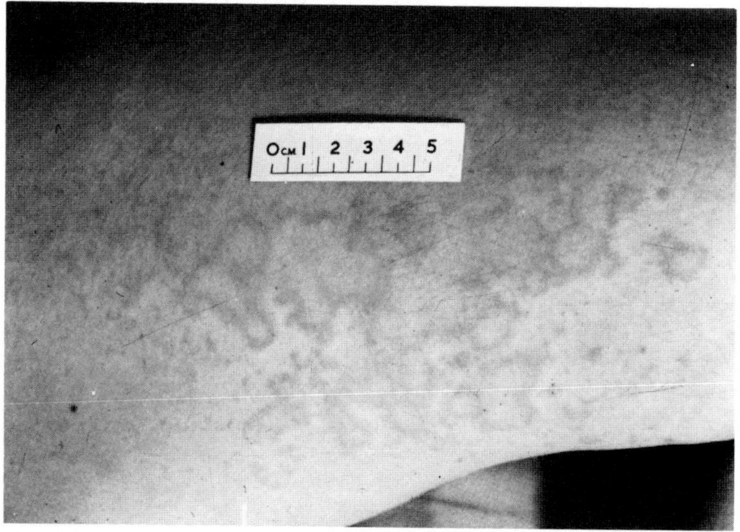

Figure 5.3. Typical erythema marginatum in rheumatic fever. Note map-like edge (see Plate 2) of the lesion which changes from hour to hour

times the onset is sub-acute with a child failing to recover after a cold or sore throat, losing energy, with some deterioration of the general health, but with only relatively minor complaints of limb pain. There may be loss of appetite and general malaise.

The characteristic rash is erythema marginatum – a large red rash with an edge (*Figure 5.3*) and, very occasionally the rash is urticarial (*Figure 5.4*). The most characteristic feature of erythema

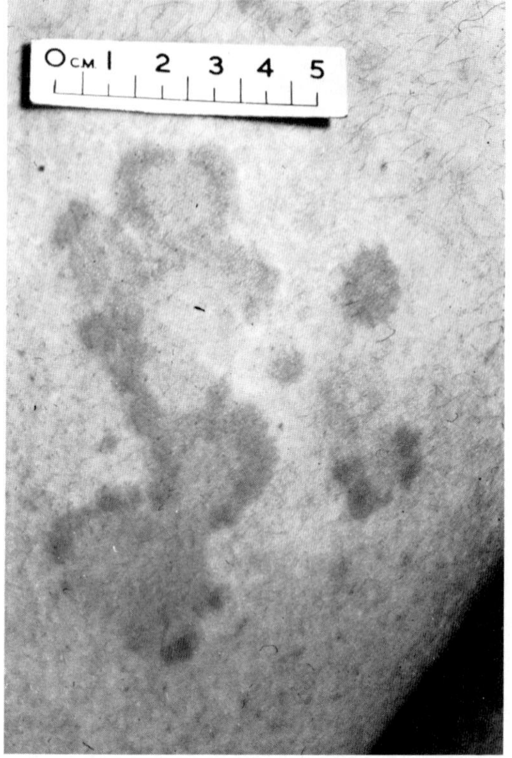

Figure 5.4. Rheumatic fever. Urticarial lesions which are raised but still retain a marginate edge; this too is mobile and transient

marginatum in rheumatic fever is its rate of spread which averages 2–4 mm/12 hours and differentiates it from fixed drug rashes, etc. Nodules tend to occur after about six weeks of illness particularly on elbows (*Figure 5.5*), knees and occasionally, on the knuckles (*Figure 5.6*), and along tendon sheaths. They are sometimes felt more easily than they are seen. Histologically, the nodules consist of granulomatous tissue intimately mixed with fibrinoid tissue; they are distinguishable from those of seropositive rheumatoid arthritis by the lack of necrosis and palissade layer as well as by the severity of the fibrinoid lattice. They seldom occur in cases without carditis, and the number of nodules appears to be roughly proportional to the severity of the disease.

In general, today in Western countries, few patients exhibit carditis, while subcutaneous nodules and erythema marginatum are extremely rare.

Carditis

Carditis is the most serious feature of the illness; its discovery incidence depends to some extent on the frequency and care with which it is looked for. Endocarditis is the most usual lesion. In the early stages this is characterised by a soft, apical pansystolic murmur. There may be, in addition, a short, soft, inconstant mid-diastolic murmur (Carey Coombs murmur) in the mitral area

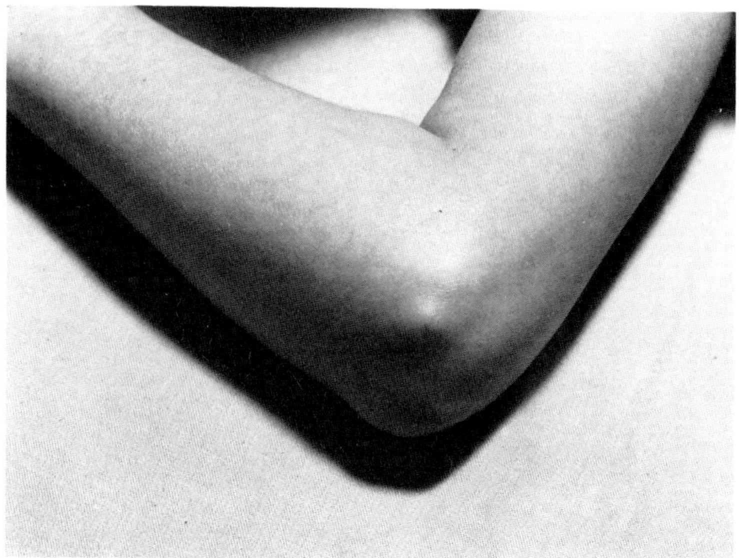

Figure 5.5. Painless nodule on elbow seen best when the skin is tightened over the elbow. With pressure they slide under the finger

and a high-pitched crescendo diastolic murmur in the aortic area, best heard on expiration at the left border of the sternum at the level of the fourth rib. These murmurs may be quite transient and the exact mechanism by which they are produced is not certain. A rising pulse, particularly while sleeping, should alert one to the possibility of carditis. Some patients will go on to develop the characteristic murmurs of established valvular disease. These must be distinguished from the innocent systolic murmurs that may be heard in up to 90 per cent of normal children. In the child who is known to have had a past attack of rheumatic fever, active heart involvement is difficult to diagnose unless fresh murmurs are heard or changes in quality occur. The electrocardiograph may

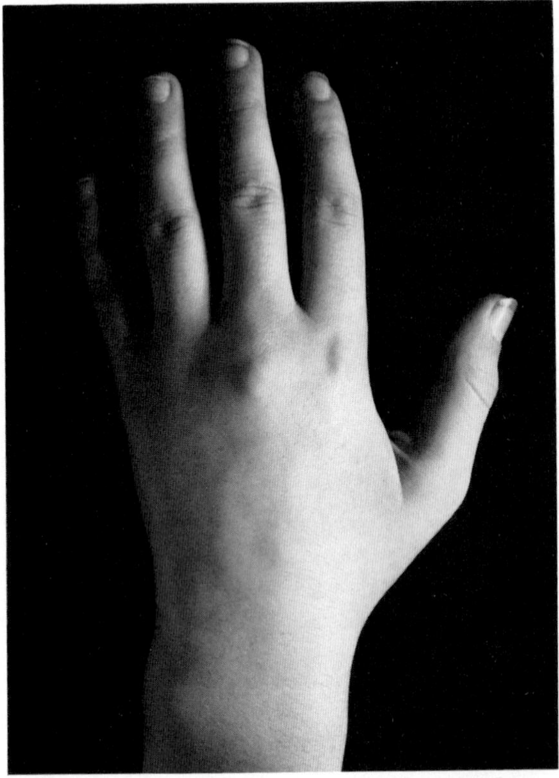

Figure 5.6. Rheumatic fever. Nodule on metacarpophalangeal joint seen and felt best when fingers are firmly flexed

show elongation of the PR interval above an arbitrary limit of 0.18 seconds; this is not necessarily associated with any other features of carditis and residual cardiac lesions seldom ensue. Very occasionally, incomplete heart block or nodal rhythm occur. Fibrillation is seldom seen except in those patients with established mitral disease.

In the early stage of rheumatic fever if pericarditis occurs it is usually dry, and manifested by a rub and sometimes electrocardiographic changes with alterations in the T-wave and the ST segment (*Figure 5.7*). Sometimes a very small effusion develops. Pericarditis developing more than four weeks from the onset of rheumatic fever is usually associated with a larger effusion and has a considerably worse prognosis. It can have a dramatic onset with sudden increase in fever, rise in sleeping pulse rate, vomiting, rise in JVP and signs at the lung bases due to accompanying pleural effusion. At other times the onset is insidious but needs to be considered in any child who is not doing well. There is usually some discomfort and a sudden enlargement of the cardiac silhouette with straightening or even bulging, along the left border. Indeed, pericarditis is the most usual cause of apparent sudden enlargement of the heart (Thomas *et al.*, 1953).

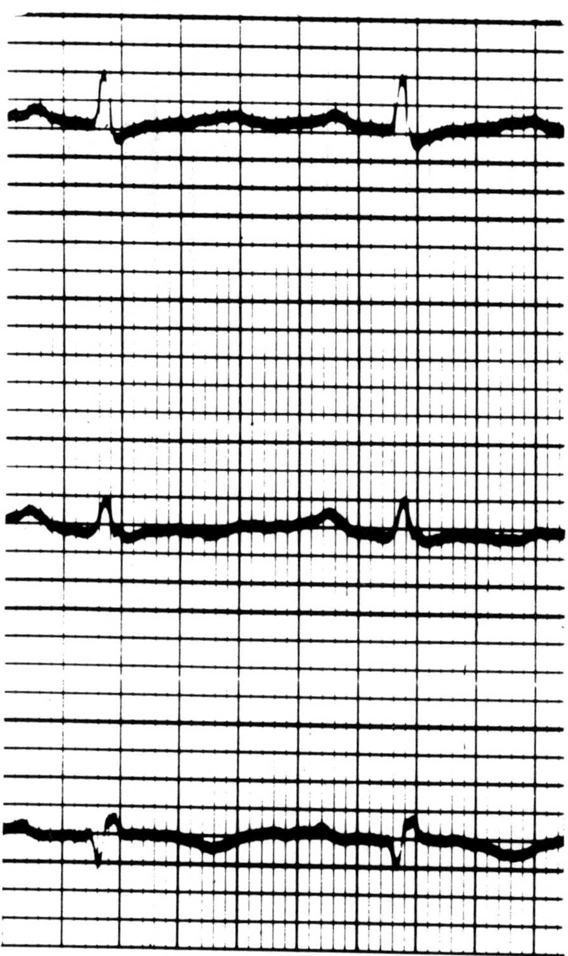

Figure 5.7. Rheumatic fever with pericarditis. ECG showing inverted T throughout and ST depression in leads 2 and 3

(a)

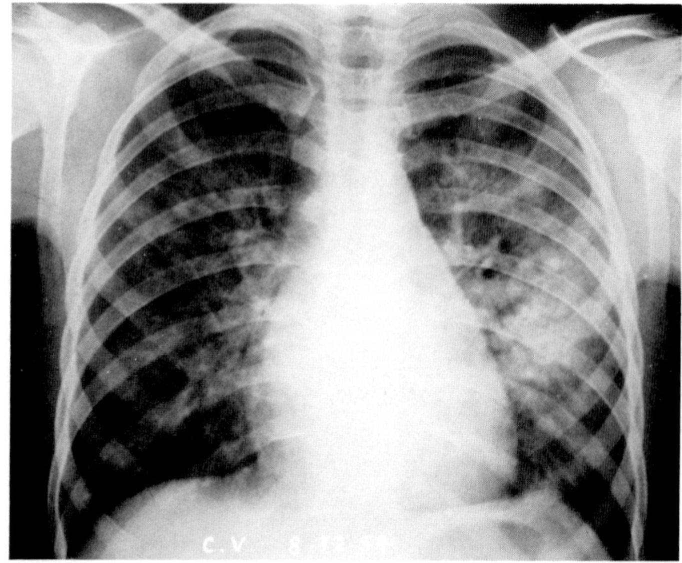

Figure 5.8a. Rheumatic fever. Chest x-rays showing a slightly enlarged heart and patchy consolidation in the lungs, probably due to fluid retention on salicylate therapy

(b)

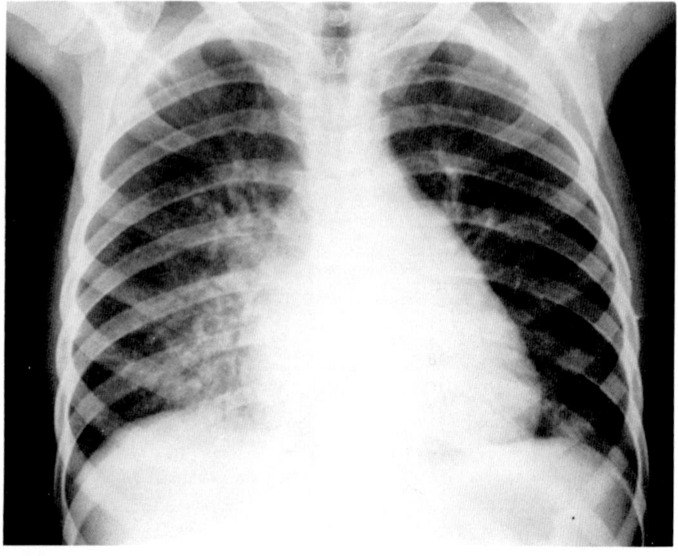

Figure 5.8b. Rheumatic fever. Some clearing of the lungs but an increasing cardiac silhouette due to pericarditis

Congestive heart failure

Congestive heart failure is relatively rare in a first attack of rheumatic fever but is more likely to occur in second and subsequent attacks. There is often little peripheral oedema. The vital capacity, however, is markedly decreased and there is an increase in respiratory rate during sleep, while a sudden increase in body weight over a short period and a rise in jugular venous pressure are helpful diagnostic features (Thomas, 1954).

Lung changes are almost invariably secondary to heart involvement, pleural effusion and basal crepitations being indicative of congestion. So-called 'rheumatic pneumonia' occurs in patients with heart failure and pericarditis and is manifested by dyspnoea, orthopnoea, cyanosis, dry cough and often blood-stained sputum. Radiologically, there is a diffuse opacity spreading out from one or both lung roots (*Figure 5.8a*). It may be associated with a high blood salicylate level and is due to increased vascular permeability and outpouring of oedema fluid (Bywaters and Thomas, 1961).

Other features

Very occasionally, abdominal pain is severe in acute rheumatic fever; this can be due to pain referred from pleura or pericardium or, possibly, even to rheumatic peritonitis. The child may then present with fever and abdominal pain mimicking acute appendicitis. Acute nephritis can accompany rheumatic fever; in our experience of some 1110 cases it was seen in 0.9 per cent of patients. These cases are particularly difficult to differentiate from systemic lupus erythematosus, Henoch–Schoenlein purpura or polyarteritis with renal involvement.

BASIC INVESTIGATIONS

It is important to emphasise that rheumatic fever is a clinical diagnosis, with investigations playing a subsidiary role. The ESR is raised in active rheumatic fever unless congestive cardiac failure is present, when it may be apparently normal. However, in such circumstances it is wise to arrange for other acute phase reactants to be studied, as the C-reactive protein remains raised despite cardiac failure. The haemoglobin may be somewhat reduced, and there may be a polymorphonuclear leucocytosis in the early acute phase. As already indicated, routine anti-streptolysin O-titres will be raised in some 80 per cent. The ECG may be of help by showing abnormalities such as prolongation of the PR interval or T-wave changes consistent with pericarditis. Chest x-ray in a first attack will usually be normal; pericardial effusion will lead to apparent cardiac enlargement and a straight left border (*Figure 5.8b*). Previous valvular involvement gives rise to typical changes (Markovitz and Kuttner, 1965).

COURSE AND PROGNOSIS

The average attack of rheumatic fever lasts about six weeks, but it can be shorter or longer than this. In the absence of specific therapy and provided cardiac failure is not present, return of the ESR to normal followed by a rise in weight indicates that the active process is at an end. Repeated attacks tend to mimic each other so that, if there is no carditis in the first attack, it is unlikely that there will be carditis in the second and subsequent attacks (Feinstein and Spagnuolo, 1960). One has, of course, to be aware that carditis can be a very transient affair with no residual lesions; but once carditis has occurred it tends to recur in subsequent attacks and may then go on to permanent valvular damage.

Among the early patients seen at Taplow five years after onset approximately half had some residual carditis and these all had had evidence of carditis during their hospital stay. The low incidence of carditis in the few cases seen more recently suggests that this is an over-estimate of the present situation.

MANAGEMENT OF RHEUMATIC FEVER

During the acute phase bed-rest is probably desirable, particularly in those patients who have carditis. Indeed, restriction of physical activity was a time-honoured method of treatment due to the assumption that a relationship existed between the work-load of the inflamed heart and the degree of residual scarring. This was based on the fact that children with unrecognised active disease, who had been ambulatory, tended to have worse cardiac damage. However, now that rheumatic fever has become milder the need for prolonged bed-rest has been seriously questioned. It is therefore, suggested that the duration of bed-rest should vary according to the severity and type of rheumatic fever present. Thus, Markowitz and Kuttner (1965, p. 112) suggest bed-rest for only one to two weeks with arthritis alone, two to four weeks with minimal carditis and several months with moderate to severe carditis, with appropriate periods of modified activity for each sub-group.

The course of rheumatic fever, once established, cannot be modified by antibiotic therapy. However, as streptococci can be present in pharyngeal tissue or tonsils even when throat cultures are negative, a course of therapeutic penicillin, e.g. 250 mg four times daily, should be given for ten days and then prophylaxis instituted (*see below*) (Stollerman, 1975).

In the absence of carditis, fever and arthritis are best treated with aspirin in some form at a dosage of 80–100 mg/kg bodyweight. This will not shorten the attack or have any effect on carditis, but will reduce pain and fever. The mode of action is not known but it has been suggested (Smith and Willis, 1971) that salicylates may act by their effect on platelet adhesiveness. The drug should be continued for about six weeks and then gradually reduced.

Corticosteroids are best reserved for those patients with moderate to severe carditis or when there is congestive cardiac failure; they are certainly very much more potent than salicylates in suppressing acute exudative inflammation. Preliminary studies with short courses of corticosteroids at low dosage suggested that there was little effect on residual carditis. The combined rheumatic fever study group (1960), using first attacks of rheumatic fever with a duration of under four weeks and giving routine dosage of corticosteroids for three months, also did not show any effect on the residual carditis at one year. However, there were few cases of severe carditis so that the mild carditis, which can regress spontaneously, may have influenced the results. Uncontrolled studies suggested that high dosage for some six to eight weeks was valuable, so the second combined rheumatic fever study (1965) of children with fever of less than 21 days' duration, used 3 mg prednisone/lb bodyweight. There was again no clear consistent demonstration that cardiac damage is prevented or minimised by steroids, even if used early in the course of the disease. Because however, steroids are more effective anti-inflammatory agents than salicylates, it is worth prescribing prednisone at 1–2 mg/kg bodyweight in those patients who have serious carditis. As the ESR falls to normal, prednisone should be gradually withdrawn to minimise rebound phenomena (Markowitz and Kuttner, 1965).

In carditis with congestive cardiac failure Stollerman (1975) suggests prednisone in a dosage of 40–60 mg daily for two to three weeks. Immediately after the introduction of the corticosteroids there will be a remarkable improvement in the response to diuretics and digitalis. As previously, slow withdrawal is desirable.

PROPHYLAXIS

In Britain, prophylaxis for rheumatic fever is generally carried out by oral penicillin V given as 125 or 250 mg twice daily but it can equally well be given as an intramuscular benzathine penicillin injection of 1.2 million units once a month. The patients do not like injections and may not return, but oral treatment may also be discontinued. In the presence of carditis some cardiologists prefer the use of oral sulphadiazine, 1 g daily, so that, should the patient develop sub-acute bacterial endocarditis, the organism is unlikely to be resistant to penicillin. Prophylaxis must be continued for at least the first year after an attack of rheumatic fever, as second attacks are most common within the first 12 months. In the presence of significant carditis it is probably wise to continue prophylaxis indefinitely, otherwise it can usually cease when the patient leaves school and exposure to sore throats is reduced. Should a sore throat due to a streptococcal infection develop despite prophylaxis, this should be vigorously treated, either with intramuscular penicillin for ten days or with erythromycin.

If there is residual carditis of any type it is extremely important that an adequate antibiotic cover for dental extractions or tonsillectomy is undertaken. This is done preferably using therapeutic doses of penicillin for five days starting just before the procedure, or by erythromycin. For genito-urinary surgery streptomycin is included in the therapy; this is to prevent sub-acute bacterial endocarditis.

Permanent scarring of the valves or myocardium may result from the first rheumatic fever episode but most serious carditis results from second or subsequent attacks, hence the importance of preventing these.

VALVULAR LESIONS: RHEUMATIC AND NON-RHEUMATIC

The validity of assigning a rheumatic aetiology to patients without a history of rheumatic fever is becoming increasingly questioned. Thus, Vendsborg *et al*. (1968) in Denmark noted no change in the incidence of patients admitted with valvular disease *without* a history of rheumatic fever while there was a marked decline in those *with* a history of rheumatic fever. There is growing concern that rheumatic heart disease may be over-diagnosed in patients without a clear-cut history of rheumatic fever. Roberts (1970) has shown that most cases with isolated aortic valve disease coming to post-mortem are non-rheumatic. In the paediatric age group more patients with various types of isolated mitral valve disease, e.g. endocardial cushion defect, are now being recognised; indeed, Schulman *et al*. (1974) suggest that streptococcal antibody patterns may help to distinguish these patients. As yet there is little direct evidence that viral infections cause endocarditis but even so, more work is required before this can be dismissed with absolute certainty.

CHOREA

Chorea minor is characterised by spontaneous movements, ataxia, incoordination and weakness; this last may be severe enough to amount to paralysis. Emotional expression may be altered or exaggerated. It is considered to be a late complication of rheumatic fever which in some patients will have been so mild that it has passed unnoticed. It occurs in girls more often than in boys and particularly in the age group 11–15. It is very important, particularly in black adolescent females, to differentiate rheumatic chorea from systemic lupus erythematosus. In rheumatic chorea the ESR is usually normal but the anti-streptolysin O-titre may still be raised; a high ESR, particularly when associated with hypergammaglobulinaemia, should lead to a search for antinuclear antibody and antibodies to DNA. There is no evidence that salicylates or corticosteroids influence the course of chorea. Recent reports on the use of tetrabenazine suggest that this may be of value in shortening the duration of chorea (Hawkes and Nourse, 1977). Prophylactic chemotherapy is required as described on p. 164.

REFERENCES

Bywaters, E. G. L. (1978). In *Textbook of Rheumatic Diseases.* Edited by Copeman. Chapter 30, *Rheumatic Fever.* London; Churchill Livingstone

Bywaters, E. G. L. and Thomas, G. (1961). Bed rest, salicylates and steroids in rheumatic fever. *British Medical Journal*, **1**, 1628

Caughey, D. E., Douglas, R., Wilson, W. and Hassall, I. B. (1975). HL-A antigens in European and Maoris with rheumatic fever and rheumatic heart disease. *Journal of Rheumatology*, **2**, 319

Combined Rheumatic Fever Study Group (1960). A comparison of the effects of prednisone on the incidence of residual rheumatic heart disease. *New England Journal of Medicine*, **262**, 895

Combined Rheumatic Fever Study Group (1965). A comparison of short-term intensive prednisone and acetyl salicylate acid in the treatment of rheumatic fever. *New England Journal of Medicine*, **272**, 63

Feinstein, A. R. and Spagnuolo, M. (1960). Mimetic features of rheumatic fever recurrences. Combined Rheumatic Fever Study Group. *New England Journal of Medicine*, **262**, 895

Hawkes, C. H. and Nourse, C. H. (1977). Tetrabenazine in Sydenham's chorea. *British Medical Journal*, **1**, 1391

Markowitz, M. and Kuttner, A. (1965). *Rheumatic fever. Diagnosis, management and prevention.* Philadelphia and London; W. B. Saunders Co

Markovitz, M. (1977). The changing picture of rheumatic fever. *Arthritis and Rheumatism*, **20**, Suppl. 2, 369

Roberts, W. C. (1970). Anatomically isolated aortic valvular disease. The case against it being of rheumatic aetiology. *American Journal of Medicine*, **49**, 151

Sanyal, S. K. (1974). The initial attack of acute rheumatic fever during childhood in North India. *Circulation*, **49**, 7

Shulman, S. T., Ayoub, E. M. and Victoria, B. E. (1974). Difference in antibody response to streptococcal antigens in children with rheumatic and non-rheumatic mitral valve disease. *Circulation*, **50**, 1244

Smith, J. B. and Willis, A. L. (1971). Aspirin selectively inhibits prostaglandin production in human platelets. *Nature New Biol.*, **231**, 235

Stollerman, G. H. (1975). *Rheumatic fever and streptococcal infection*, New York; Grune and Stratton

Strasser, T. (1978). Rheumatic fever and rheumatic heart disease in the 1970s. *WHO Chronicle*, 18

Thomas, G. (1954). Heart failure in children with acute carditis. *British Medical Journal*, **2**, 205

Thomas, G. T. (1961). Five-year follow-up on patients with rheumatic fever treated by bed rest, steroids and salicylate. *British Medical Journal*, **1**, 1635, p. 2

Thomas, G., Besterman, E. and Hollman, A. (1953). Rheumatic pericarditis. *British Heart Journal*, **15**, 29

Vendsborg, P., Heusen, L. F. and Olsen, K. H. (1968). Decreasing incidence of a history of acute rheumatic fever in chronic rheumatic heart disease. *Cardiologia*, **53**, 332

CHAPTER 6

The Rarer Connective Tissue Disorders

The rarer connective tissue disorders include systemic lupus erythematosus, dermatomyositis and polymyositis, scleroderma, the mixed connective tissue disease syndrome, Sjögren's syndrome and various forms of arteritis. They have in common pathological changes in blood vessels and a tendency to multi-system involvement.

All can present as limb pain, arthralgia or arthritis, with or without fever, while Raynaud's phenomenon is an extremely common feature of these disorders. Indeed, Raynaud's phenomenon, which is characterised by vasospasm on exposure to cold causing the fingers to go blue then white, is extremely uncommon in childhood except as part of one of these conditions (Emery and Schaller, 1977).

It is the combination of clinical findings that will suggest the correct diagnosis. Thus, in systemic lupus erythematosus there is multi-system involvement with marked immunological abnormalities. By contrast, in dermatomyositis the rash is characteristic while muscle weakness is usual but the laboratory findings will only be confirmatory. The mixed connective tissue syndrome can have features of scleroderma, dermatomyositis and systemic lupus erythematosus; indeed, it may well be a variant of the last. The different forms of scleroderma are particularly puzzling in childhood and dermatomyositis can end up looking like scleroderma, while the various forms of arteritis need to be differentiated. Because of this, each disorder is described in some detail, particularly with reference to joint manifestations.

SYSTEMIC LUPUS ERYTHEMATOSUS

The *most common* age of onset is in the adolescent years, 60 per cent of childhood cases occurring between the ages of 11 and 15, with girls being more commonly affected than boys; it is excessively rare before the age of five although it has been recorded in children as young as one year. It tends to be more prevalent in Negroes.

Clinical features

The presenting features are usually arthralgia, arthritis, skin rash and fever. Intermittent, often severe, arthralgia may precede overt arthritis. The arthritis itself varies from a symmetrical polyarthritis, often affecting the hands and clinically indistinguishable from

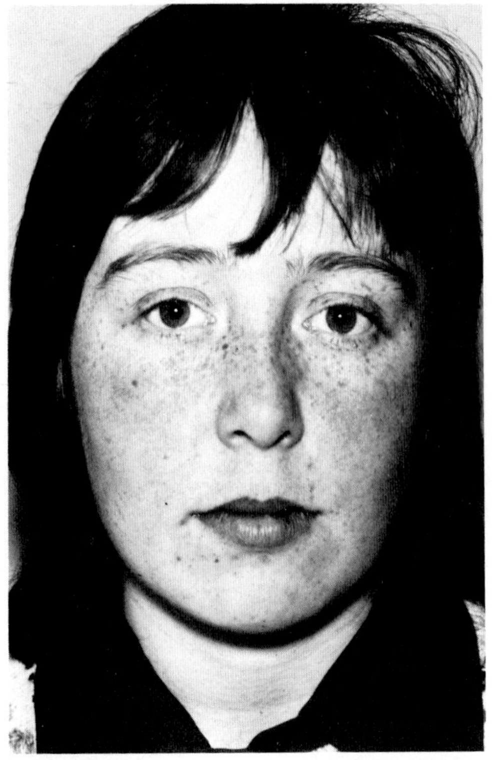

Figure 6.1. Systemic lupus erythematosus. Rash on face — typical

that of juvenile chronic arthritis, to a migratory arthritis more like that of rheumatic fever. At times pain is not localised to the joints but presents as discomfort in the extremities. Weakness and muscle fatigue are frequent complaints and may be associated with transient swelling along the muscles.

The characteristic skin rash is facial, appearing as erythema covering the malar area of the face and extending over the bridge of the nose in a butterfly distribution (*Figure 6.1*). At times, the facial lesions may become vesicular or even bullous. The rash can become progressive and involve the entire face (*Figure 6.2*), scalp, neck, chest and upper arm. Papular vesicular lesions may appear

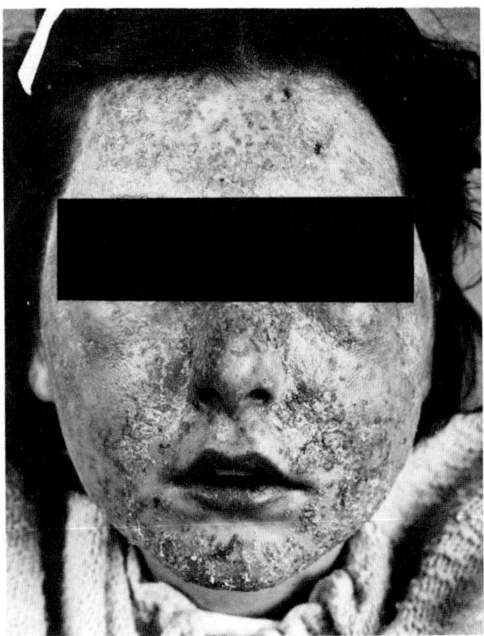

Figure 6.2. Systemic lupus erythematosus. Rash — exfoliative

on the extremities as well as on the face; these are usually surrounded by markedly erythematous lesions. In the fingers there may be sub-ungual haemorrhages, nail-fold thromboses (*Figure 6.3*), inflammation of the cuticle or paronychia. Areas of infarction due to vasculitis may occur in the palms of the hands (*Figures 6.4* and *6.5*). In many children, involvement of the oral mucous membranes is a prominent feature, as is palatal erythema;

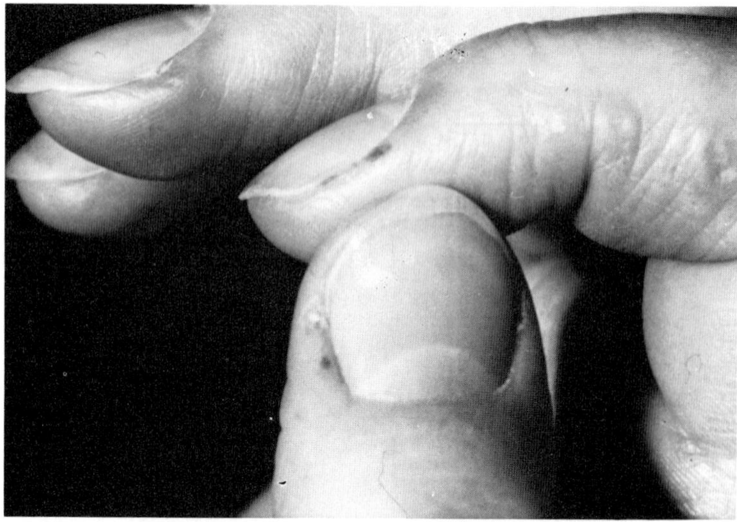

Figure 6.3. Systemic lupus erythematosus. Nail-fold thromboses in a girl of 14 who presented with arthritis

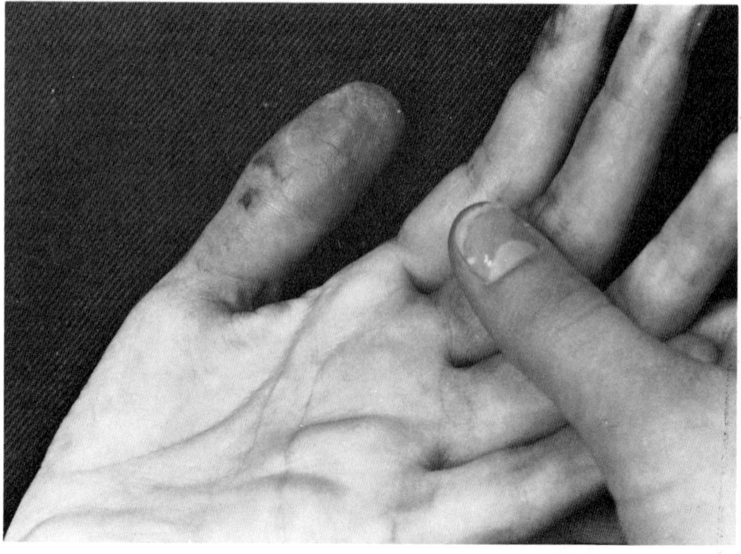

Figure 6.4. Systemic lupus erythematosus. Vasculitic lesions in the hand

these lesions can vary from ulcers in the mouth to quite extensive bullous lesions on the hard palate (Kornreich, 1976). Petechiae and purpuric lesions may appear without accompanying thrombocytopenia.

Fever may be a prominent feature, which, although occasionally intermittent, tends to be sustained; at times it can be quite low

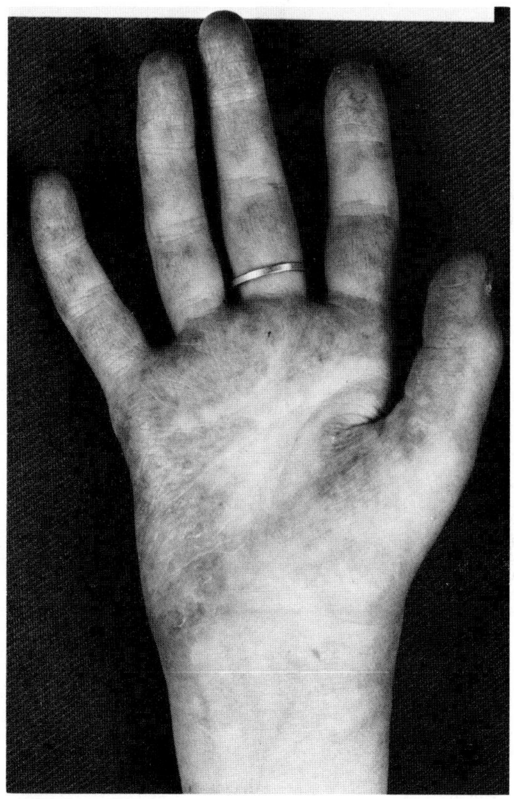

Figure 6.5. Systemic lupus erythematosus. Extensive vasculitic rash on the palm in a girl of 12 presenting as pericarditis with fever. Note the early pulp atrophy over terminal phalanx 2

grade. Non-specific complaints such as fatigue, weight loss, hair loss (*Figure 6.6*) which can go on to alopecia, headache and night sweats, often accompany these symptoms.

Less commonly, the onset of systemic lupus erythematosus is manifested by the nephrotic syndrome, complaints of abdominal pain and Raynaud's phenomenon. The clinical symptoms are variable and unpredictable with any number of organ systems eventually becoming involved (*Table 6.1*). Similarly, the course can be acute and fulminating, sub-acute or chronic, while a low grade onset may be followed by an episode of acute fulminating disease.

Renal involvement in systemic lupus erythematosus should be suspected on evidence of proteinuria, haematuria, abnormal Addis counts or a rising blood urea as well as by the onset of a

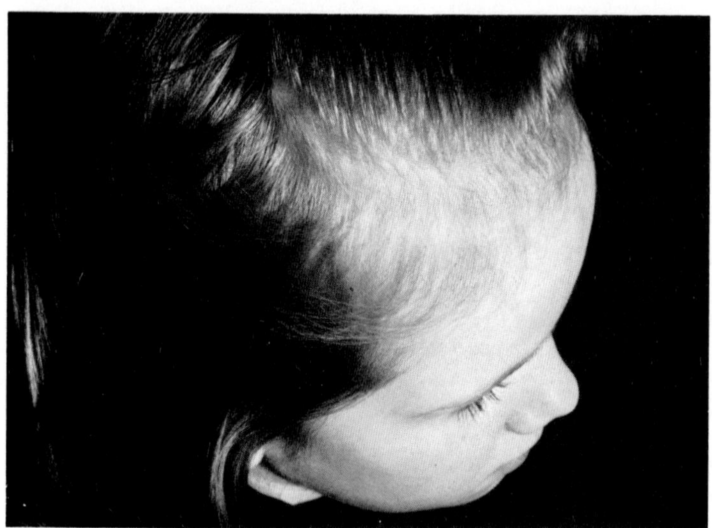

Figure 6.6. Systemic lupus erythematosus. Loss of hair in an eight year old presenting with fever and arthritis

nephrotic syndrome. Renal biopsies may show mild glomerulitis and/or focal segmental nephritis, which suggest a good prognosis, or a diffuse proliferative glomerulonephritis or membranous lesions; patients with these last are more likely to become azotemic, hypertensive and ultimately die (Koster-King *et al.*, 1977). *Abdominal pain* is present in up to one-third of children, while occasionally hepatitis and pancreatitis are seen.

In contrast to adult disease, *hepatosplenomegaly* is frequent in childhood systemic lupus erythematosus (Meislin and Rothfield, 1968), while *pulmonary disease* is somewhat less common but includes pleurisy, pleural effusions, interstitial infiltrates mimicking pneumonia and pulmonary haemorrhagic lesions. *Cardiac* abnormalities include pericarditis, endocarditis, cardiomegaly due to myocarditis as well as arrhythmias. *Central nervous system involvement* varies in its frequency in different series, as does its

TABLE 6.1
Major systems involved in 108 children with systemic lupus erythematosus

System involvement	*% patients affected between onset and diagnosis*
Joints	78.7
Cutaneous	70.4
Renal	61.1
Haematopoietic	46.3
Lymphadenopathy	38.9
Hepatosplenomegaly	27.8
Palatal exanthem	21.3
Pulmonary	19.4
GI tract	18.5
Cardiac	16.7
CNS	13.0

(From Koster-King *et al.*, 1977)

extent; chorea (Kukla *et al.*, 1978) and seizures are the most common during childhood but psychosis, vascular accidents and peripheral neuropathy are all occasionally seen.

Laboratory investigations

The ESR is raised, usually to very high levels, the haemoglobin is often slightly low and the white blood count reduced, usually below 5000 and often below 3000 particularly in the presence of high fever. Thrombocytopenia may be demonstrated, as may circulating anticoagulants, decreased factor 2, anti-factor 8 and 9 and Coombs positivity. This last can, but rarely, be associated with life-threatening haemolytic anaemia. Hypergammaglobulinaemia is usual, while IgA deficiency is occasionally observed. Blood cultures are negative, an important method of distinguishing those patients with fever, vasculitic lesions, splenomegaly and sometimes cardiac involvement, from those with sub-acute bacterial endocarditis.

IgM rheumatoid factor may be present in the serum, as well as a false positive WR test result. In addition, immune complexes can be detected by a variety of techniques. The hallmark of systemic lupus erythematosus is, however, the presence of antibodies against a wide variety of nuclear cytoplasmic and serum protein antigens. While antibodies against nuclei are not specific, their presence in very high titres in suspicious cases should lead to the estimation of antibodies to DNA, which are raised in active disease, as well as to the estimation of levels of complement; particularly in renal lupus, reduction of C3 is common. In the presence of any clinical evidence of nephritis it is wise to perform a renal biopsy to establish the type of lesion present.

Aetiology

The aetiology is probably multifactorial. There may well be a genetic component as suggested by reports on familial incidence, including monozygotic twins.

Inherited defects in the complement system have also been implicated in adults, particularly inherited defects in the synthesis of C2 component of complement suggesting that C2 deficiency represents a significant defect in the host defence mechanism (Schur, 1975; Schaller *et al.*, 1977). As yet no definite relationship with any particular HL-A group has been reported.

It has been suggested that an impairment of the regulatory suppressor lymphocytes may lead to a defect in tolerance and loss of control of auto-antibody production (Bresnihan and Jason, 1977); other possibilities include viral infection and this is supported by studies with animal models (Whaley, Hughes and Webb, 1976). A number of drugs have also been implicated in children, the most frequent being the anti-convulsants – ethosuximide, hydantoins, trimethadione (Miller, 1977). Antibiotics, particularly Septrin, may cause a hypersensitivity reaction in the skin looking like lupus (*Plate 5*). It is therefore extremely important to get an adequate history in suspected cases. Many of these young patients are photosensitive, it is therefore desirable that excessive exposure to sun is avoided.

Prognosis

The course of systemic lupus erythematosus in childhood is highly variable and unpredictable. In children under 12 it was usually fatal but the increasing and better use of corticosteroids appears to be improving the outlook. Of 90 patients followed up for 15 years,

24 had died; the incidence of complete remission, however, was low – in only 14 patients – the remainder requiring constant therapy and monitoring (Kornreich, 1976). Prognosis relates closely to renal involvement. Mesangial deposits are common to all patients with systemic lupus erythematosus. Certain specific immunological events are probably responsible for focal proliferative, diffuse proliferative and membranous lupus nephritis. Renal disease tends to occur in the first year and remain typical for that patient. Both diffuse proliferative and membranous nephritis, which account for two-thirds of patients with renal involvement, tend to have continued activity and progressive glomerular damage. Fish *et al.* (1977) have suggested that children and adolescents with lupus nephritis might have a better prognosis than adults.

Management

The aims of treatment are to relieve incapacitating symptoms, prevent progressive tissue damage and thereby prevent early death from the complications of the disease, as well as prevent death from complications of therapy, particularly infection. At the same time it is important to provide a lifestyle for the child which allows normal growth and development. At the time of diagnosis the majority of patients are systemically ill and will usually require treatment with corticosteroids.

This is particularly important in the presence of a diffuse proliferative glomerulonephritis or membranous nephritis; there is little doubt that this is due to deposition of antigen–antibody complexes in the kidney. The starting dose of prednisone needs to be in the order of 1.5–2 mg/kg bodyweight daily in those patients with renal involvement; it should be given as a single daily dose each morning. Whether to introduce cytotoxic therapy from the beginning in such patients is still controversial.

Although trials have not been conclusive there is a suggestion that they are helpful in renal disease and certainly allow reduction in corticosteroid therapy to acceptable levels (Decker, 1975). Cyclophosphamide is probably more potent than azathioprine but with more side effects. Thus, in general, azathioprine is most frequently used at 2.5–3 mg/kg bodyweight daily. When the overall disease appears to be improving and the renal state controlled as shown by a fall in urinary sediment, reduction in proteinuria, rise in C3 and fall in antibodies to DNA, corticosteroids should be reduced to alternate days using two and a half times the expected dose as a single morning dose every 48 hours. If the period on daily steroid therapy has been long it is sometimes better to give almost the full dose every 48 hours, reserving from between 5 and 10 mg for the alternate day as, again, a single morning dose. As the child improves the dosage of corticosteroids is further reduced (*Figure 6.7*).

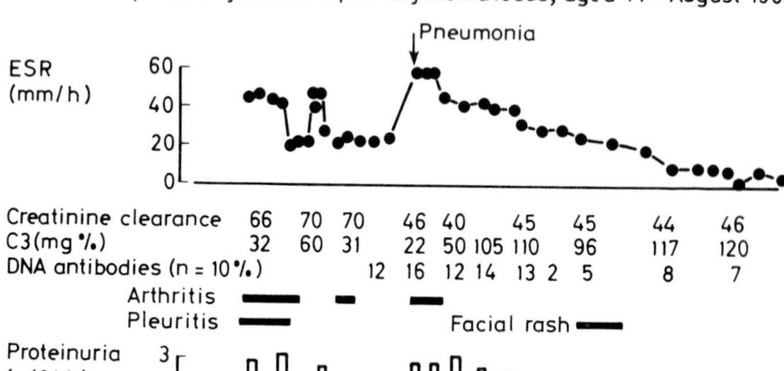

Figure 6.7. Systemic lupus erythematosus. Course of a 14 year old girl with severe renal disease

For those patients without serious renal involvement or evidence of other serious visceral problems, it is wiser to start on an alternate-day regime even though it may be necessary to give small doses of steroid on the alternate day. It is particularly in this group that the administration of an anti-malarial drug such as chloroquine or hydroxychloroquine in the usual childhood dosage can often allow a reduction in the steroid dose (Meislin and Rothfield, 1968).

The question of treatment with immunosuppressive drugs will need consideration in (a) those patients whose disease remains uncontrolled, (b) those who require frequent hospital admissions because of exacerbations, as well as (c) those who cannot be maintained either on an alternate-day regime or on small daily doses of steroid and particularly in the presence of side effects from corticosteroid therapy, even in the absence of renal disease. In general azathioprine is the first drug to be used, although encouraging reports with chlorambucil in adults make this an alternative if azathioprine is not tolerated or is ineffective. Another interesting drug that may be considered in severe cases which are resistant to therapy is levamisole which appears to be immunostimulating (Rosenthal, 1978). As yet, there have been no formal trials in systemic lupus.

As intercurrent infections may be associated with exacerbations of disease, they warrant prompt treatment by appropriate antibiotics, taking care to avoid any containing the penicillin ring or Septrin if the patient is sensitive to them. Care should be taken over exposure to sunlight, particularly if the child has been demonstrated as sun sensitive. Exacerbations associated with high fever require monitoring for infection before assuming that the fever is due to the disease process itself. However, should they occur, and particularly if there is a sudden deterioration of renal function, pulsing with methylprednisone will need to be considered (Levinsky *et al.*, 1977).

DERMATOMYOSITIS

Dermatomyositis affects children of both sexes and its commonest age of onset is between the ages of four and ten years. The two features which set childhood dermatomyositis in a separate class from that of the adult disease are the presence of vasculitis (Banker, 1975) and the late development of calcinosis.

Clinical features

In 50 per cent the onset is acute with *pain*, not just muscular, but also in the hands and feet, together with fever, loss of weight and general malaise.

Peripheral oedema of the hands and feet may occur and be difficult to distinguish from arthritis; synovitis of knees and flexor tendons may also be present.

A violaceous hue of the face may be present within a few hours, or certainly days of onset. Ultimately, a rash occurs in the majority. The typical facial rash consists of a dusky heliotrope eruption in the peri-orbital region and occasionally on the forehead (*Plate 6a*). Involvement of the neck, shoulders, front and back of the chest can occur. On the upper eyelid a dusky suffusion can be detected, ultimately accompanied by telangiectasia. In conjunction with the facial erythema, a scaling rash can occur on the extensor surfaces and down the front of the legs (*Figure 6.8*), again purplish in colour. With the rash there may be acute intradermal and subcutaneous oedema. Dusky red patches which are slightly elevated, smooth or scaly, occur over the knuckles, (*Plate 6b*) knees, elbows and medial maleoli. Eventually, these areas become shiny, red, and somewhat atrophic with the skin tending to flake; they are then referred to as collodion patches

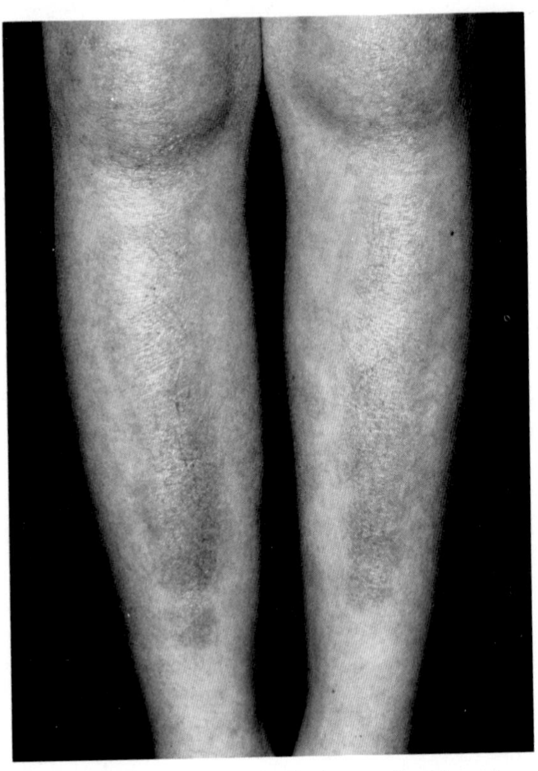

Figure 6.8. Dermatomyositis. Rash extending down from the knees, mauve in colour

(*Figure 6.9*). Around the nail beds there is characteristic telangiectasia (*Figure 6.10*). Severe skin ulceration may occur particularly in the axillae and groins, but also at any site (*Figure 6.11*). Its high incidence presumably relates to the vasculitis present.

Mucous membranes can also be involved and dysphagia is not uncommon; associated with this there may be ulceration of the oesophagus. Ulceration in other parts of the intestine as a result of

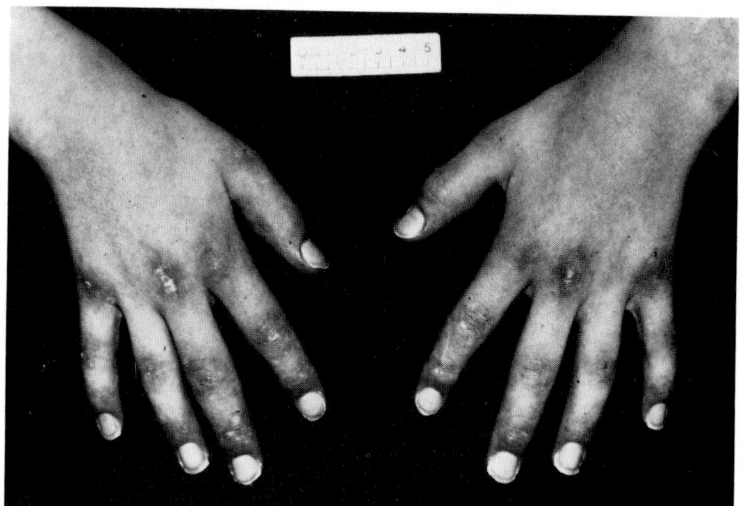

Figure 6.9. Dermatomyositis. Rash over knuckles and joints with collodion patches(see also Plate 6b)

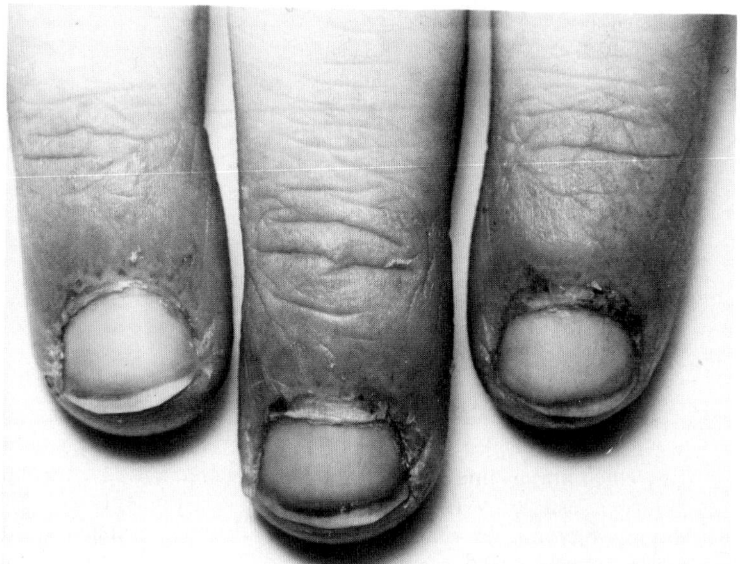

Figure 6.10. Dermatomyositis. Telangiectasia around nail-fold edge

infarction can give rise to abdominal pain, haematemesis and melaena.

The *retinitis* which occasionally occurs is characterised by extensive 'cotton-wool' exudative deposition mimicking (*Figure 6.12*) the cytoid bodies of systemic lupus erythematosus, with haemorrhages (Fruman *et al.*, 1976).

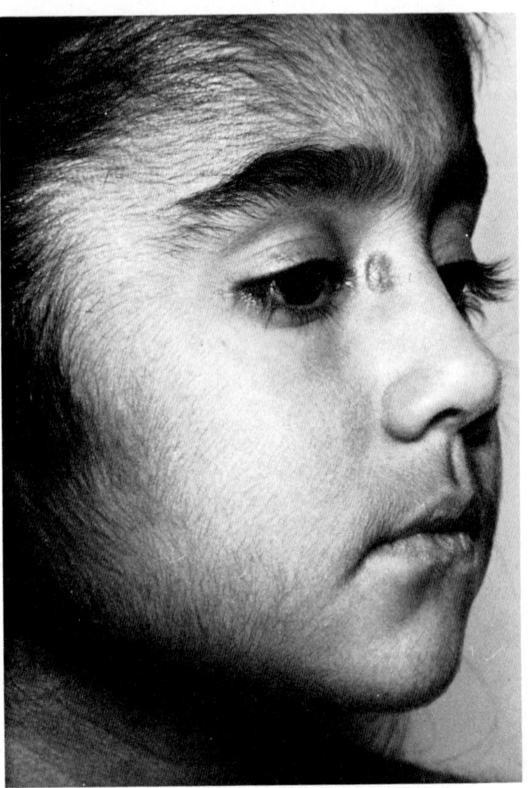

Figure 6.11. Dermatomyositis. Healing ulcer at side of nose in a four year old Indian girl who had been ill for nine months

At this early stage, weakness may be the clue to diagnosis as the child is often unable to sit up in bed when asked. He may resent palpation of muscles because of pain and not be able to attempt to abduct the shoulders or raise the legs against resistance. Weakness of the posterior pharyngeal muscles gives rise to a picture of partial bulbar palsy with dysphagia, dysphonia and often a marked nasal voice.

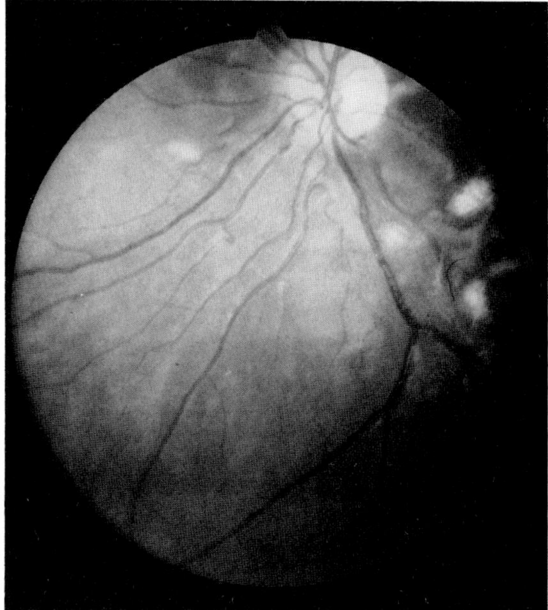

Figure 6.12. Dermatomyositis. 'Cotton-wool' exudate in the retina

Acute *pulmonary manifestations* can occur (Park and Nyhan, 1975), similarly myoglobinuria with acute renal failure has been recorded (Sloan *et al.*, 1978) as has cardiac involvement. Very occasionally, in rapidly advancing cases, progressive involvement of the respiratory muscles can prove fatal, as can progressive oedema of face, neck and chest giving a 'bull-neck' appearance.

Insidious onset and differential diagnosis

Clinical diagnosis is more difficult in the 50 per cent of children who have an insidious onset. The picture can vary from a rash, through minor synovitis of joints and flexor tendons, tendon nodule formation, Raynaud's phenomenon, to muscle weakness of varying degree. Occasionally, this is so mild as not to be recognised, so that a child presents with calcinotic nodules and a story of episodes of repeated falling for perhaps three or four months or longer some years previously. In general however, the onset of muscular weakness is sufficient to allow one to suspect the diagnosis. This weakness usually affects the pelvic girdle first causing a tendency to fall, or difficulty in rising without assistance and ultimately difficulty in climbing stairs, getting in and out of a bath and sitting up in bed. The shoulder muscles tend to be involved later, but anterior neck muscles may be involved relatively early. Occasionally a sub-acute onset is followed by a very acute illness. Ultimately, contractures due to muscle shortening will develop. The most common sites are the elbows, due to involvement of biceps brachialis, the wrist extensors preventing full extension of the wrists, and the hamstrings and quadriceps causing contractures of hips and knees. Muscular atrophy is a late event.

Polymyositis alone, without skin involvement, is relatively uncommon in childhood although a rash can be difficult to recognise in children of Indian or Jamaican origin. The nature and pattern of the rash, together with the muscle weakness, allows a fairly confident diagnosis from systemic lupus erythematosus to be made. In the absence of rash, other disorders must be considered. These will include viral infections, toxoplasmosis (McNicholl and Flynn, 1978) and trichinosis. This last can cause muscle pain, weakness and often general symptoms; early there is an eosinophilia; it is caused by ingesting larvae of *Trichinosis spiralis* in undercooked pork, so biopsy will show encysted larvae as well as an inflammatory response. Proximal myoglobinuria can usually be excluded on the story of its paroxysmal nature and the rapid recovery after ceasing exercise. In those with a less acute onset the more difficult differential diagnoses are from atypical muscular dystrophy, scleroderma and the mixed connective tissue syndrome. For the 30 per cent of cases with arthritis, differential diagnosis is from juvenile chronic arthritis. Chronic polymyositis particularly in young children will have to be differentiated from limb girdle dystrophy.

Laboratory investigations

The ESR tends to be low or normal. The white blood count may be raised and predominantly polymorphonuclear. The antinuclear antibody is not infrequently positive but antibodies to DNA and complement are normal. If the antinuclear antibody shows a speckled patterning, mixed connective tissue syndrome should be seriously considered and extractable nuclear antigen searched for. The enzyme creatine phosphokinase (CPK) is usually raised in the acute phase of dermatomyositis, but a proportion of patients never have a raised enzyme level and some are already so wasted that even in an exacerbation the CPK level does not rise. Other enzymes should also be investigated as they too may show modest elevations, while cardiac involvement is usually associated with a rise in hydroxybutyric acid. Electromyography may show abnormality in muscle function but it does not give the clue as to the aetiology of this.

A muscle biopsy will show a mixture of degeneration of muscle fibres, regenerative activity, infiltrates of chronic inflammatory cells particularly near blood vessels, phagocytosis of necrotic fibre substance, interstitial fibrosis and a variation in cross-sectional diameter of the adjacent muscle fibres. The outstanding feature of childhood dermatomyositis is the *involvement of intramuscular blood vessels*. This angiopathy results in multiple thrombus formation and infarction of muscle. Histochemical staining can be of value in differentiating lower motor neurone disease from primary muscle disorders (Dubowitz, 1978). Biopsy of the skin shows epidermal atrophy, degeneration of basal cells, vascular dilatation and lymphocytic infiltration in the dermis; mucin deposits resembling acid mucopolysaccharides have also been noted.

The diagnosis of dermatomyositis is therefore based on the clinical features of symmetrical weakness of the limb girdle muscles and typical skin rashes, and is confirmed by elevation of serum muscle enzymes, abnormal electromyography and/or a muscle biopsy showing inflammatory myositis.

Prognosis

In general, in dermatomyositis of childhood there are no associated disorders but it has been recorded in leukaemia (Hanson and Kornreich, 1967) and in hypogammaglobulinaemia (Gotoff *et al.*, 1972). The appearance of such children is somewhat different from typical dermatomyositis in that they get a gradual thickening and hardening of the muscles with progressive contracture and somewhat atypical rash. However, it is of particular interest that Echo virus has been grown from the cerebrospinal fluid and the muscles in more than one such case (Webster *et al.*, 1978).

The prognosis of dermatomyositis is good, the duration of the acute phase varying from a few months with complete reversal of physical signs and symptoms, to recurrent periods of activity with eventual recovery over two to three years. Recovery from the acute phase in childhood and young adult life may be associated with interfascial muscle plane calcinosis (*Figure 6.13*) which can at times cause impairment of muscle function as well as the more common subcutaneous lesions. In our experience, (Sewell *et al.*, 1978) calcinosis has been seen as early as six months when it may develop as acute red hot swelling (*Figure 6.14*) mimicking sepsis and as late as 15 years (*Figure 6.15*). The subcutaneous lesions are particularly common at elbows and knees but may also occur in the tendo Achillis and on the buttocks. Subcutaneous lesions tend to

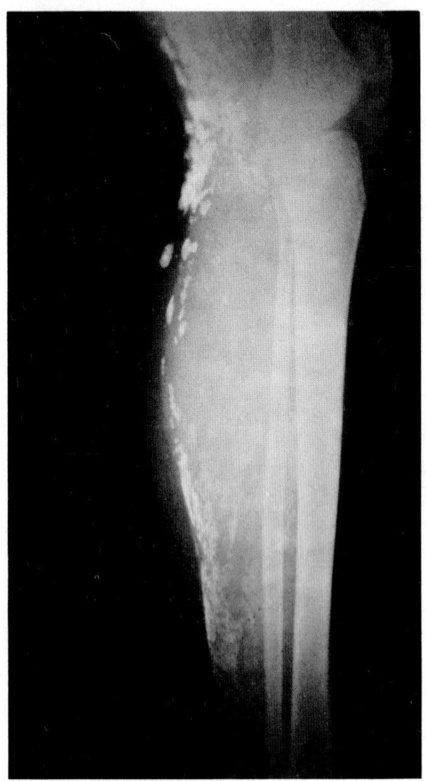

Figure 6.13. Dermatomyositis. X-ray of interfascial plane and subcutaneous calcification

regress as the years pass. Usually there are no demonstrable alterations in serum levels of calcium, phosphate or alkaline phosphatase although occasionally transient rises in the latter are seen in adolescents with multiple deposits.

A very small proportion of children go on over many years with continuing activity, extensive muscle wasting, severe contractures

Colour Plate Section

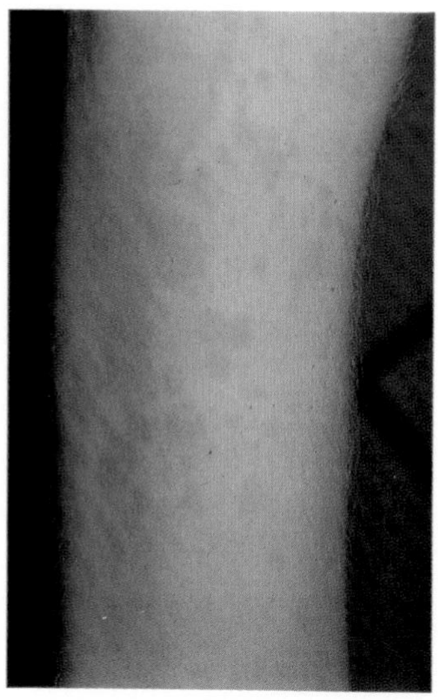

Plate 1. Juvenile chronic arthritis: rash showing a mixture of small and large lesions – the latter becoming confluent

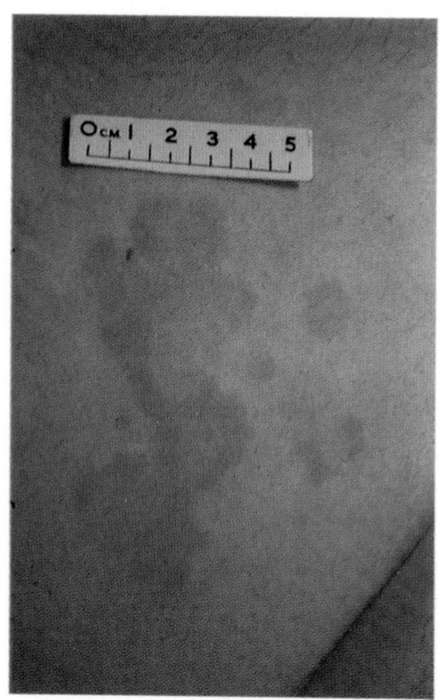

Plate 2. Erythema marginatum. characteristic of rheumatic fever. This needs to be differentiated from the rash of systemic juvenile chronic arthritis

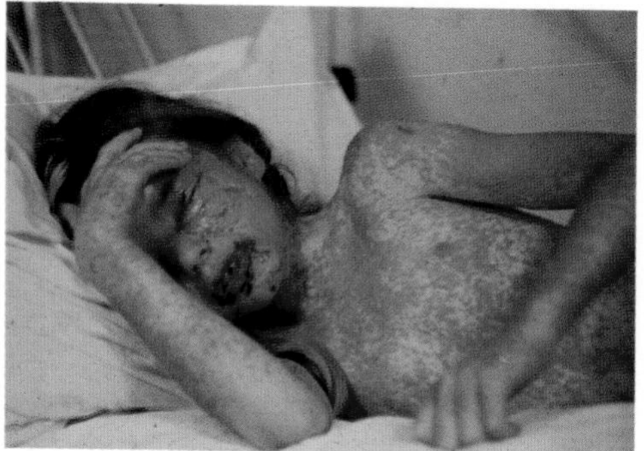

Plate 3. Stevens-Johnson syndrome – typical appearance

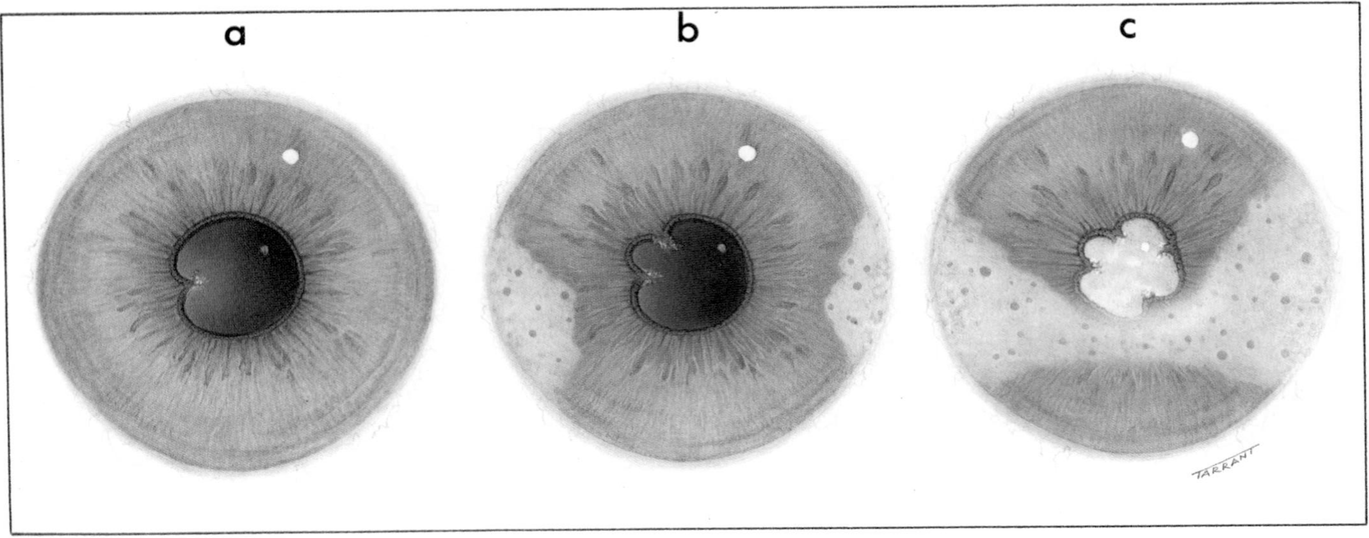

Plate 4. Progressive eye involvement in juvenile chronic arthritis

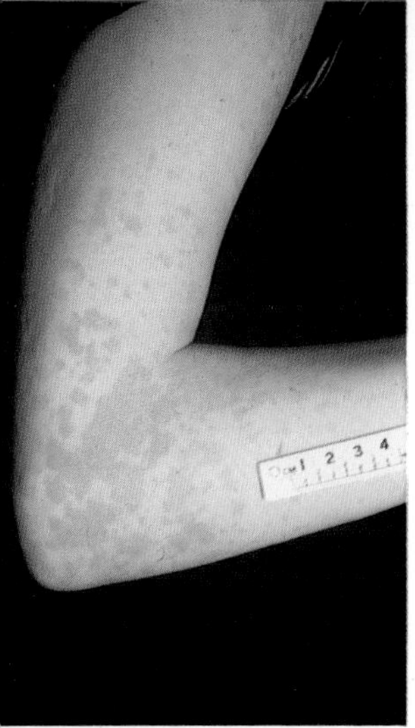

Plate 5. Hypersensitivity rash on the arm. It also appeared on the face where it mimicked systemic lupus erythematosus and on the trunk where it was somewhat like juvenile chronic arthritis

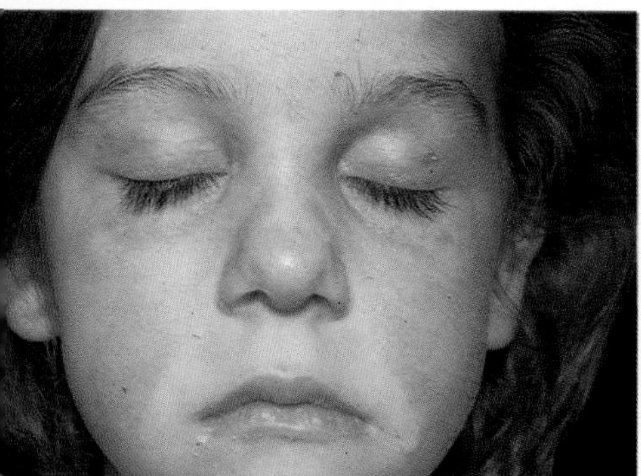

Plate 6. Dermatomyositis: (a) facial rash; (b) typical hands with collodion patches

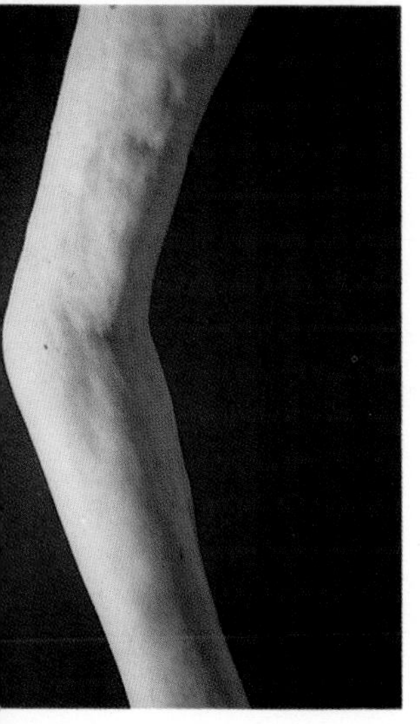

Plate 7. Scleroderma: eosinophilic fasciitis showing rivulets

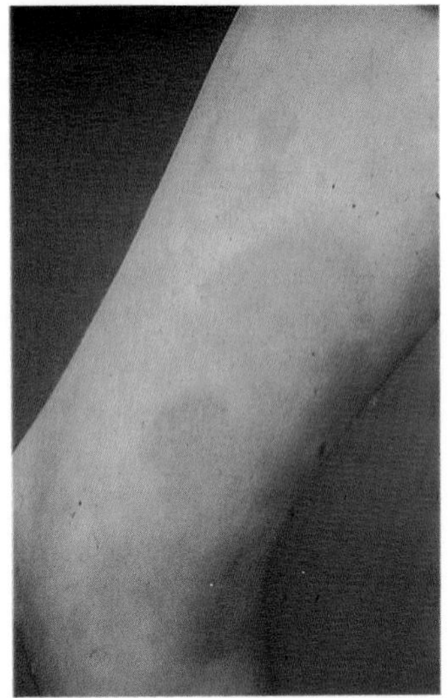

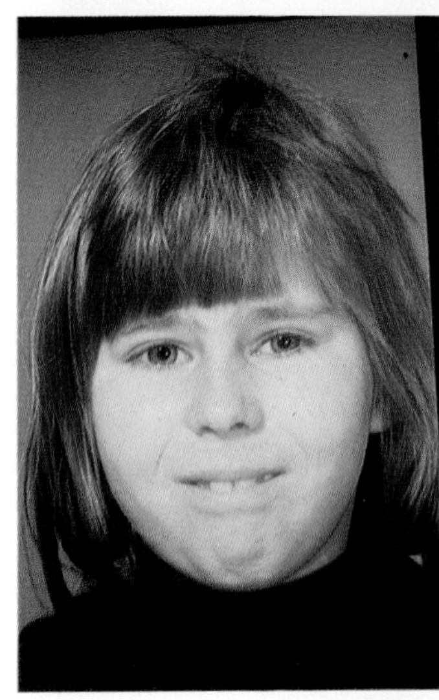

Plate 8. Mixed connective tissue syndrome: (a) rash on leg, suggesting bruising; (b) parotid swelling

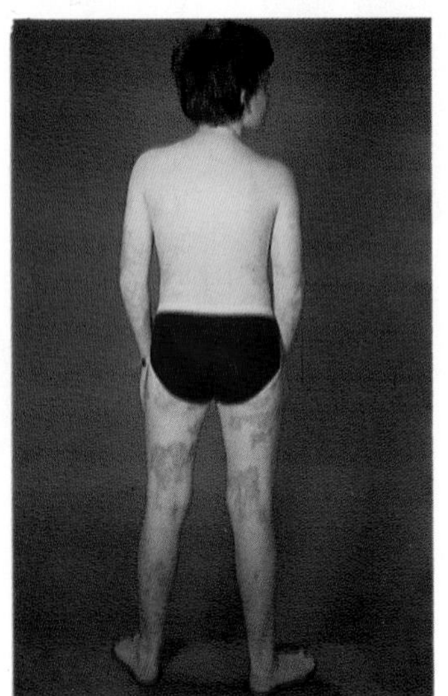

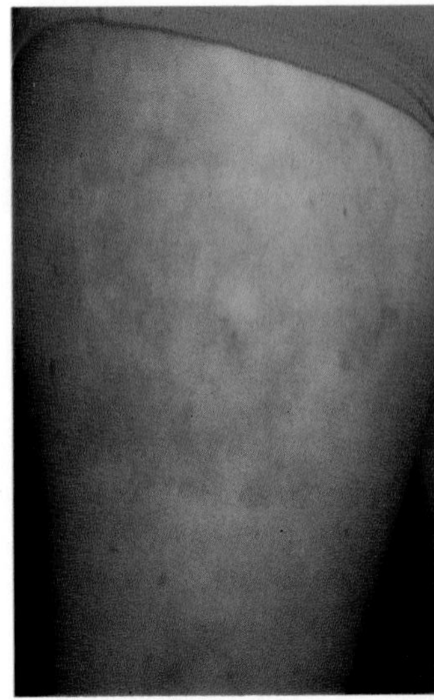

Plate 9. Polyarteritis (a) skin affecting thighs and calves; (b) close-up of calves

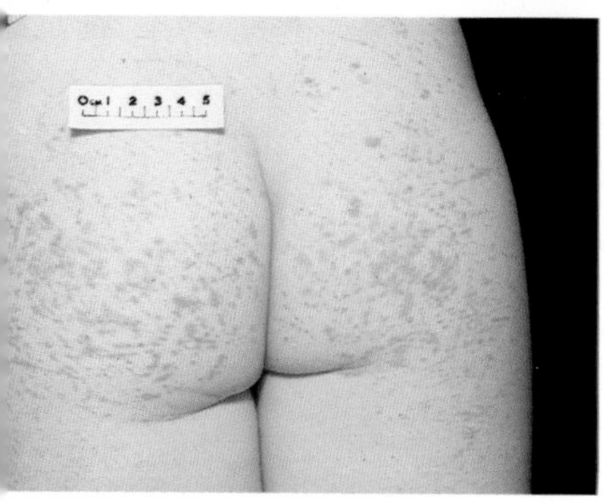

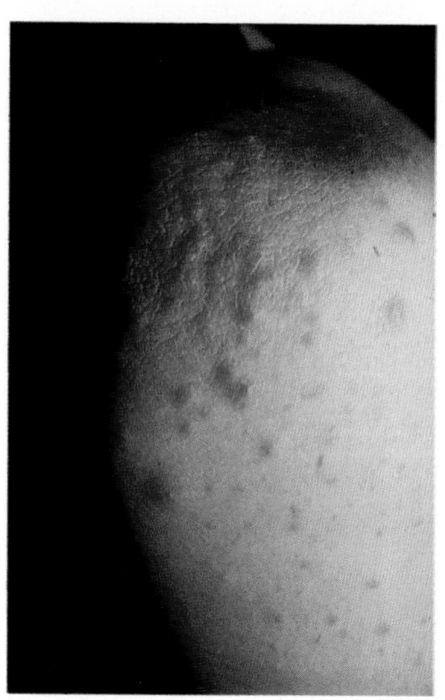

). Henoch–Schoenlein purpura: (a) rash on buttocks; (b) elbow nodule

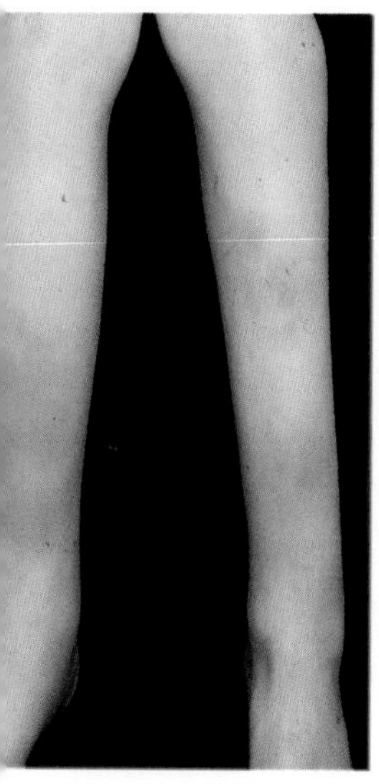

Plate 11. Erythema nodosum

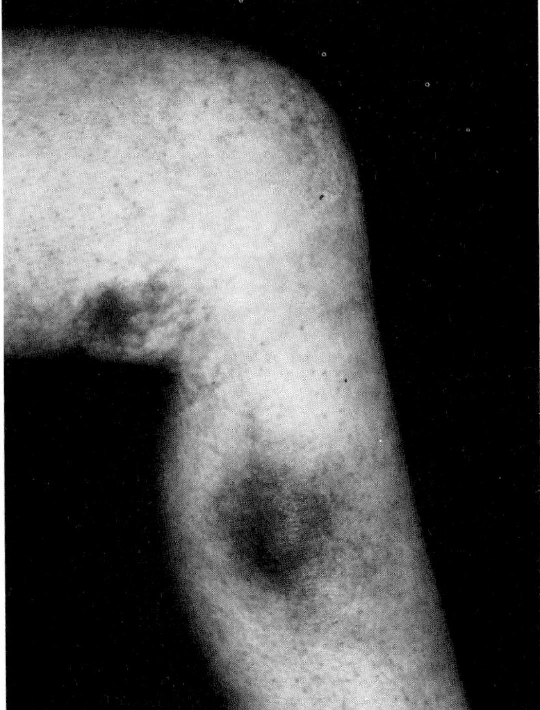

Figure 6.14. Dermatomyositis. Acute calcinosis which produced fever with red tender lesions

and widespread calcinosis (Miller and Koetler, 1977). Occasionally, recovery from the acute phase of the disease may be followed by an appearance like scleroderma (Ansell, 1978).

Management

During the acute phase of the disease, bed-rest is imperative and it is important that the limbs are maintained in a good position. To prevent the development of contractures plastazote is useful for splinting as it is soft and will not damage inflamed skin. Only as the inflammatory element subsides should assisted exercises commence and even then, care should be taken to avoid overstretching weak muscles. Once all inflammation has subsided a more active physiotherapeutic regime can be introduced. Special problems will include the occasional requirement of semi-solid

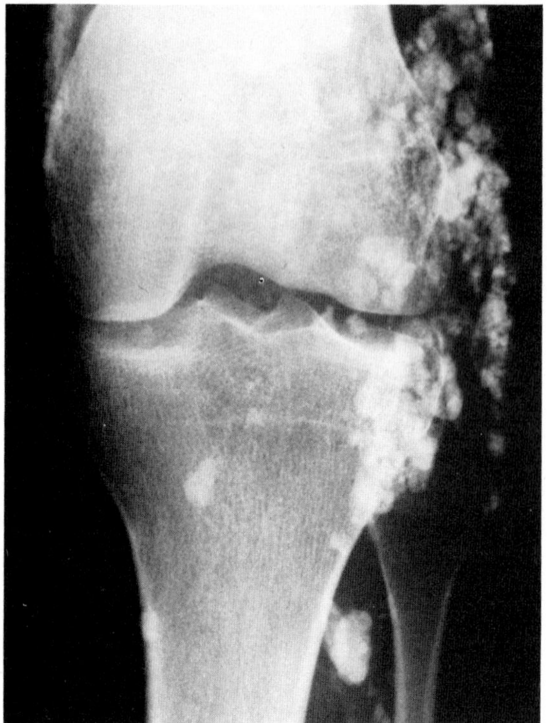

Figure 6.15. Dermatomyositis. Extensive subcutaneous calcinosis some 15 years from onset and 13 years after recovery from the acute illness

food for dysphagia, a respirator for intercostal muscle weakness or tracheostomy for bull neck due to oedema.

Corticosteroids at approximately 1.5–2.0 mg/kg bodyweight have proved to be the first effective therapy capable of suppressing disease activity (Dubovitz, 1976). In severe acute illness it will be necessary to use this therapy daily but even so it is advisable to give it as a single morning dose, rather than in divided doses; once the acute phase has been controlled it is desirable to reduce the dose to an alternate-day one. The use of alternate-day therapy from the onset may be considered in mild cases (*Figure 6.16*), to reduce complications. Monitoring of drug therapy by serum creatine phosphokinase, vital capacity and regular assessment of muscle function is essential. It has been suggested that corticosteroid side effects are relatively rare, however, this is not our experience, so it is imperative to get the children on to the lowest possible dose that controls the inflammation as quickly as possible because of the risk of osteoporosis with multiple crush fractures of vertebrae, diabetes, steroid cataract and growth failure, while a secondary steroid myopathy can be confused with weakness due to dermatomyositis.

Cytotoxic drugs are best reserved for the case that does not respond to reasonable doses of corticosteroids or has run into side effects on corticosteroids which cannot be easily withdrawn because of persistent activity. The first such drug to receive particular attention was methotrexate; originally it was given intravenously and because of this there is little experience in

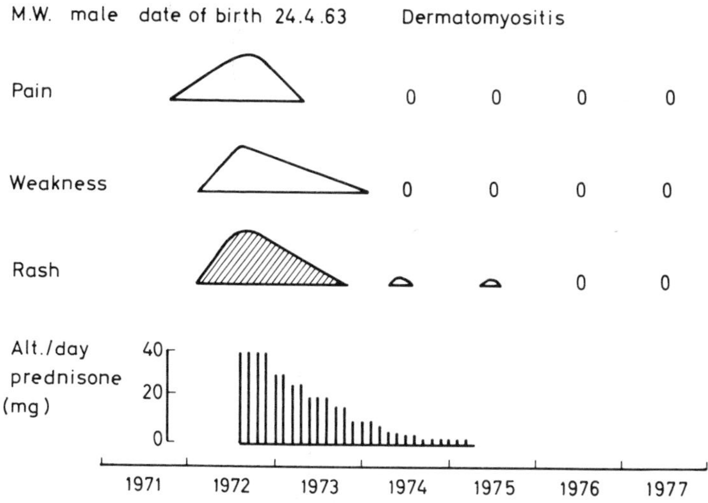

Figure 6.16. Dermatomyositis. The use of an alternate-day corticosteroid regime in a patient who had a sub-acute onset of disease

childhood (Jacobs, 1977). The side effects are liver damage, stomatitis, sore throat, skin rash, purpura, fever and gastro-intestinal problems. The maximum effect comes on in about ten weeks and continues thereafter. Azathioprine in a dose of 1.5–2.5 mg/kg bodyweight and adjusted to just depress the blood count appears to be equally successful. At Taplow we originally used cyclophosphamide in a dosage up to 4 mg/kg bodyweight as oral therapy; seven juveniles so treated have done well (Ansell, 1978) (*Figure 6.17*). Because of hair loss we have now started to use chlorambucil in a dosage of 0.5–1.0 mg/kg bodyweight; this appears equally successful. It is important that these cases are followed carefully so that the patients are kept on the lowest possible dosage of appropriate drugs. The acute deposition of hydroxyapatite crystals has been successfully treated by colchicine at 0.65 mg twice or three times daily (Tabourne *et al.*, 1978). This needs to be continued for a prolonged period to suppress the local and systemic inflammation of calcinosis universalis. Numerous remedies have been suggested for management of calcinosis

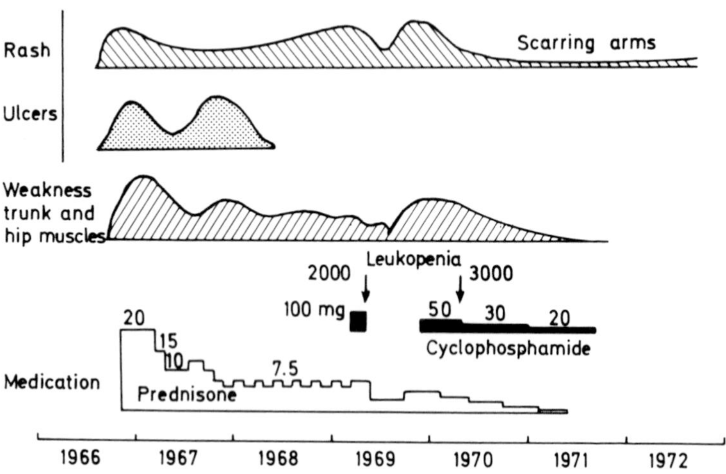

Figure 6.17. Dermatomyositis. Even these moderate doses of prednisone had caused slowing of growth and the disease was continuing active, so cyclophosphamide was introduced with benefit

(Ansell, 1978). Our original suggestion that Benemid (probenecid) might be useful in subcutaneous calcinosis must be reconsidered in the light of the decrease in calcinosis seen in our long-term follow-up (Sewell *et al.*, 1978).

Intercurrent infection will require prompt treatment, calcinotic nodules may need to be removed surgically and above all, from time to time morale will need to be boosted.

SCLERODERMA

The relationship between systemic sclerosis and other forms of diffuse or localised scleroderma is seen at its most confusing in childhood at an age when systemic sclerosis is rare and localised forms are common (Ansell *et al.*, 1976). Progressive systemic sclerosis is a very rare but serious disease usually affecting girls (Cassidy *et al.*, 1977).

Clinical features – localised scleroderma

It is generally considered that morphea, linear scleroderma in the limbs and scleroderma *en coup de sabre,* as on the face, have no systemic manifestations, but in a proportion of children, symptoms related to the musculoskeletal system at a distance to the local patch of scleroderma do arise. This can occur throughout childhood; the majority of children present mimicking juvenile chronic polyarthritis with stiffness rather than joint pain, although occasionally some slight soft tissue swelling of joints is seen. The limitation of movement of joints is not accounted for by the local skin lesions (*Figure 6.18*). Loss of movement is particularly

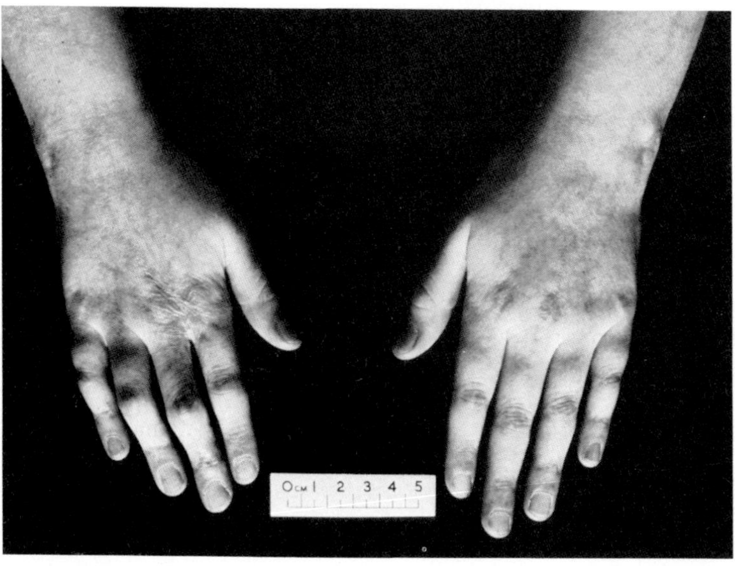

Figgure 6.18. Scleroderma. Local lesion on the hand and finger causing contracture was associated with stiffness in the other hand, knees and feet

common at wrists and elbows but is also seen at ankles and feet and knees. Widespread tendon nodule formation (*Figure 6.19* and *6.20*) is common in such cases. Indeed, the outstanding feature of the group studied by us was the high incidence of tendon nodule formation with associated difficulty in movement (*Figure 6.21*). Kornreich *et al*. (1977) indicate that localised scleroderma does not involve just skin and subcutaneous tissue but can involve muscle, bone and synovial tissue and in rare instances, internal organs.

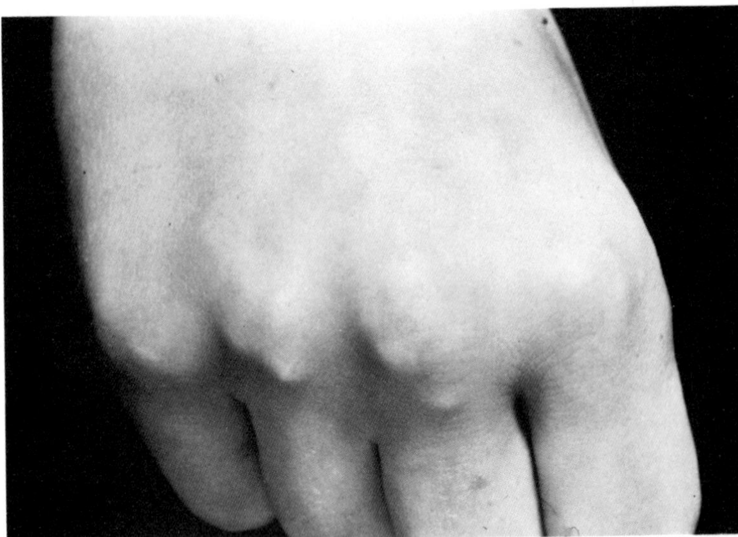

Figure 6.19. Scleroderma. Nodules in the tendons over the metacarpal joints in an 11 year old girl

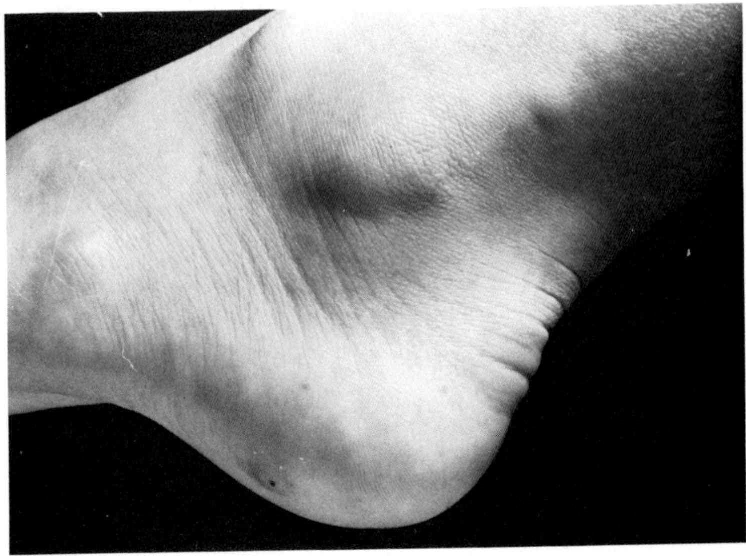

Figure 6.20. Scleroderma. Nodules over the lateral malleolus in the girl shown in Figure 6.19

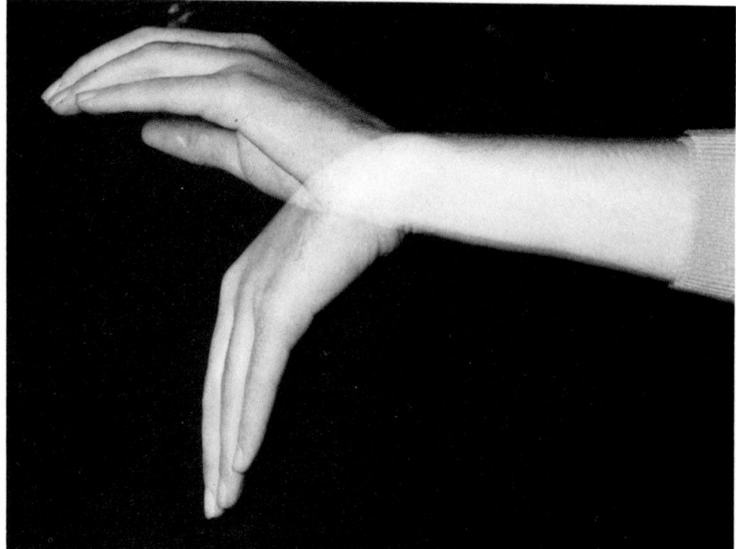

Figure 6.21. Scleroderma. Loss of movement due to tendon lesions. Hand movement is almost full when palmar flexed but markedly limited when dorsiflexed

Linear scleroderma (*Figure 6.22*) may be associated with patches of morphea elsewhere as well as tendon nodules and joint symptoms.

Prognosis

There may be some loss of movement subsequent to tendon fibrosis – this being particularly common in the hands. The bands of cutaneous sclerosis tend to progress slowly ultimately causing loss of function in the affected limb with marked growth defects. Facial lesions can lead to subcutaneous atrophy and pigmentary change with severe cosmetic problems. Rarely localised skin lesions are associated with diffuse sclerosis of internal organs although this tends to be milder than in progressive systemic sclerosis.

Clinical features of systemic sclerosis

Raynaud's phenomenon frequently heralds the onset of systemic sclerosis together with stiffness of the hands, contractures of the fingers, tightening of the skin and vague joint discomfort. Very

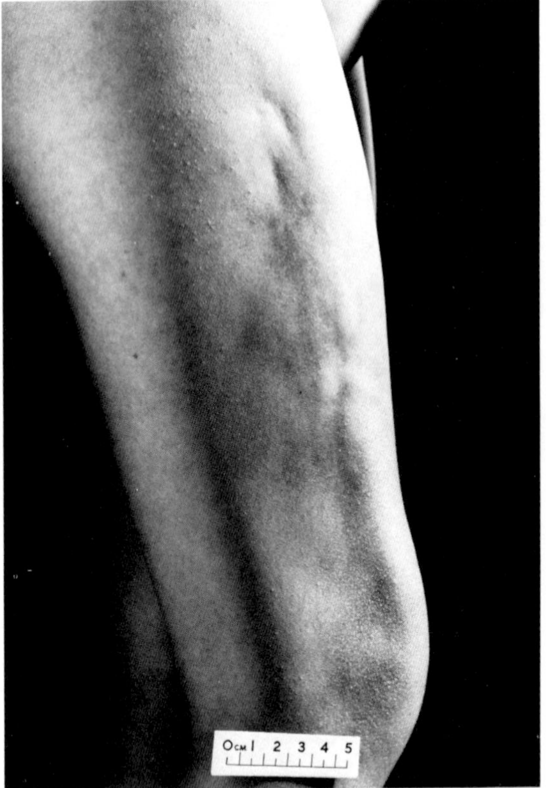

Figure 6.22. Scleroderma. Linear scleroderma in a boy who presented with pain and discomfort in hands and feet as well as difficulty in extending the knee on the affected side. (By courtesy of Annals of Rheumatic Diseases)

occasionally diffuse sclerodermatous change in the skin occurs without apparent systemic involvement (Ansell *et al.*, 1976). It is, however, important to check the oesophageal, pulmonary, cardiac and renal status in all cases. Indeed, it is usually only on direct questioning that dysphagia, muscle weakness and dyspnoea come to light. There tends to be a relatively symptomless advance of both cutaneous and visceral lesions so that ultimately pigmentation with depigmentation, ulceration of the skin, telangiectasia and subcutaneous calcification develop, together with radiological evidence of absorption of terminal phalanges. Abnormalities of mobility of the oesophagus, and finally constriction, is not uncommon while other gastro-intestinal lesions such as colonic sacculations and dilatation of the duodenum are less common. Although the vital capacity is frequently reduced and diffusion abnormal, symptoms are relatively mild. However, cardiac and pulmonary disease are usually responsible for the mortality, immediate causes of death commonly relating to myocardial fibrosis or cardiac failure secondary to lung involvement. Renal involvement tends to be subtle in its progression and is difficult to detect, but is also another cause of death.

Prognosis

In general then, it is important to regard progressive systemic sclerosis as a serious disorder in childhood despite the fact that occasionally, as in adults, the disease in children may improve spontaneously, but the presence of renal, cardiac and pulmonary involvement must cause a guarded prognosis.

Laboratory investigations

The ESR is usually normal. Rheumatoid factor in our group was negative but Hanson *et al*. (1974) have reported weak positive rheumatoid factors in this group. Antinuclear antibodies may be present in as high a percentage as 50 per cent without rise in antibodies to DNA or change in complement. Slight rises in IgG are not uncommon. These changes are particularly likely in children with multiple skin lesions, who are also more likely to have joint symptoms.

Histological changes in the local lesions are typical of scleroderma; showing increasing thickness and density of the collagen in the dermis, flattening of the retepegs and the presence of mononuclear cells, infiltrates of lymphocytes and macrophages around small blood vessels and skin appendages. The nodules histologically show a fibrinoid material without inflammatory reaction, collagen bundles of varying size with some round cells.

Fasciitis and eosinophilia

In juveniles, as in adults this very rarely reported disorder closely mimics scleroderma (Schulman, 1974). Our first case (Ansell *et al*., 1976) was diagnosed retrospectively. At age 14 he presented with stiffness and pain in the hands and knees and when seen three months from onset, in addition to widespread joint limitation, was noticed to have extensive flexor and extensor tendon nodule formation. Pitting oedema of the skin in some sites with thickening in others was noted at this time and, although scleroderma was suggested, a raised ESR, and negative antinuclear factor made us think this was an atypical onset of juvenile chronic arthritis. He did, however, have 21 per cent eosinophils in a white blood count of 9700. Over the next six months he developed progressive tightness of the skin over the arms and legs looking very much more like scleroderma. His ESR continued to be raised and he continued to have eosinophilia.

Reviewing the biopsy retrospectively, it passed from normal epidermis into a layer of collagenous thickening typical of scleroderma but extending into the fatty tissue down to the deep fascia of muscle. The new tissue was cellular, the fascial plane showed numerous inflammatory cells, the fibroblasts were plumper and more numerous than usual and there were numbers of lymphocytes, and an occasional eosinophil. Subsequent treatment with corticosteroids produced improvement generally but he has residual deformities of his hand joints. Two subsequent cases diagnosed more promptly (*Plate 7*) regressed over one and one and a half years respectively without any clinical or radiological residua.

Other diagnostic problems

In addition to the different types of scleroderma described, multiple joint contractures particularly of the hands, with the skin often thick, tight and waxy, mimicking scleroderma, have been seen to occur in a high proportion of juvenile diabetic children (Grgic *et al.*, 1976). In the few cases personally seen, the diabetes had commenced early in childhood and had been particularly difficult to control. Severe flexor tendon involvement was present in one teenager, which responded well to a local corticosteroid injection.

Following streptococcal infection scleroderma is occasionally seen in childhood, in this the skin tends to pit and the site of involvement is often atypical for scleroderma. The prognosis for the disorder is excellent, remission occurring quickly and completely.

A relatively recent association with scleroderma has been phenylketonuria (Lasser *et al.*, 1978).

Management

In *local scleroderma* due to morphea, penicillamine at low dosage has been shown to be of use (Moynihan, 1977); while agreeing that the morphea improved there has been relatively little objective evidence of improvement in tendon nodules with this therapy. However, function can be maintained by the appropriate use of physiotherapy and an exercise programme designed to maintain, and possibly improve function. It is accepted that in linear scleroderma, while some patients may ultimately improve, atrophic changes and growth changes are usual. We therefore decided to try the use of penicillamine in a relatively low dose (250 mg daily); over two years there appears to be improvement in the linear band in two patients allowing the contracture to straighten and restoration of normal function in the knee. One patient who was not started on treatment until very late, i.e. already with severe growth defect and contracture of an arm, has not deteriorated as might have been expected but restoration to normal function has not occurred. Because of the seriousness of this situation, Kornreich *et al.* (1977) have treated five patients with immunosuppressive therapy, either azathioprine or cyclophosphamide with some improvement but as yet it is too early to judge the long-term effect. There is certainly no evidence that corticosteroids affect the localised types of scleroderma.

In *progressive systemic sclerosis* our experience with corticosteroids first and subsequently with penicillamine has been as disappointing as others. It therefore seems reasonable to consider cytotoxic therapy in such patients. To date we have used chlorambucil, over a three-year period in one such patient with apparent benefit. The improvement witnessed could have been spontaneous; it is encouraging enough to warrant studies on further patients.

Fasciitis with eosinophilia would appear to be an acute problem which, in contrast to the other forms of scleroderma, responds promptly to corticosteroids. Prednisone needs to be given daily at approximately 1.5–2.0 mg/kg bodyweight until all acute symptoms have subsided; it can then be gradually withdrawn with little difficulty.

MIXED CONNECTIVE TISSUE DISEASE IN CHILDREN

Sharp and his colleagues (1969) drew attention to the presence of an antibody to ribonuclear protein in patients who had overlapping features suggestive of systemic lupus erythematosus, systemic sclerosis, polymyositis and rheumatoid arthritis. A retrospective review by Singson *et al.* (1977) allowed them to identify ten children out of a paediatric rheumatic disease population of 2000. That it is not rare is suggested by the fact that five children have been diagnosed by us in the last two years (Peskett *et al.*, 1978). Their age tends to be towards double figures. The onset is usually

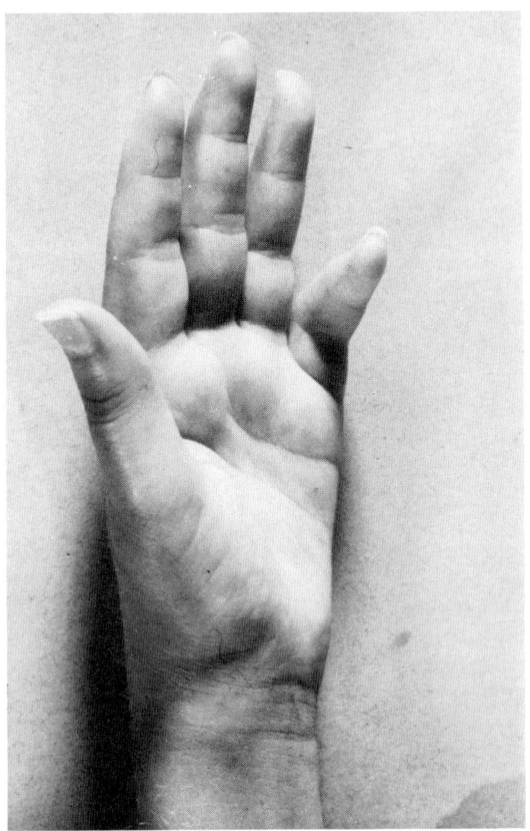

Figure 6.23. Mixed connective tissue syndrome. Acute flexor tenosynovitis in a ten year old with Raynaud's phenomenon and intermittent parotid swelling

as a polyarthritis with particularly marked involvement of the small joints of the fingers and very marked involvement of flexor tendons (*Figure 6.23*), and sometimes also extensor tendon involvement, with a tendency to contractures of the fingers (*Figure 6.24*). Skin changes consistent with scleroderma with tightness of the skin over the fingers is also common, as is Raynaud's phenomenon. At times, symptoms of muscle pain, with tenderness and a slightly raised CPK are found, while very occasionally rashes mimicking those of dermatomyositis are seen. More usually the rash is non-specific, often leaving areas like bruising (*Plate 8a*). Muscle involvement tends to be transient. At times a facial rash may suggest systemic lupus erythematosus. Other features include lymphadenopathy, hepatosplenomegaly, splenomegaly as well as abnormal oesophageal mobility. Pericarditis occurs occasionally as does parotid swelling (*Plate 8b*). Two of the patients reviewed

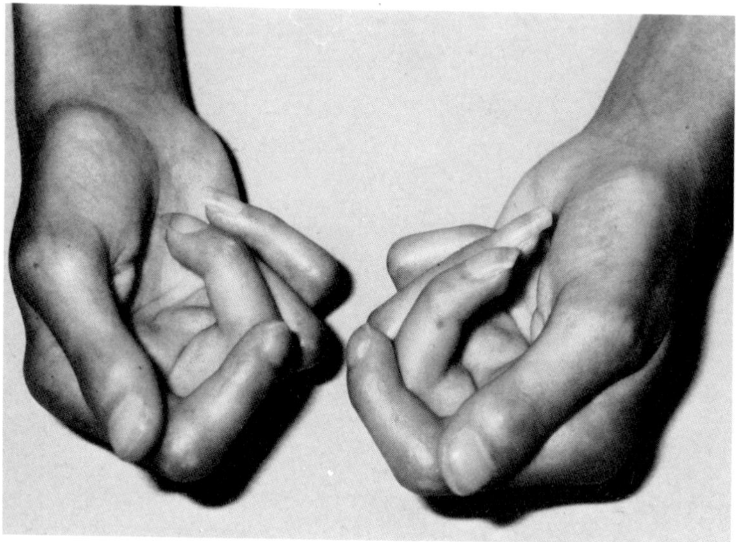

Figure 6.24. Mixed connective tissue syndrome. Contracture of hands in a 13 year old girl who had developed Raynaud's phenomenon two and a half years earlier followed by multiple nodules over forehead, elbows and knees and progressive stiffening of joints

retrospectively by Singson *et al*. (1977) had evidence of pulmonary involvement, while thrombocytopenia, neurological and also renal involvement were seen in them.

The disorder should be suspected when a child appears to have features of more than one of the connective tissue disorders, particularly when they are developing sequentially. It is supported by the presence of a strongly positive antinuclear antibody with nucleolar staining, negative antibodies to DNA and normal complement; the presence of extractable nuclear antigen of the ribonuclear protein variety confirms the diagnosis. The ESR is usually raised and rheumatoid factor tests may be variably positive.

Is it of importance to recognise this syndrome? In the past the majority of affected children have been labelled as having juvenile chronic arthritis. Firstly, however, it does not seem to have the prognosis of juvenile arthritis, as apparently this entity can slowly develop with new features being added as the years go by. Secondly, the majority of the patients may warrant corticosteroid therapy to maintain function, which it will be necessary to continue for a prolonged period of time. Three of our patients with marked nodule and tendon involvement are doing well on gold.

SJÖGREN'S SYNDROME

Sjögren's syndrome is a chronic inflammatory disease characterised by infiltration of lymphocytes and plasma cells into the salivary glands particularly but also into the lacrimal glands and at other sites, when glandular insufficiency results.

In childhood the syndrome usually presents as recurrent parotid swelling. It is, however, extremely rare. The majority of cases that one has suspected ultimately developed into either systemic lupus erythematosus or mixed connective tissue syndrome; to date I have only one child with recurrent parotid swelling and a positive antinuclear antibody who has not declared other features of a connective tissue disorder.

Our experience is at variance with Bernstein *et al.* (1977) in that in our cases, in addition to the above symptoms, dry eyes are occasionally seen in association with severe chronic iridocyclitis. Also a typical kerato-conjunctivitis sicca without other manifestations has now been seen in a number of juvenile rheumatoid arthritics who carry IgM rheumatoid factor; and in all their illness had begun in the early teens and followed a pattern similar to that of adult rheumatoid arthritis.

VASCULITIC SYNDROMES

Polyarteritis

At present, the clinical variants of polyarteritis seem to depend on the location and size of affected vessels. As yet, no classification has proved entirely satisfactory, so that given in *Table 6.2* aims to help the practising clinician. Histological appraisal of case reports of polyarteritis in childhood shows that various pathological processes have been described.

TABLE 6.2
Types of polyarteritis

		Associations
(1) Infantile (under 2 years) ? Kawasaki syndrome synonymous		
(2) Older children 6–16		
(a)	Cutaneous with systemic features	Streptococcal
(b)	Generalised }	Streptococcal
(c)	Renal }	hepatitis B antigen

Infantile polyarteritis

Is infantile polyarteritis, which is completely different from polyarteritis seen in older children, the same as the recently described mucocutaneous lymph node syndrome (Kawasaki *et al.*, 1974) (Ahlstrom *et al.*, 1977)? Taking two years of age as the upper limit of onset, Roberts and Peterman (1963) analysed the characteristics of 20 cases of infantile polyarteritis. The chief features were prolonged fever and rash, while cough and conjunctivitis were observed in half of the infants and signs of central nervous system disease in 30 per cent. Gangrene of the extremities was noticed in two. Coronary arteritis was the most usual cause of death. The average duration from first symptom to death was 27 days. Among laboratory investigations leucocytosis was usual and abnormal urinalysis was found in three-quarters of patients. Radiologically, cardiomegaly was common and six out of seven ECGs performed were abnormal. At autopsy the coronary arteries were involved in 18 of the 20 children, including multiple aneurysms which were filled with thrombi. Myocardial abnormalities were present in nine. Arteritis was also reported in the kidneys, spleen, mesentery and extremities but in the skeletal muscle in only one child. Histologically, the coronary artery disease in these infants was characteristic of polyarteritis nodosa. An immunopathogenic mechanism is suspected by more recent work where high levels of IgE have been reported in the serum of two such infants and a low serum complement in one.

Mucocutaneous lymph node syndrome (Kawasaki's disease)

This syndrome was first described in Japan by Kawasaki *et al.* (1974); from there many thousands of cases have now been reported. The next big series came from Hicks (1977) in Hawaii; it was interesting that a large number of her patients were of Japanese background and she had no Caucasians in the series. Subsequently numerous cases have been reported from all over the world, including more than one in a family (Lyen and Brook, 1978). Have we been calling the extreme end of the spectrum infantile polyarteritis nodosa and ignoring the ones who recovered or passing them off as viral infections? The syndrome is now being recorded not only in infants but also in children of three, four, five and six years of age; but it does appear to be the very young who fare worst from the cardiological point of view, consistent with our view of infantile polyarteritis nodosa.

Clinical features (Table 6.3)

The characteristic features consist of a mild upper respiratory infection followed by a spiking fever which lasts approximately seven to 21 days. The children appear moderately ill (*Figure 6.25a*) and an erythematous skin rash (*Figure 6.25b*) is usually seen; occasionally this is transient. Conjunctival injection is usual, the oropharynx shows a diffuse erythema with a magenta hue, and ultimately prominent papillae on the tongue resemble a strawberry tongue. Soon after the onset of the fever the hands and feet become diffusely indurated and swollen; the skin and underlying

TABLE 6.3
Kawasaki syndrome

Principle features	*Subsidiary features*	*Complications*
Fever spiking 7–21 days	Pyuria	Cardiac involvement
Conjunctival injection	Diarrhoea	Aseptic meningitis
Erythema of oropharynx		Arthralgia and arthritis
Erythematous rash		
Induration of palms and soles		
Desquamation		
Cervical lymphadenopathy		

tissue developing a woody firmness resembling scleroderma. Children are unwilling to use their hands or stand on their feet at this time.

After two to three days the oedema and induration disappear with striking desquamation on the tips of the fingers (*Figure 6.25c*), at times there can be a generalised desquamation. Other changes consist of dryness around the mouth and fissuring at the edge of the lips. Cervical lymphadenopathy occurs in the majority.

During the acute phase the urine may contain some protein and pus cells and diarrhoea may be present. Other described features include aseptic meningitis and quite severe arthralgia and arthritis. During the second and third week of the illness, cardiac involvement may be detected, by softening of the heart sounds, cardiac enlargement and ECG change. In the 26 patients described by Hicks (1977) two died in the third week and were shown at autopsy to have massive coronary thrombosis; the microscopic examination was consistent with polyarteritis nodosa. Kato (1977) using coronary angiography noticed an incidence of coronary involvement of 31 per cent.

During the acute phase the ESR is raised and there is a marked leucocytosis. At times, thrombocytosis is also present. Transient rises of serum lactic dehydrogenase in some patients suggest that myocarditis may be occurring. Serial electrocardiograms have only been done in one or two series, notably that of Hicks (1977) who reported five out of 26 showing non-specific abnormalities. The aetiology of this condition is not known although an infection is suspected. Kawasaki reported rickettsial-like particles in the skin and lymph node specimens but these have not yet been confirmed by other workers. In determining the differential diagnosis, intercurrent infection, and particularly a prolonged viral infection, together with serum sickness and Stevens-Johnson syndrome will need to be considered.

Therapy is symptomatic. However, in view of the reported high incidence of thrombocytosis, persisting into the third week, at which time occlusion of coronary vessels is common, it is perhaps wise to continue giving aspirin during this period even though the fever and other features have subsided (Kato *et al.*, 1979).

Childhood polyarteritis

Childhood polyarteritis tends to occur from about six years of age upwards and males are affected more frequently than females. The usual presentation is with fever and abdominal pains, limb pain

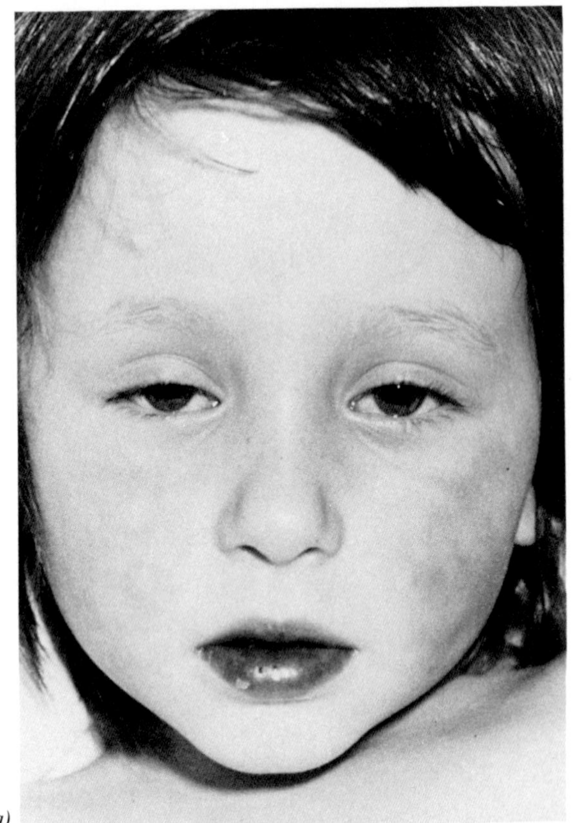

(a)

Figure 6.25. Mucocutaneous lymph node syndrome. (By courtesy of Dr M. L. Liberman.) (a) A five year old girl with persistent fever, general toxic appearance with cracking of the lips and rash on the face

and arthralgia (*Table 6.4*). Because of the non-specific nature of the symptoms the disease can mimic a number of entities including rheumatic fever, erythema nodosum and Henoch–Schoenlein purpura. In general the pain is in the limbs and although there may be oedema of the hands and feet, synovitis is relatively mild and the arthralgia does not usually have the flitting pattern of rheumatic fever.

Cutaneous polyarteritis is characterised by a variety of cutaneous lesions clinically, necrotising arteritis histologically, and a benign although often prolonged course. It is not strictly a cutaneous

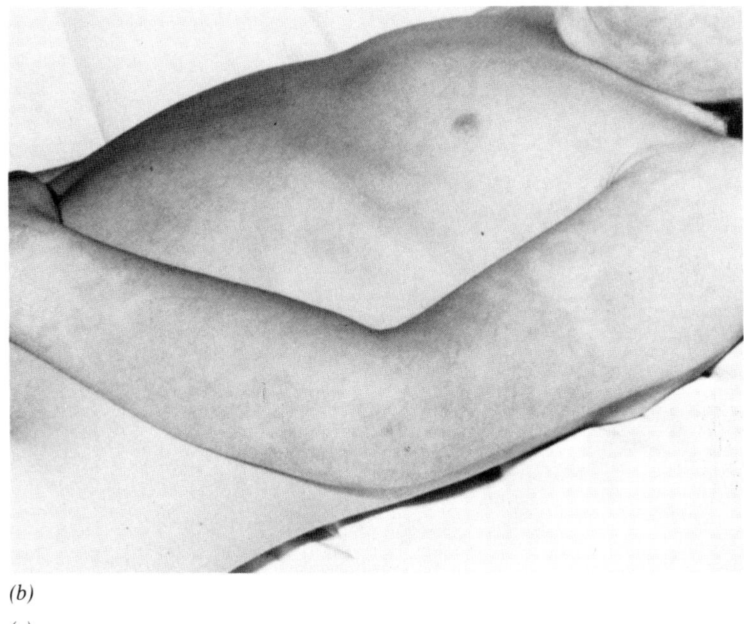

(b)

(c)

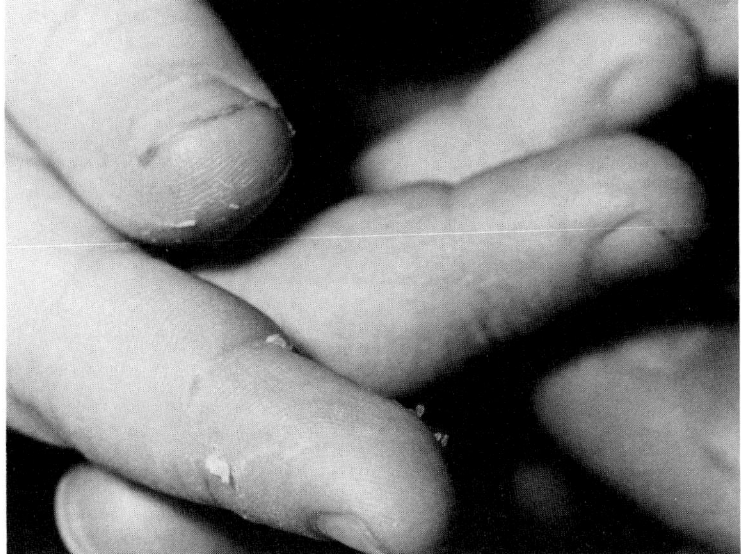

Figure 6.25. (b) She rapidly developed an erythematous rash and limbs that were painful to touch; (c) skinning of the fingers on subsidence of the swelling of the hands, and rash

TABLE 6.4
Childhood polyarteritis

Non-specific features	
Fever	
Abdominal pain	
Limb pain	
Arthralgia/arthritis	
'Cutaneous'	'Systemic'
Nodules, cutaneous and subcutaneous	Raynaud's phenomenon
	Asthma
	Neuropathy
	Cardiac involvement
	Hepatic involvement
	Renal involvement

disease as arthralgia, arthritis and fever may also occur. The painful subcutaneous nodules may suggest erythema nodosum but the nodules are smaller and much more widespread and considerably more indurated. The site however, is at times similar along the pretibial surface of the shin but the nodules also occur in the calves, thigh and at other sites (*Plate 9a* and *b*). It is also not uncommon to get associated small vasculitic lesions elsewhere. As this form of vasculitis is frequently associated with a recent history of streptococcal infection, together with rising anti-streptolysin O-titres, the initial differential diagnosis from erythema nodosum can be very difficult. However, in general the child with polyarteritis is much more sick and the nodules are very much more extensive than in erythema nodosum. As already indicated, the joint features lack the typical extremely painful red flitting arthritis of rheumatic fever.

Generalised polyarteritis which may present with Raynaud's phenomenon, as well as fever and myalgia and sometimes pulmonary infiltrates and asthma, can mimic systemic lupus erythematosus; while at times the severity of limb pain makes one wonder about dermatomyositis. Skin rashes of many types may occur, including purpura without thrombocytopenia, erythema, erythematous patches and involvement of small vessels of the skin. The most serious of the visceral involvements would appear to be renal (Reimold *et al.*, 1976). As the characteristic feature histologically is focal necrosis of the walls of small and medium-sized arteries it can affect the arcuate arteries or the small renal vessels and the glomeruli causing a prolific glomerulonephritis.

In suspected polyarteritis the urine should be regularly monitored, as should the blood pressure. Neuropathy, coronary, mesenteric and hepatic involvement do occur but are relatively rare.

Management

In patients in whom there is a preceding streptococcal infection it might be wise to consider penicillin prophylaxis as there is a very real risk of relapse with further streptococcal infection (*Figure 6.26*). In general, the prognosis for those with predominantly cutaneous lesions is good although relapses are not uncommon;

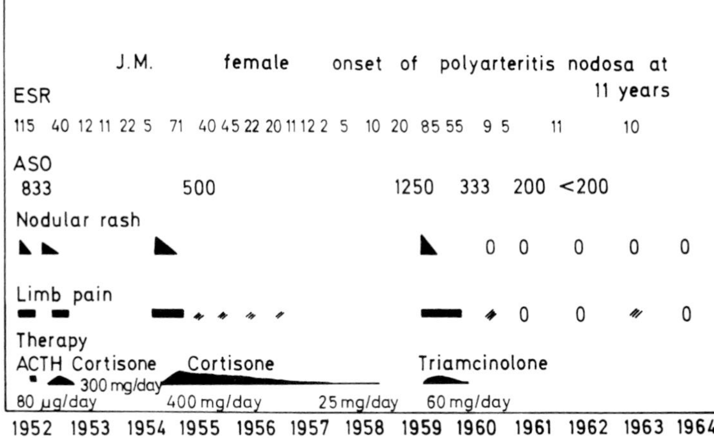

Figure 6.26. Polyarteritis. Chart of course of 11 year old girl who had cutaneous polyarteritis with systemic features. Note the relapses after streptococcal infection of the throat causing rise in ASO titres

corticosteroids may, however, be required to control fever and the general constitutional features. Indomethacin is helpful in controlling joint symptoms.

In those patients with more sinister lesions, such as renal involvement, if they fail to improve rapidly on a high-dose steroid, on our present evidence it would appear advisable to go on to cytotoxic drugs, of which most experience appears to be with cyclophosphamide (Reimold *et al.*, 1976).

HENOCH–SCHOENLEIN PURPURA

Children of both sexes are affected by Henoch–Schoenlein purpura and while usually beginning at about the age of three, it can occur throughout childhood and into adult life.

Clinical features

The outstanding clinical feature is the rash which begins as red macules or papules together with purpura which is non-thrombocytopenic. Characteristically this affects buttocks (*Figure 6.27* and *Plate 10a*), legs and feet (*Figure 6.28*) and at times, the trunk, head and arms. There may be extensive ecchymoses; very rarely the lesions proceed to vesiculation and skin necrosis can then occur.

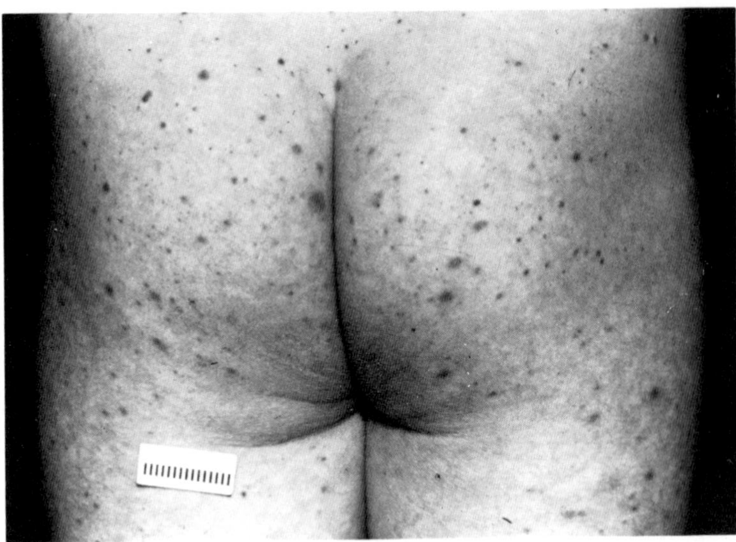

Figure 6.27. Henoch–Schoenlein purpura. Purpuric rash on buttocks (see also Plate 10a)

Joint involvement consists of transient, non-migratory arthritis with the ankles, knees, wrists and elbows most commonly affected. As oedema, particularly of the hands and feet is not uncommon, this mimics synovitis. Patchy oedema may also develop at other sites, the face and the scrotum being not uncommon sites. Small intracutaneous nodules on the elbows are seen in about a quarter of children and are diagnostic (*Plate 10b*).

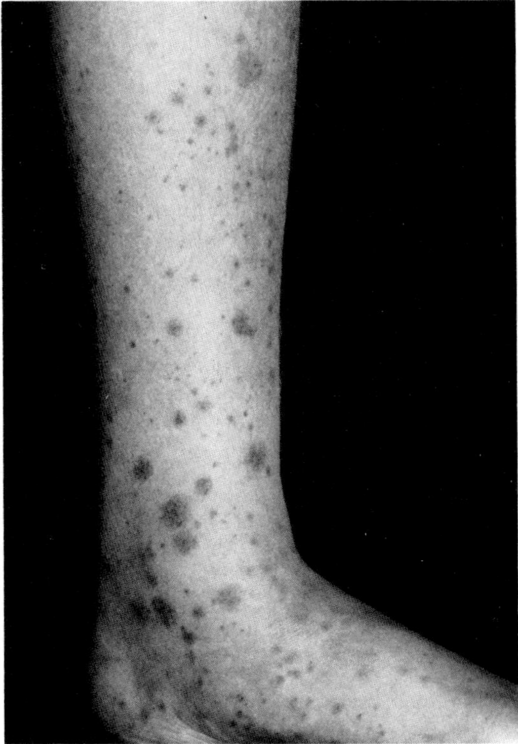

Figure 6.28. Henoch—Schoenlein purpura. Purpuric and maculopapular eruptions on leg of a seven year old who presented with swelling of hands and feet

Abdominal pain, usually colicky, indicates gastro-intestinal involvement which is due to oedema and haemorrhage of the gut wall; there may be overt intestinal haemorrhage or intersusception. Bleeding has occasionally been reported at other sites, intracranial and ocular.

The serious problem in this disorder results from renal involvement. The frequency with which renal involvement is found depends to a considerable extent on how carefully it is looked for, i.e. how often the urine is examined. There has been an occasional case reported where the renal biopsy has been abnormal with a normal urinary sediment. In most series acute glomerulonephritis is seen in about 50 per cent of patients, although this is only of serious significance in the order of 10 per cent in the acute phase. Long-term follow-up studies suggest that late sequelae are not uncommon (Counahan *et al.*, 1977).

Pathology

The basic *pathology* consists of a widespread vasculitis involving arterioles and small capillaries, associated with a perivascular accumulation of polymorphonuclear neutrophils and erythrocytes. Increased vascular permeability leads to the development of oedema and in the serum of children with Henoch–Schoenlein purpura. IgA rises early, while IgG is usually normal and IgM may rise later; IgE is also normal.

IgA immune complexes have been detected as well as IgG complexes: these last are particularly associated with renal disease.

Aetiology

The aetiology is unknown. It has been variously attributed as an allergy to a number of possible agents, including streptococci and various foods. Despite the combination of arthritis, vasculitis, enteritis and nephritis mimicking serum sickness, evidence that it is an immune complex disease is still inconclusive. Immunoglobulins and complement components have been shown by immunofluorescence in affected vessels; thus, deposits of IgA and complement C3 and C4 or only C3 have been shown simultaneously in capillary walls in both cutaneous and renal biopsies. Deposition of C3 and properdin in the absence of $C1_q$ suggests that the C3 in the mesangium of these patients results from the alternative complement pathway (Garcia-Fuentes *et al.*, 1978). A recent study by Nakamoto *et al.* (1978) showed that the immunohistology of primary IgA glomerulonephritis and Henoch–Schoenlein purpura nephritis were identical.

Why IgA is deposited is uncertain, but it may be as part of an immune complex. The recent report on the presence of cryoglobulins at a considerably raised level (Garcia-Fuentes *et al.*, 1977) in the sera of patients with acute Henoch–Schoenlein purpura and those with chronic nephritis, but not in those who had recovered, supports the concept that both the underlying disease and the chronic nephritis could have an immune complex pathogenesis. IgA and properdin were found in the cryoglobulins, suggesting that complement has been activated by the alternative pathway. However, isolated cryoglobulins capable of splitting C3 *in vitro* did so by the classic pathway.

The role of IgA in Henoch–Schoenlein purpura remains unclear. It could be present as an antibody against an infectious organism or other antigen which entered via the respiratory or gastro-intestinal mucosa. Alternatively, the IgA might be altered by an infectious organism so that it becomes antigenic and causes immune complex formation; and certainly the experimental evidence suggests this is a possible pathogenesis as IgA can activate complement via the alternative pathway or classic pathway, as can IgA, IgG or IgM cryoglobulin. From the high prevalence of glomerular properdin and IgA in patients with Henoch–Schoenlein nephritis and indirectly, from the occurrence of Henoch–Schoenlein purpura in patients with C2 deficiency (Gelfand *et al.*, 1975), it is postulated that the alternative pathway of complement is more likely to be the *in vivo* mechanism. C2 deficiency in Henoch–Schoenlein purpura would, however, appear to be rare.

Investigations

The initial investigations may show a normal ESR even in the presence of an increased level of IgA. The haemoglobin, white count and platelets are also normal and occult blood may be present in the stools. The presence of red cells in the urine and proteinuria will occur in 50 per cent of patients.

Therapy

The patient should be managed by rest in bed and given supportive care. Corticosteroids can be used but there has been no controlled trial; they do not appear to have any effect on the skin lesions, the duration of the illness or the development of renal complications. They may, however, be helpful in reducing localised soft tissue swelling within 24–48 hours and sometimes appear to give relief of colicky abdominal pain.

The prognosis of the renal lesion is variable. At one time it was thought to be linked with the time of onset, developing during the illness, and the degree of haematuria and proteinuria, but this is not longer entirely tenable (Counahan *et al.*, 1977). A clinical presentation with a combination of acute nephritis and nephrotic syndrome and a high proportion of crescents in renal biopsy is associated with a poor prognosis. The best management of the serious renal lesion of Henoch–Schoenlein purpura is still not certain. It is generally agreed that even high dose corticosteroids have little to offer and an MRC controlled trial (1971) showed that in the chronic renal disease, azathioprine and prednisone had no effect. Uncontrolled observations on the use of cytotoxic drugs in proliferative glomerulonephritis have suggested that some benefit may be derived from early therapy. It would therefore seem reasonable that in those patients who have the nephrotic syndrome, nitrogen retention, heavy proteinuria or hypertension, biopsy should be performed early and if they fall into the category known to have bad prognosis, the combination of cytotoxic therapy with a high dosage corticosteroid and possibly also anticoagulants needs to be considered.

RARER FORMS OF ARTERITIS

Wegener's granulomatosis

Wegener's granulomatosis is a very rare condition characterised by destructive granulomatous lesions of the upper and lower respiratory tract, glomerulonephritis and disseminated small vessel vasculitis. The relationship of this syndrome both to other forms of vasculitis such as polyarteritis nodosa and to purely granulomatous disorders is not clear. It is excessively rare in childhood. Absolute diagnosis is based on biopsy. It requires intensive treatment with cytotoxic therapy and corticosteroids (Baliga *et al.*, 1978).

Takayasu's arteritis

Since its first description by Takayasu 70 years ago, this rare condition has been described under a number of names, with the term 'pulseless disease' suggested by Shimizuk and Sano (1951) being the one most generally accepted nowadays. Pathologically it is a panarteritis of unknown causation involving the aorta and its branches, which leads to thrombosis, areas of stenosis and aneurysm formation (*Figure 6.29*). These may ultimately rupture.

It affects girls predominantly, tending to occur from the age of nine or ten years. Its presenting features include fever, myalgia, arthralgia, fatigue, deterioration in general health, pleurisy with effusion abdominal pain. At times, intermittent claudication mimics involvement of muscles. On examination, the outstanding feature is lack of pulsation in major vessels, tenderness of arterial trunks and the presence of bruits particularly in carotids and sometimes femorals. The ESR is raised, as is the IgG, but other findings such as low haemoglobin and leucocytosis are non-specific (Warshaw and Spach, 1965).

It may be confused with rheumatic fever, systemic juvenile chronic arthritis and myositis. A rise in blood pressure when renal vessels are involved may also suggest polyarteritis nodosa.

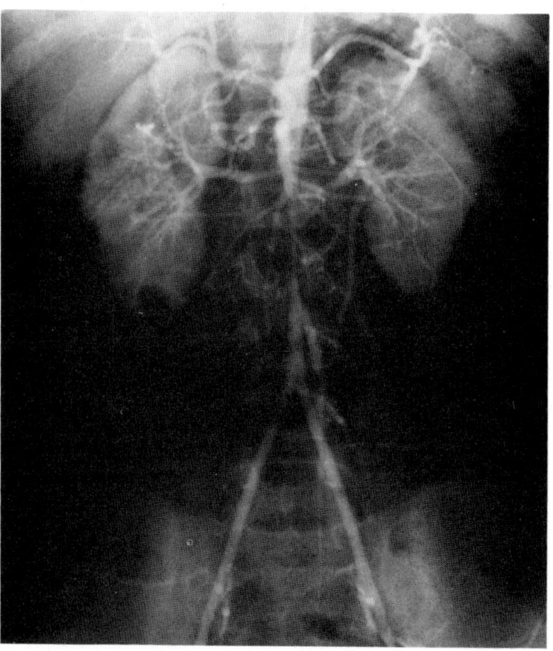

Figure 6.29. Takayasu's arteritis. X-ray showing extensive involvement of the abdominal aorta in a girl who presented with pain in the legs. (By courtesy of Dr R. Wilkins)

Immunosuppressive drugs may be valuable as can be steroids. Anticoagulants seem to have little effect. Very occasionally surgery may be required for established vascular stenoses. The prognosis is not good as even if healing occurs, there is the problem of growth in children with narrowed fibrosed arteries.

Giant cell arteritis

McEnery (1977) described a child who presented with joint pains for several months after an intercurrent infection which was followed by an abacterial meningitis, then fever, a palpable spleen, chronic iridocyclitis and pains in the calves, i.e. mimicking systemic juvenile chronic arthritis. It was not until occlusion of the left femoral artery, which led to amputation of the leg, that a diagnosis of giant cell arteritis was made. This would appear to be the first juvenile case of giant cell arteritis on record. The course has been difficult with involvement of an arm and the other leg necessitating lumbar sympathectomy despite corticosteroids and cytotoxic therapy.

Goodpasture's syndrome

This serious condition, characterised by haemoptysis, anaemia and nephritis, appears to have some overlap with polyarteritis. It can occur in late childhood but is rare (Trygstad, 1976).

REFERENCES

Ahlström, H., Linström, N. P., Tortensson, W., Östberg, G. and Lantorp, K. (1977). Infantile periarteritis nodosa or mucocutaneous lymph node syndrome. *Acta Paediatrica Scandinavia*, **66**, 193

Ansell, B. M. (1978). Dermatomyositis and polymyositis. *Copeman's Textbook of the Rheumatic Diseases*. London; Churchill Livingstone

Ansell, B. M., Nasseh, G. A. and Bywaters, E. G. L. (1976). Scleroderma in childhood. *Annals of the Rheumatic Diseases*, **35**, 189

Baliga, R., Chung-Ho, C., Bidani, A. K., Perrin, E. V. D. and Fleischmann, L. E. (1978). A case of generalised Wegener's granulomatosis in childhood: successful therapy with cyclophosphamide. *Pediatrics*, **61**, 286

Banker, B. Q. (1975). Dermatomyositis of childhood; ultrastructural alterations of muscle and intramuscular blood vessels. *Journal of Neuropathology and Experimental Neurology*, **34**, 46

Bernstein, B., Koster-King, K., Singsen, B., Kornreich, H. K. and Hanson, V. (1977). Sjögrens syndrome in childhood. *Arthritis and Rheumatism*, **20**, (2), 361

Bresnihan, B. and Jason, H. E. (1977). Suppressor function of peripheral blood mononuclear cells in normal individuals and inpatients with systemic lupus erythematosis. *Journal of Clinical Investigation*, **59**, 106

Cassidy, J. T., Sullivan, D. B., Dabich, L. and Petty, R. E. (1977). Scleroderma in children. *Arthritis and Rheumatism*, **20**, (2), 361

Counahan, R., Winterborn, M. H., White, R. H. R., Heaton, J. M., Meadow, S. R., Bluett, N. H., Swetschin, H., Cameron, J. S. and Chantler, CC. (1977). Prognosis of Henoch–Schönlein nephritis in children. *British Medical Journal*, **2**, 11–14

Decker, J. J. (1975). Cytotoxic agents in the management of systemic lupus erythematosus. *Clinics in Rheumatic Diseases*, **1**, 665

Dubovitz, V. (1976). Treatment of dermatomyositis in childhood. *Archives of Diseases in Childhood*, **51**, 494

Dubovitz, V. (1978). Muscle disorders in childhood. *Major Problems in Clinical Paediatrics*. **16**, Philadelphia; W. B. Saunders

Emery, H. and Schaller, J. C. (1977). Raynaud's phenomenon in childhood. *Arthritis and Rheumatism*, **20**, (2), 363

Fish, A. J., Blau, E. B., Westberg, N. G., Burke, B. A., Vernier, R. L. and Michael, A. F. (1977). Systemic lupus erythematosus within the first two decades of life. *American Journal of Medicine*, **62**, 99

Fruman, L. S., Sullivan, D. B. and Petty, R. E. (1976). Retinopathy in juvenile dermatomyositis. *Journal of Pediatrics*, **88**, 267

Garcia-Fuentes, M., Chantler, C. and Williams, D. G. (1977). Cryoglobulinaemia in Henoch–Schoenlein purpura. *British Medical Journal*, **2**, 163

Garcia-Fuentes, M., Martin, A., Chantler, C. and Williams, D. G. (1978). Serum complement components in Henoch–Schoenlein purpura. *Archives of Diseases of Childhood*, **53**, 417

Gelfand, E. W., Clarkson, J. E. and Mista, J. O. (1975). Selective deficiency of the second component of complement in a patient with anaphylactoid purpura. *Clinical Immunology and Immunopathology,* **4,** 269

Gotoff, S. P., Smith, R. D. and Sugar, O. (1972). Dermatomyositis with cerebral vasculitis in a patient with agammaglobulinaemia. *American Journal of Diseases of Children*, **123**, 53

Grgic, A., Rosenbloom, A. L., Weber, F. T., Giordano, B., Malone, J. I. and Shuster, J. J. (1976). Joint contracture – a common manifestation of childhood diabetes mellitus. *Journal of Pediatrics*, **88**, 584

Hanson, V., Drexler, E. and Kornreich, H. (1974). Rheumatoid factor (anti-gammaglobulins) in children with focal scleroderma. *Pediatrics*, **53**, 945

Hanson, V. and Kornreich, H. (1967). Systemic rheumatic disorders ('collagen disease') in childhood: lupus erythematosus, anaphylactoid purpura, dermato-cyositis, and scleroderma I. *Bulletin of Rheumatic Disease*, **17**, 435

Hicks, R. M. (1977). Mucocutaneous lymph node syndrome in Hawaii. *Arthritis and Rheumatism*, **20**, (2), 389

Jacobs, J. C. (1977). Methotrexate and azathioprin in the treatment of childhood dermatomyositis. *Pediatrics*, **59**, 212

Kato, H. (1977). *Vascular Lesions of Collagen Diseases and Related Conditions*. Tokyo; University of Tokyo Press

Kato, H., Koike, S. and Yokoyama, T. (1979). Kawasaki disease: effect of treatment on coronary artery involvement. *Pediatrics*, **63**, 175

Kawasaki, T., Kosaki, F., Okawa, S., Shigematusi, I. and Yanagawa, H. (1974). A new infantile acute febrile mucocutaneous lymph node syndrome (MLNS) prevailing in Japan. *Pediatrics*, **54**, 271

Kornreich, H. (1976). Systemic lupus erythematosus in childhood. *Clinics in Rehumatic Diseases*, **2**, 429

Kornreich, H. K., Koster-King, H., Bernstein, B. H., Singsen, B. H. and Hanson, V. (1977). Scleroderma in childhood. *Arthritis and Rheumatism*, **20**, (2), 343

Koster-King, K., Kornreich, H. K., Bernstein, B. H., Singsen, B. H. and Hanson, V. (1977). The clinical spectrum of systemic lupus erythematosus in childhood. *Arthritis and Rheumatism*, **26**, (2), 287

Kukla, L. F., Reddy, C., Silkalns, G. and Prasad, M. (1978). Systemic lupus erythematosus presenting as chorea. *Archives of Disease of Childhood*, **53**, 345

Lasser, A. E., Schultz, B. C., Beaff, D., Bielinski, S. and Kirschenbaum, B. (1978). Phenylketonuria and scleroderma. *Archives of Dermatology*, **114**, 1215

Levinsky, R. J., Cameron, J. S. and Soothill, J. F. (1977). Serum immune complexes and disease activity in lupus nephritis. *Lancet*, **1**, 564

Lyen, K. R. and Brook, C. G. D. (1978). Mucocutaneous lymph node syndrome in two siblings. *British Medical Journal*, **1**, 1187

McEnery, G. (1977). Giant cell arteritis with gangrene in a child. *Archives of Disease in Childhood*, **52**, 733

McNicholl, B. and Flynn, J. (1978). Acquired toxoplasmosis in children. *Archives of Disease in Childhood*, **53**, 414

Medical Research Council Working Party (1971). Controlled trial of azathioprine and prednisone in chronic renal disease. *British Medical Journal*, **2**, 239

Meislin, A. G. and Rothfield, N. F. (1968). Systemic lupus erythematosus in childhood; analysis of 42 cases with comparative data on 200 adult cases followed concurrently. *Pediatrics*, **42**, 37

Miller, J. J. (1977). Drug-induced lupus-like syndromes in childhood. *Arthritis and Rheumatism*, **20**, (2), 308

Miller, J. J. and Koehler, J. P. (1977). Persistence of activity in dermatomyositis of childhood. *Arthritis and Rheumatism*, **20**, (2), 332

Moynihan, E. J. (1977). Penicillamine and disorders affecting dermal collagen. *Proceedings of the Royal Society of Medicine*, **70**, (3), 73

Nakamoto, Y., Asano, Y., Dohi, K., Fujioka, M., Iida, H., Kida, H., Kibe, Y., Hattori, N. and Takeuchi, J. (1978). Primary IgA glomerulo-nephritis and Schönlein–Henoch purpura nephritis; clinicopathological and immunohistological characteristics. *Quarterly Journal of Medicine*, **47**, 495

Park, S. and Nyhan, W. L. (1975). Fatal pulmonary involvement in dermatomyositis. *American Journal of Diseases of Children*, **129**, 723

Peskett, S. A., Ansell, B. M., Fiszman, P. and Howard, A. (1978). Mixed connective tissue disease in children. *Rheumatology and Rehabilitation*, **17**, 245

Reimold, E. W., Weinberg, A. G., Fink, C. W. and Battles, N. D. (1976). Polyarteritis in children. *American Journal of Diseases of Children*, **130**, 534

Roberts, F. B. and Fetterman, G. H. (1963). Polyarteritis nodosa in infancy. *Journal of Pediatrics*, **63**, 519

Rosenthal, M. (1978). A critical review of the effect of levamisole on rheumatic diseases other than rheumatoid arthritis. *Journal of Rheumatology*, **5**, (4), 97

Schaller, J. G., Gilliland, B. G., Ochs, H. D., Leddy, J. P., Agodoa, L. C. Y. and Rosenfeld, S. I. (1977). Severe systemic lupus erythematosus with nephritis in a boy with deficiency of the fourth component of complement. *Arthritis and Rheumatism*, **20**, 1519

Schur, P. H. (1975). Complement in lupus. *Clinics in Rheumatic Diseases*, **1**, 519

Sewell, J., Liyanage, B. and Ansell, B. M. (1978). Calcinosis in juvenile dermatomyositis. *Skeletal Radiology*, **3**, 137

Sharp, G., Irvin, W., Holman, H. and Tan, E. (1969). A distinct rheumatic disease syndrome associated with antibody to a particular nuclear antigen and unusual responsiveness to corticosteroid therapy. *Clinical Research*, **17**, 359

Shimizu, K. and Sano, K. (1951). Pulseless disease. *Journal of Neuropathology and Clinical Neurology*, **1**, 37

Shulman, L. E. (1974). Diffuse fasciitis with hypergammaglobulinaemia and eosinophilia; a new syndrome. *Journal of Rheumatology*, **1**, (1)

Singsen, B. H., Kornreich, H. K., Koster-King, K., Brink, S. J., Bernstein, B. H., Hanson, V. and Tan, E. M. (1977). Mixed connective tissue disease in children. *Arthritis and Rheumatism*, **20**, (2), 355

Sloan, M. F., Franks, A. J. Exley, K. A. and Davison, A. M. (1978). Acute renal failure due to polymyositis. *British Medical Journal*, **1**, 1457

Taborne, J., Bole, G. G. and Thompson, G. R. (1978). Colchicine suppression of local and systemic inflammation due to calcinosis universalis in chronic dermatomyositis. *Annals of Internal Medicine*, **89**, 648

Trygstad, C. W. (1976). *Clinical Pediatric Nephrology*, Ch. 10, p. 187. Edited by Lieberman, E. Philadelphia; J. B. Lippincott & Co.

Warshaw, J. B. and Spach, M. S. (1965). Takayasu's disease (primary aortitis) in childhood; case report with review of literature. *Pediatrics*, **35**, 620

Webster, A. D. B., Tripp, J. H., Hayward, A. R., Dayan, A. D., Doshi, R., Macintyre, E. H. and Tyrrell, D. A. J. (1978). Echovirus encephalitis and myositis in primary immunoglobulin deficiency. *Archives of Disease of Childhood*, **53**, 33

Whaley, K., Hughes, G. R. V. and Webb, J. (1976). Systemic lupus erythematosus in man and animals. In *Recent Advances in Rheumatology*. Edited by Buchanan, W. W. and Dick, W. C. Edinburgh; Churchill Livingstone

CHAPTER 7

Musculoskeletal Aspects of Blood Dyscrasias

The musculoskeletal system may be the presenting site in a number of haematological disorders. The mechanisms involved include bone infarction (as in the haemoglobinopathies), bleeding into joints (as in haemophilia) and over-production of cells within the marrow (as in leukaemia). Not infrequently, bones are involved early in malignant disease and symptoms can precede radiological manifestations.

THE HAEMOGLOBINOPATHIES

The abnormal haemoglobins may exert no obvious clinical effect, especially when present in the heterozygous state, but in the homozygous state they may cause severe clinical disorders. Musculoskeletal symptoms result from bone trabecular changes associated with the expansion of the bone marrow, and from bone infarction which, in children, can cause alterations of growth and infection. The most common and best documented haemoglobinopathy affecting bone is that of sickle cell disease.

Sickle cell disease

Haemoglobin S is inherited as a mendelian dominant; as the sickle cell trait it is fairly common among Negroes, the homozygous state is by no means rare. In Britain the disorder is seen predominantly in West Indians. Hyperplasia of the bone marrow causes the 'hair on end' appearance in the skull x-ray together with cortical thinning of bones particularly noticeable in the pelvis and ribs but at times affecting long bones. Thrombosis of small vessels causes infarction in bone. It is also considered to be the cause of bone pain in a sickle cell crisis. Patients with sickle cell disease are particularly susceptible to bacterial infection, so that osteomyelitis and septic arthritis are seen much more frequently than in patients with normal haemoglobin. While many organisms have been incriminated, the most common is *Salmonella*, particularly in the joints and somewhat less so in bones. The reduction in complement mediated serum opsonising activity for *Salmonella* may be responsible for this predisposition (Hand and King, 1978). Multiple sites can be involved; at such times it may be difficult to distinguish between a crisis and an infection, while at times both can occur together. If in doubt it is better to investigate and treat for infection as otherwise further severe destruction of bone can occur. In general, septic arthritis is much less frequent than osteomyelitis.

Clinical features

Any child with Negro ancestry who presents with pain localised to bones or joints should be investigated for the presence of sickle cell disease. Symptoms can arise from any of the previously described mechanisms (Schumacher, 1975).

Sickle cell crisis

During a sickle cell crisis the young patient can experience severe pain around the joints and along the shafts of the bones; the joints themselves may be swollen, hot and tender with occasionally an effusion. The severity of the anaemia may give rise to a cardiac murmur. The patient is often ill with a high fever and a leucocytosis. In such circumstances, and unless this condition is thought of, the patient may be mistakenly diagnosed as having rheumatic fever or systemic juvenile chronic arthritis. Diagnosis is suspected by identification of sickle cells *in vitro*, by the use of a reducing agent, and established by starch or cellulose acetate haemoglobin electrophoresis.

Hand/foot syndrome

This is seen in children aged from six months to two years and may be the first manifestation of sickle cell disease. There is a general, diffuse, symmetrical, extremely tender warm swelling of hands or feet or both. As fever and a peripheral leucocytosis up to about 50 000 are usual, the condition can mimic systemic juvenile arthritis. However, the swelling tends to last only one to three weeks, subsiding without residua. Initially the bone x-rays are normal but towards the end of the first week densities may be visualised within the marrow and elevation of the periosteum. Rarefaction of the medulla can occur (*Figure 7.1*). By between one

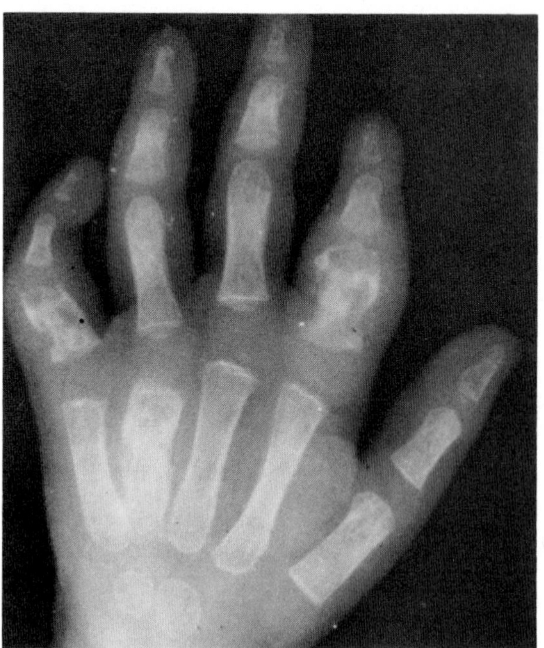

Figure 7.1. Sickle cell disease. Multiple episodes of infarction are present in the small bones of the hand; note the varying age of the lesions. (By courtesy of Dr P. Renton)

and four months the radiological changes have usually regressed. It is considered that infarction of the marrow, or possibly of the cortical bone and periosteum, is the most likely underlying mechanism. Repeated episodes can lead to permanent radiological changes.

Bone infarction

This results from sickling and thrombosis in small blood vessels. When this affects the epiphyseal plate it gives rise to failure of bone growth and subsequent localised deformity. This is common in the hand. The hip is a frequent site of avascular necrosis as the

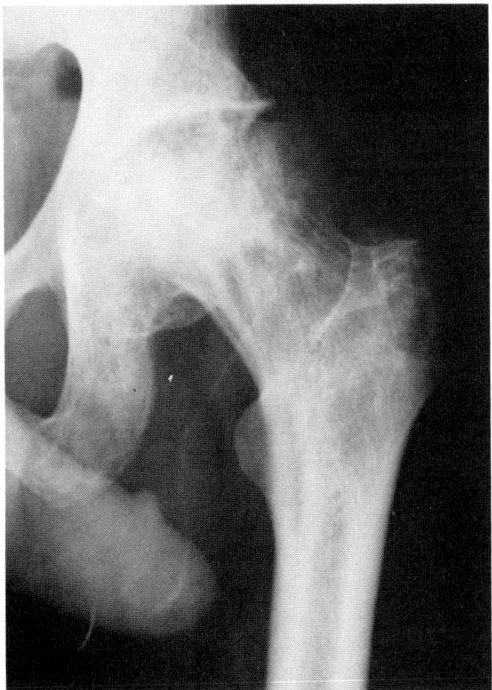

Figure 7.2. Sickle cell disease. Femoral head avascular necrosis with collapse in a teenager; note the change in the femoral neck and evidence of infarction in the epiphysis of the greater trochanter and femoral shaft. (By courtesy of Dr P. Renton)

circulation of the femoral head is particularly vulnerable. There may be severe pain, but symptoms can be trivial so that the patient merely presents with a limp. The radiological appearances, which initially resemble Perthes' disease, may be unilateral or bilateral and the necrosis can be segmental or complete (Chung and Raltsin, 1969). The outcome depends on the age of onset and the amount of femoral head involved (Lloyd-Roberts, 1978). Thus, segmental necrosis in the young child is more likely to end with a reasonably sized and shaped femoral head than in an older child

(*Figure 7.2*). Other sites of aseptic necrosis include the humeral head and tibial condyles.

It should be remembered that low oxygen tension, e.g. anaesthetic administered without due precaution, is important in the pathogenesis of bone infarction.

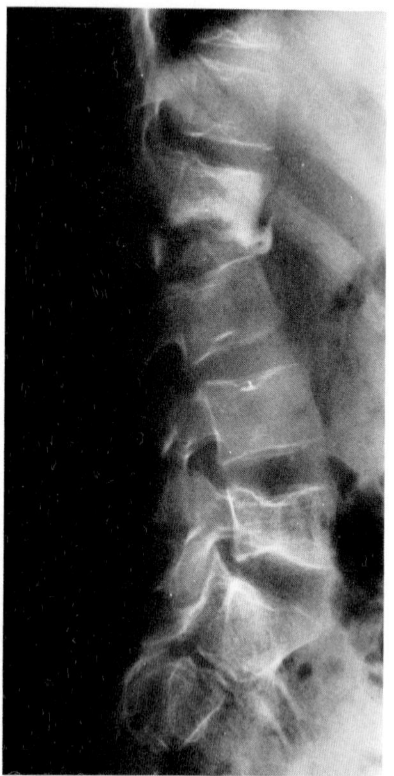

Figure 7.3. Sickle cell disease. To show typical changes in several vertebrae with coarsening of the trabeculae and the central cup-like indentation; in addition osteomyelitis (Salmonella typhimurium) has caused collapse of L1 and 2

Vertebral changes

The vertebral bodies show distinctive radiological changes, with coarsened trabeculae, most often vertical, and a characteristic central cup-like indentation. This rarely gives rise to symptoms unless there is superimposed infection (*Figure 7.3*).

Joint effusions

These are most commonly seen in the knees but can occur at other sites. Usually only one or two joints are involved and the swelling subsides in a few days. Effusions may be associated with pain, warmth and tenderness; this last may extend into the bone. This is helpful in the differential diagnosis of the cause of the effusion in such a patient.

The persistence of symptoms should make one suspect infection.

Thalassaemia

In thalassaemia haemoglobin A is not produced in adequate amounts so that fetal haemoglobin persists; this is associated with abnormally shaped cells which have a reduced survival. It is particularly common in people of Mediterranean extraction. Many types of thalassaemia exist, depending on which polypeptide chain, alpha or beta, is depressed.

For practical purposes it is beta thalassaemia major (where there are no beta chains) that gives rise to the skeletal problems. It is usually recognised early in life because of anaemia, splenomegaly and hepatomegaly. Marrow hyperplasia occurs and this gives rise to the characteristic cranial radiological features of wide separation of the skull sutures, thinning of both tabes (*Figure 7.4a*) and with thin spicules of periosteal bone causing the classic 'hair on end' appearance. The face is said to be 'mongoloid' as a result of thickening of the bones of the cranium with apparent sinking of the nose. This can occur in any type of haemolytic anaemia where there is a marked increase in red cell production in the bone marrow, as can the orthodontic problems due to deformities of the maxillae. Generalised cortical thinning of bones can affect hands (*Figure 7.4b*), feet and long bones (*Figure 7.4c*). This can lead to pathological fractures.

Clinically, episodes of joint pain, swelling and stiffness lasting for short periods and interfering with normal exercise are not uncommon. A few patients have severe symptoms, particularly in the lower limbs, with swelling and tenderness around the ankles. Radiologically there is osteoporosis, widening of the medullary spaces, thin cortices with trabeculation, and evidence of microfractures (Gratwick *et al.*, 1978).

Beta thalassaemia minor is perhaps the most widespread haemoglobinopathy but causes little disability, and skeletal changes, if present, are of a mild type.

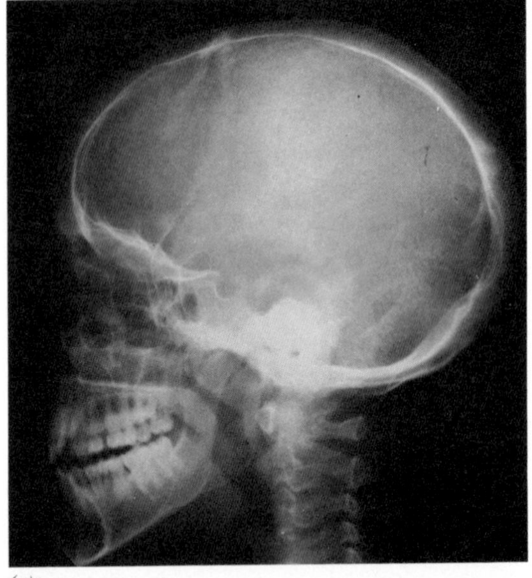

(a)

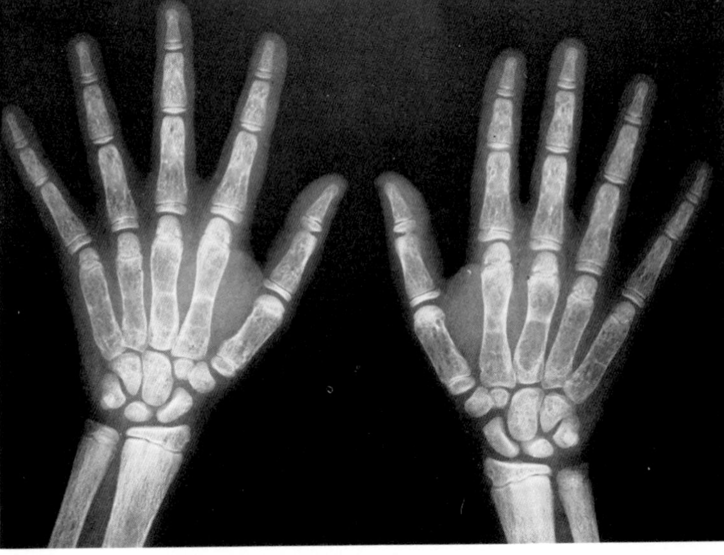

(b)

Figure 7.4 (By courtesy of Dr B. Liyanage.) Thalassaemia. (a) The skull shows very marked separation of the sutures and a thinning of both tables. (b) Generalised thinning of the bones in the hands, but no localised areas of infarction

(c)
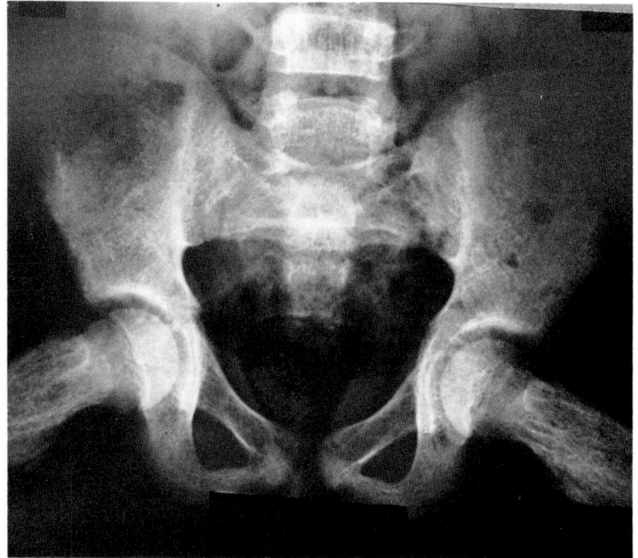

Figure 7.4(c). Thinning of the femora

HAEMOSTATIC DISORDERS

The *hereditary disorders* of haemostasis can give rise to major involvement of the musculoskeletal system. *Haemophilia*, Factor VIII deficiency, affects males but is transmitted by females; in some 30 per cent there is, however, no positive family history. *Christmas disease*, or Factor IX deficiency, is clinically indistinguishable from haemophilia and also affects males, is sex-linked and is recessive in its inheritance. In contrast to these two disorders is *Von Willebrand's disease*, which is characterised by prolongation of the skin bleeding time and reduced Factor VIII level in the blood probably due to a primary defect in Factor VIII related protein. It affects both sexes equally, is inherited as an autosomal dominant, and does not usually cause bleeding into joints; very occasionally haemarthroses, particularly of the knees, occur but usually in association with injury.

As the manifestations of Factor VIII and Factor IX deficiency do not differ, they will be considered together. The severity of the bleeding varies with the level of the Factor present in the blood. This tends to remain fairly constant in a given family. Therefore, if a child has a grandfather with severe deficiency, he is likely to be severely affected. In haemophilia, when there is less than 1 per cent of Factor VIII, spontaneous haemarthroses and intramuscular haemorrhages with consequent contractures are common. When the level is 1–5 per cent there may be occasional spontaneous bleeding and haemarthroses. If the level is between 5–20 per cent bleeding is only likely after injury or surgery.

In severe haemophilia (less than 1 per cent Factor VIII), when the child starts to crawl, excessive bruising, particularly of the head and buttocks, which are prone to injury at this stage, is noticed; then as he starts to walk haemarthroses occur. Eighty per cent of severe haemophiliacs have haemorrhages into their joints; in such patients there is often no history of preceding trauma. The joints most commonly affected are knee, ankle and elbow although the reason for this is not certain; of course, other joints can be affected. It has been suggested that the bleeding tends to occur in cycles and some people have even suggested a seasonal incidence, but this has not been substantiated (Duthie and Rizza, 1975).

The origin and nature of *spontaneous joint haemorrhage* is unknown. In the majority of cases it appears that the bleeding is intracapsular. Haemorrhage both into the extracapsular tissues and into the joint cavity occurs, as a rule, only with direct trauma. Within a few hours of the haemorrhage a cellular reaction, with exudate, polymorphonuclear leucocytosis and increase in the synovial lining cell population takes place. In a few days hyperplasia of the synovial cells occurs and the inflammatory cells presenting in the synovial membrane now include lymphocytes and histiocytes as well as polymorphonuclear cells; haemosiderin pigment is soon present. After repeated bleeding into a joint there is a generalised hypertrophy and hypervascularity of the synovium.

Acute haemarthrosis

Many patients comment on warmth or ‘pricking’ in the joint before overt signs and all subjects should be forewarned. Intelligent parents will get used to acting on these premonitory symptoms and seek immediate advice. The most disabling complaint in acute haemarthrosis is pain, which is due either to the local irritant effect of blood, or to acute joint distension. Patients who have had a number of bleedings into a joint may develop fibrosis, so that even a small haemarthrosis can cause severe pain.

Distension of the joint is usually the first visible sign. This is easy to detect in the knee where it usually occurs anteriorly, in the ankle below the malleoli and posterolaterally in the elbow. In the shoulder it tends to occur anteriorly. In the hip distension is difficult to palpate; the differentiation between an iliacus haematoma and a bleed into the hip joint is particularly difficult: a femoral nerve palsy suggests iliacus haematoma. An haemarthrosis is usually apparent on x-ray as joint distension.

The joint affected is held in an attitude of flexion. Examination should be very carefully undertaken, noting with the eye the extent of the joint swelling. The knee can easily be measured with a tape measure and compared with the other side. Acute haemarthroses are always tender and often feel warm. The range of movement should not be tested at the initial examination, indeed, the examination must be very gentle in suspected haemarthrosis. Unless there have been previous bleeds an x-ray will merely demonstrate the degree of joint distension.

Deciding that acute swelling is due to a haemarthrosis is easy in a known haemophiliac but, if this is not known, infection may be suspected because haemarthroses can be accompanied by fever. Points in favour of a haemarthrosis are the well-being of the patients and the rapidity of onset, as well, of course, as the rapid response to treatment.

Treatment

Because of the potentially crippling effect of bleeding into joints, urgent management is required. The aim of treatment is to stop the bleeding, relieve pain, maintain and restore joint function and prevent chronic joint damage. The joint is best immobilised by a light splint. Clotting factor should be replaced immediately.

One aims to raise the patient's Factor VIII level to between 5–15 per cent of normal for several hours. In calculating the dose of therapeutic material required to maintain the patient's Factor VIII about the desired level it is important to remember that the half-life of transfused Factor VIII in the circulation of the haemophiliac is approximately 12 hours. Early 'on demand' treatment for joint and muscle haemorrhage is now accepted. In many centres the relatives of known cases are being trained to give the transfusions of anti-haemophiliac factor in their own home (Biggs, 1978). An indication that the bleeding has stopped is the relief of pain and relaxation of muscle guarding.

If the spontaneous haemorrhage into joints and muscles is treated soon after the onset of the bleeding, the response is usually good. A large, tense, acute haemarthrosis which does not settle rapidly after institution of clotting factor replacement may occasionally need to be treated additionally by aspiration. Once the pain and spasm go, non-weight bearing exercises to remobilise the joint may begin. For the knee it is particularly important that the quadriceps are in good condition before full mobility is allowed, otherwise walking can further damage the joint and cause a fresh haemarthrosis. If necessary, particularly for the knee and ankle, some type of support may be required, i.e. brace or cosmetic caliper. If treatment is not undertaken early, subsequent major orthopaedic problems may develop.

Sub-acute arthropathy

Following one or more bleeding episode the involved joint can remain tense, swollen and painful and, on palpation, has a doughy, semi-solid consistency. This usually means that the haemarthrosis has clotted. The condition can arise in several ways: firstly, the patient has not reported early for treatment; secondly, the joint haemorrhage has been inadequately treated, either because of insufficient dosage or duration of Factor replacement; thirdly, failure to recognise and treat a recurrence of the haemarthrosis; or fourthly, antibodies to Factor VIII have developed.

Conservative management of the joint will depend on immobilisation in a plaster splint with periodic examination and measurement over a few weeks to obtain a slow resolution of the joint swelling. Unfortunately, organisation of the clot can produce intra-articular adhesions and permanent joint stiffness. Should antibody to Factor VIII be present in the blood there is really no alternative to such management, but, if this is not present, aspiration under appropriate cover or even arthrotomy to clean out the joint may need to be considered. If adequate movement is to return, mobilisation of the joint should be achieved within two weeks of surgery; remobilisation of the patient with lower joint problems usually requires a brace or support for weight-bearing initially.

Chronic haemophilic arthropathy

After several acute apisodes of bleeding the joint does not return to its normal configuration and so there tend to be recurrent bleedings. The synovium will appear thickened and there may be a small effusion. After several months in the above state radiological

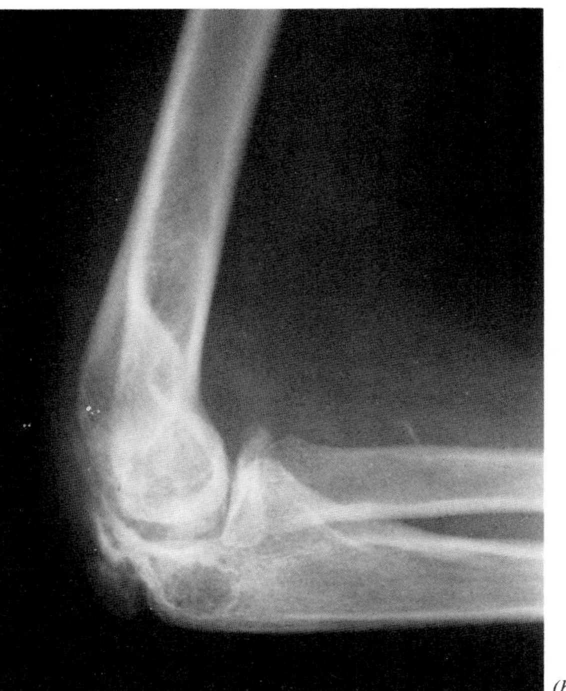

(a) 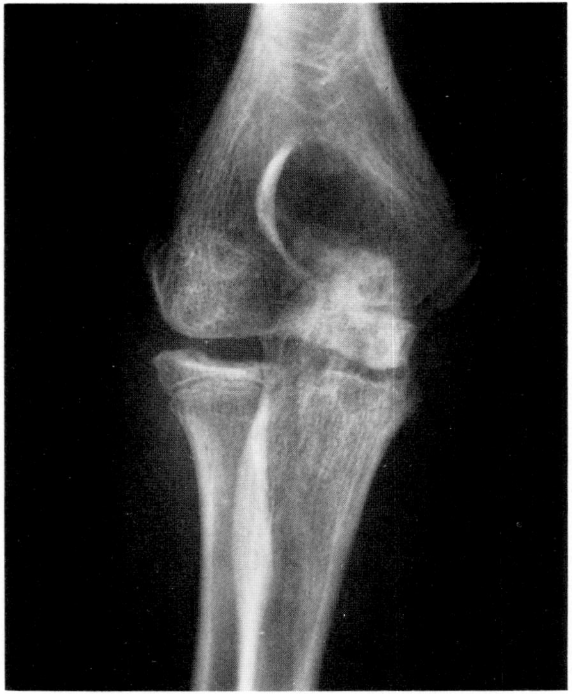 (b)

Figure 7.5(a). Haemophilia. Posterior-anterior view of elbows shows some relatively minor changes in the radial head with slight overgrowth but joint space doubtfully affected. (b) The lateral view confirms alteration in the growth of the radial head, but also marked cystic formation in the ulna with joint space narrowing and some loss of cartilage

abnormalities occur including overgrowth, particularly of the femoral epiphysis, patella and radial head (*Figure 7.5a* and *b*). While this is usually seen in known haemophiliacs who have had overt recurrent bleeding, occasionally a child with a persistent monarticular arthritis that commenced with trauma and then recurred after numerous minimal traumatic episodes is found to have typical radiological changes and somewhat reduced levels of Factor VIII. Initially the condition is one of recurrent effusions often punctuated by occasional bleeding; eventually fibrosis supervenes with a tendency to contracture at knees and elbows.

Exactly how the bleeding causes the chronic joint change is not certain (Arnold and Hilgartner, 1977). Certainly the persistence of blood in the joint space maintains a cellular reaction of the synovium, with an increase in number of synovium lining cells and of macrophages and lymphocytes probably due to the presence of haemosiderin pigment. This leads to a thickening of the synovial membrane and the formation of many thickened villae. The synovial fluid and synovial tissue have increased acid phosphatase levels similar to those seen in rheumatoid arthritis. Cathepsin D and acid phosphatase are also increased in the synovial fluid. After some time the phagocytic reaction is partially replaced by fibroblastic activity; in addition there are often patchy areas of necrosis of the synovium, probably the result of mechanical trapping of the nodular projections and this in itself may be the cause of recurrent haemorrhages. In addition, fragments of cartilage and necrotic bone may sometimes be found lying within the hyperplastic synovia or immediately beneath it, probably due to the disintegration of cartilagenous and bony tissues as a result of a chronic haemarthrosis. Eventually the joint surface cartilage may be covered partially or wholly by fibrous tissue in which there are deposits of haemosiderin and a variable number of inflammatory cells of chronic type. Underneath the cartilage is irregularly pitted and the cartilage cells may undergo necrosis and autolysis. Prolapse of the cartilage into the sub-chondral bone, shearing away from the bone and necrosis eventually occur. Haemosiderin pigment is often present in the fibrous tissue covering the articular cartilage but is not usually found within the articular cartilage itself.

Radiological changes

Initially in acute haemorrhage distension of the joint cavity is the only abnormality seen on the x-ray. Subsequently there is loss of cartilage space, sub-chondral collapse, cystic changes (*Figure 7.5*) and osteophyte formation. Avascular necrosis with loss of the weight-bearing segment is seen most commonly in the femoral head but can also occur in the humeral head. The radiological changes in the knee have been well reviewed by Gilbert and Cockrin (1972). Repeated bleeding is associated with squaring of the patella particularly the inferior pole; ultimately there is narrowing of the joint space and loss of congruity of the patello–femoral compartment. In the tibio–femoral joint condylar squaring, tibial plateau depression, narrowing of the cartilage space and joint incongruity occur. These changes tend to be more marked in the medial than in the lateral compartment, where there is often overgrowth of the medial femoral condyle. Osteoporosis, which is more marked in the epiphysis and the shaft, causes resorption of the trabeculae giving an open lattice-work pattern, while after repeated bleeding Harris lines are seen in large numbers. Epiphyseal over-growth is common particularly at elbow and knee. Ultimately cartilage destruction with irregular cyst formation at the joint surface occurs (*Figure 7.5b*).

Clinical aspects

The most common feature is loss of movement and this can occur long before gross deformity. In the knee it is initially extension, as it is in the elbow; restriction of ankle movement is less marked than at the knee and elbow. Ultimately particularly at the knee valgus and rotational deformities are frequent. Loss of function is the chief complaint; pain is felt early and is usually due to further bleeding; later this may also result from cartilage damage.

Management

In the management of chronic haemophilic arthropathy the most important requirement is prevention of residual joint deformity, and this is best achieved by the early treatment of acute bleeding with Factor VIII replacement. Aspirin in any form is best avoided as an analgesic but ibuprofen has proved satisfactory. The most important aspect of the physiotherapeutic management is the maintenance of good muscle power. The use of calipers or plastic splints to protect knees and ankles subject to recurrent haemarthrosis is often helpful and they are particularly useful in supporting lower limbs when there is already some arthropathy present; but a balance needs to be achieved between the degree of external bracing and the maintenance of adequate muscle function. Correction of fixed deformities is usually best achieved by wedging plasters, and the redevelopment of muscles to control the joint. Once muscle function is improving hydrotherapy is of enormous benefit. The maintenance of good muscles by regular swimming should be encouraged.

Provided adequate levels of anti-haemophilic globulin can be produced in the blood, when pain and disability are interfering with the patient's life, it may be necessary to consider soft tissue release, joint stabilisation or even, arthroplasty (Arnold and Hilgartner, 1977).

Muscle bleeding

Bleeding into the muscle, although much less common than bleeding into joints, is probably even more serious because of pressure on nerves and blood vessels. In the upper limbs it is usually manifest in the anterior flexor musculature, while in the lower limbs it tends to be in the iliacus and triceps surie. It rarely recurs except in the iliacus; this is because the healing of the muscle haematoma by fibrous tissue usually obliterates the bleeding site. The cause is usually trauma – this includes intramuscular injections! Bleeding into the muscle produces necrosis of the muscle fibres around the haematoma; very occasionally a large encysted haematoma occurs which causes progressive necrosis or atrophy.

Pain produced by bleeding into muscle is less acute than that produced by bleeding into joints, often taking two to three days before it becomes severe. The swelling is hard and tense; there is protective spasm and a contracture can develop. Peripheral nerve pressure, particularly on the femoral nerve in association with an iliacus haematoma can occur. A lesion resembling Volkmann's ischaemic contracture can also occur. The basic principles of management of intramuscular bleeding are the same as those for haemarthrosis, with immobilisation and adequate dosage of Factor VIII or IX.

LEUKAEMIA

Leukaemia is divided into two broad groups, acute and chronic, which are then sub-divided according to the type of predominant cell. Except for the adolescent and, to a lesser extent, the infant, in whom myeloid leukaemia is more common, childhood leukaemia is usually of the acute lymphoblastic type.

Frequency and mode of presentation of bone and joint involvement

Among 173 children studied the incidence of osteo-articular leukaemia was 13.9 per cent (Silverstein and Kelly, 1963). Those who present with musculoskeletal symptoms but little else, are among the more difficult to diagnose. The most common symptom is pain, which is more usual in the lower rather than the upper limbs, with the knee a frequent referral site. The initial presentation as an 'irritable hip' has been seen on a number of occasions (Ansell, 1978). A single red-hot joint due to secondary gout is a less common mode of monarticular presentation.

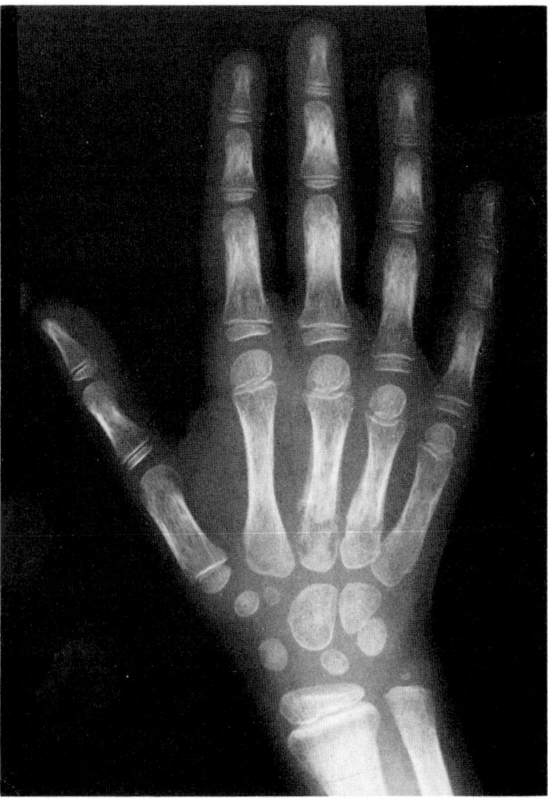

Figure 7.6. Leukaemia in a six year old girl presenting as arthritis affecting both wrists, carpi, ankles and tarsals and with an enlarged spleen and lymphadenopathy. There is a well marked translucent line at the end of the radius, and extensive osteolytic lesions in the bases of the metacarpals associated with a periosteal reaction

Where there is widespread joint involvement, particularly with the hands and wrists affected (*Figure 7.6*) it closely mimics juvenile chronic arthritis. The picture can be further confused by the finding of rheumatoid-like nodules and a positive latex test in leukaemia (Schaller, 1972). At other times arthralgia and arthritis can be fleeting, suggesting rheumatic fever.

Clinical findings

At any site of pain there may be considerable limitation of movement. Clinically there can be soft tissue swelling and sometimes effusions into the joints; histologically the synovitis is mild and non-specific. There may be marked tenderness over bones which are the site of infiltrative lesions, out of all proportion to the radiological changes present, and such a finding should lead to a check for bony tenderness in the lower part of the sternum, which is often found in acute leukaemia.

At times muscles appear to be affected, so that children can present with muscle pain even mimicking polymyositis (*see* p. 183). Haemorrhage can also occur into the muscles, particularly if there is thrombocytopenia or coagulation factor deficiency.

Other clues, such as undue lymphadenopathy and hepatosplenomegaly, will also make one suspect the diagnosis; an unexpected rise in serum uric acid, a low haemoglobin early in the course of arthritis, some atypical white cells in the peripheral blood smear, all warrant further investigation which will usually include a bone marrow examination. The diagnosis depends finally on bone marrow examination and sometimes a lymph gland biopsy.

X-ray findings

The demonstration of bone lesions radiologically is often extremely helpful in distinguishing leukaemia from diseases such as juvenile chronic arthritis, rheumatic fever, brucellosis, reticulosis and other types of malignant tumours including neuroblastoma or local malignancy of bone. The most usual site for bone destruction in leukaemia is the metaphyseal end of the femur and tibia, the proximal end of the humerus (*Figure 7.7*) and the distal end of the radius.

Four types of radiological lesions have been described. The commonest, which unfortunately is not diagnostic, is a thin translucent line in the juxta-metaphyseal area of a long bone. The next is osteolytic lesions which are fairly common and eventually lead to a moth-eaten appearance of bone (*Figure 7.8*). At this stage it can be difficult to distinguish leukaemia from deposition due to neuroblastoma. The two least common appearances are the elevation of periosteum along the shaft of a long bone, and osteosclerosis occurring as a result of an osteoblastic reaction

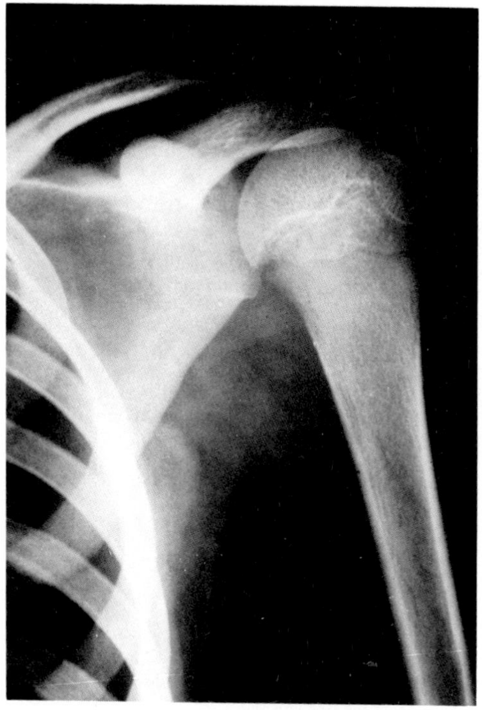

Figure 7.7. Leukaemia. A 13 year old boy with acute pain and loss of movement in first one and then the other shoulder. An osteolytic lesion is shown in the upper end of the shaft of the humerus just below the epiphysis

(*Figure 7.9*). Infection is not uncomon in childhood leukaemia, so that if a patient has been misdiagnosed as juvenile chronic arthritis and treated with corticosteroids, presentation as a sub-acute osteomyelitis in one site can occasionally be seen. The radiological pictures then become even more confusing, with a very profuse localised periostitis at the site of the infection.

Diagnosis

Bone marrrow examination is usually diagnostic, although in the early stages of the disease this may not be so; occasionally patients with a hypoplastic marrow and very few blast cells can cause difficulty, as can a marrow so full of blast cells that aspiration is dificult. If the bone marrow is not satisfactory lymph node biopsy may be required. In this latter group a trephine biopsy may be necessary.

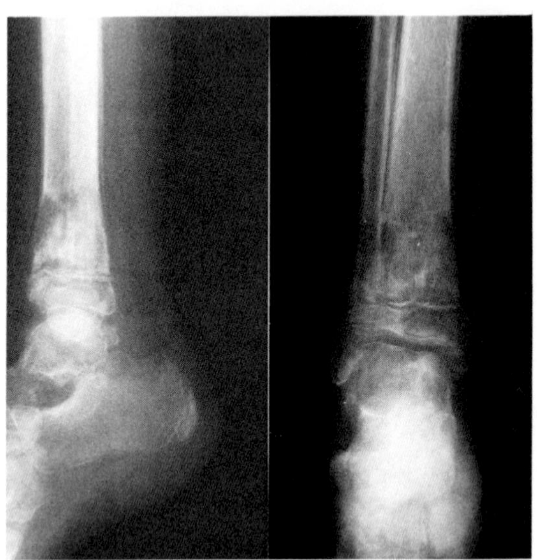

Figure 7.8. Leukaemia. An eight year old girl with widespread arthritis and subcutaneous nodules was managed as arthritis for many months before leukaemia was diagnosed. Note widespread osteolytic lesions and moth-eaten appearance of the bone

The two most difficult differential diagnoses are from juvenile chronic arthritis on the one hand and neuroblastoma (*see* p. 236) on the other; estimation of the excretion rate of vanillyl mandelic acid (VMA) in the urine is important in excluding neuroblastoma.

Other problems in the diagnosis of leukaemia include that of the juvenile form of atypical granulocytic leukaemia (Hardisty *et al.*, 1964). Here, joint involvement occasionally occurs and this, together with lymphadenopathy and an erythematous rash, also closely mimics a late-onset juvenile chronic arthritis. The rash, however, is not typical while the characteristic fever pattern of

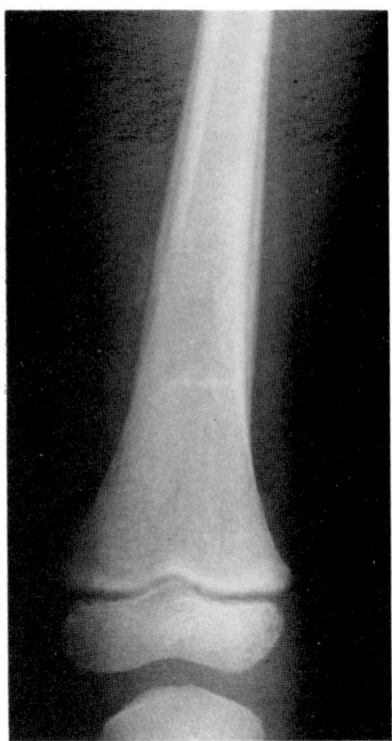

Figure 7.9. Leukaemia. This boy presented with pain in the leg and a progressive anaemia. Note marked periosteal reactions along the lower end of the femur together with an area of apparent new bone formation

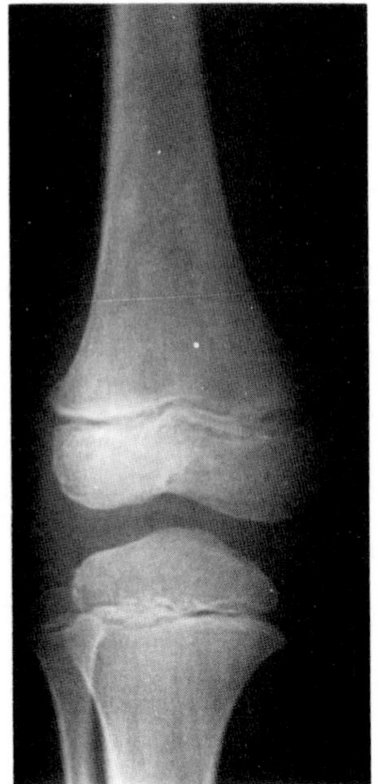

Figure 7.10. Neuroblastoma. This boy was referred with persistent pain in the knees, no evidence of synovitis but marked bony tenderness in the lower femur; x-ray shows mild periostitis. Diagnosis was made by bone marrow and lymph node biopsy

systemic juvenile chronic arthritis is not seen. There are also tumour-like growths usually arising from the sub-periosteal region of the bones of the skull, but occasionally from the sternum, ribs, vertebrae and long bones, often called chloromas (Wiernick and Serpick, 1970).

Neuroblastoma

Differentiation of patients with neuroblastoma from those with leukaemia can be very difficult. It is most commonly seen under the age of three years but can occur in older children. The most

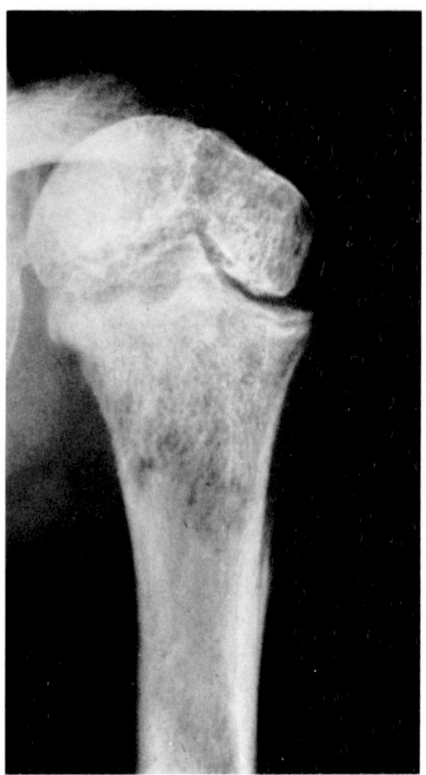

Figure 7.11. Neuroblastoma. This girl presented with transient recurrent effusions into several joints associated with intense pain. The clue to her diagnosis was bony tenderness which preceded the illustrated radiological changes of periostitis and mottled osteoporosis due to infiltration

usual clinical picture is that of a child with widespread bony metastases (Bond, 1975) who complains of pain on standing or walking and markedly dislikes joint movement because of pain. Initially the radiological change is that of a mild periosteal reaction (*Figure 7.10*), but ultimately bony changes become more obvious (*Figure 7.11*). Diagnosis is based on the increased urinary excretion of vanillyl mandelic acid (VMA) as well as the presence of tumour cells in bone marrow or lymph gland.

REFERENCES

Haemoglobinopathies

Chung, S. M. and Raltsin, E. L. (1969). Necrosis of the femoral head associated with sickle cell anaemia and its genetic variants. *Journal of Bone and Joint Surgery*, **51A**, 33

Gratwick, G. M., Bullock, P. H., Bohne, W. H. O., Markenson, A. J. L. and Petersone, M. (1978). Thalassemic Osteoarthropathy. *Ann. Int. Med.*, **88**, 494

Hand, W. L. and King, N. L. (1978). Serum opsonisation of salmonella in sickle cell anaemia. *American Journal of Medicine*, **64**, 388

Lloyd-Roberts, G. (1978). In *Hip Disorders in Childhood*, Chapter 7, p. 226. London; Butterworths

Schumacher, H. R. (1975). Rheumatological manifestations of sickle cell disease and other hereditary haemoglobinopathies. *Clinics in Rheumatic Diseases*, **1**, 37

Haemophilia

Arnold, W. D. and Hilgartner, M. W. (1977).Haemophilic arthropathy; concepts of pathogenesis and management. *Journal of Bone and Joint Surgery*, **59A**, 277

Biggs, R. (1978). *Treatment of Haemophilia A and B and Von Willebrand's Disease*. Oxford; Blackwell

Duthie, J. B. and Rizza, C. R. (1975). Rheumatological manifestations of the haemophilias. *Clinics in Rheumatic Diseases*, **1**, 53

Gilbert, M. and Cockrin, J. (1972). The evaluation of the radiological changes in the haemophiliac arthropathy of the knee. *Proceedings of the 7th Congress of the World Federation, Haemophilia, Teheran*. Amsterdam; Excerpta Medica

Leukaemia

Ansell, B. M. (1978). Case Report 40. *International Skeletal Journal*, **2**, 113

Bond, J. V. (1975). Clinical features of neuroblastoma. *British Journal of Hospital Medicine*, **14**, 543

Hardisty, R. M., Speed, D. E. and Till, M. (1964). Granulocytic leukaemia in childhood. *British Journal of Haematology*, **10**, 551

Schaller, J. (1972). Arthritis as a presenting manifestation of malignancy in children. *Journal of Pediatrics*, **81**, 793

Silverstein, M. N. and Kelly, P. J. (1963). Leukaemia with osteoarticular symptoms and signs. *Ann. Int. Med.*, **59**, 637

Wiernick, P. H. and Serpick, A. A. (1970). Granulocytic sarcoma chloroma. *Blood*, **35**, 361

CHAPTER 8

Some Soft Tissue Lesions

In this chapter a number of conditions affecting predominantly the soft tissues are described. The first group consists of nodules in skin and subcutaneous tissue which, with the exception of erythema nodosum, are uncommon. Rarer conditions such as algodystrophy, arthrogryphosis and fibrous dysplasia ossificans progressiva, all of which can mimic a rheumatic state, follow. Finally, the mucopolysaccharidoses, where Scheie's syndrome with its normal mentality, minor radiological change and contracting joints is the most difficult to differentiate from juvenile chronic arthritis. However, as it usually takes months if not years for the characteristic features of the other syndromes to be obvious, presentation of the Hunter–Scheie syndrome with stiff shoulders or Hurler's syndrome with bent fingers requires prompt recognition if only to allow prenatal diagnosis of other sibs.

'PSEUDO' RHEUMATOID NODULES; GRANULOMA ANNULARE

Histologically the lesions show central areas of fibrinoid necrosis surrounded by palisades of histiocytes and mononuclear cells and thus resemble the nodules of adult rheumatoid arthritis. When the lesions are intracutaneous they are often referred to as granuloma annulare; these last may show only patchy degeneration of collagen fibres and very little in the way of a palisade. They may contain an occasional giant cell and there is often an infiltrate of lymphocytes around the newly formed blood vessels nearby

(Fassbender, 1975). Both forms occur in children without any associated rheumatic illness and they do not portend the later development of serious rheumatic disease.

In granuloma annulare the nodules are in the skin, but they can be in the subcutaneous tissue as well and can even be fixed to deeper tissues. They occur at various sites, particularly the pretibial area (*Figure 8.1*), the dorsum of the feet, scalp, hands and elbows. It

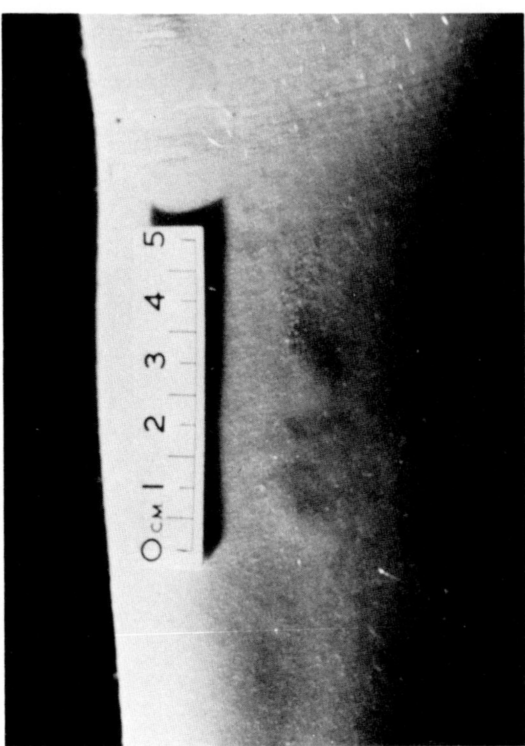

Figure 8.1. Granuloma annulare in ten year old girl. These are on the shin and had been recurring over one year. She was a keen cyclist

has been suggested that they may be traumatic in aetiology, though why they should persist or recur after removal has not been established (Burrington, 1970). Very occasionally, new crops repeatedly develop after sore throats. When these are associated with rising anti-streptolysin O-titres it is wise to use prophylactic penicillin. The lesions regress spontaneously; widespread excision only leads to scar formation.

ERYTHEMA NODOSUM

Erythema nodosum is rare in children under the age of six years; girls are particularly affected. It is characterised by the development of painful, indurated, elevated, red shiny nodules, usually distributed over the anterior surfaces of the shins (*Figure 8.2* and *Plate 11*). Associated with the lesions there may be fever, general

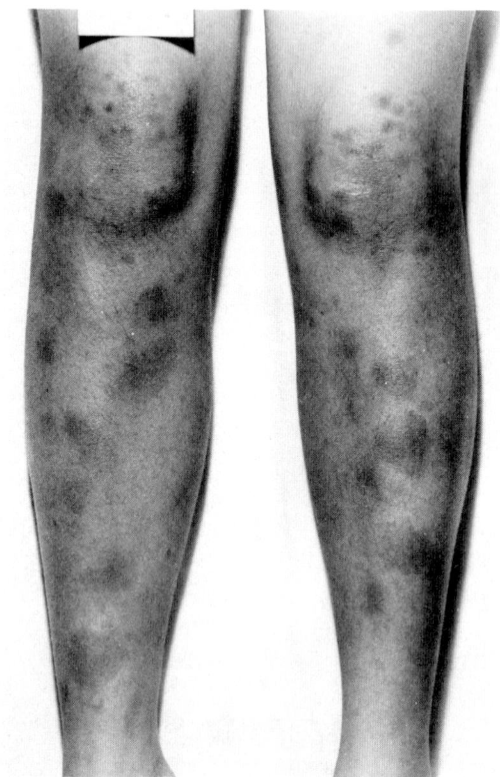

Figure 8.2. Erythema nodosum which developed two weeks after a streptococcal sore throat in a boy of nine years. (See also Plate 11)

malaise and arthralgia; very occasionally there is a symmetrical arthritis involving knees, ankles and wrists, with occasional involvement of the small joints of the hands. In children it is rare for arthritis or arthralgia to precede the onset of the typical lesions, so diagnosis is usually straightforward. The lesions themselves are from 1 to 3 or 4 cm in diameter, very tender to touch, raised from the surface and, whilst they occur predominantly on the shins, they can occur in the calves, thighs and forearms. They tend to persist for approximately one to two weeks, gradually subsiding and leaving a bruised-looking area, but may recur in crops for several weeks. Differentiation is required from nodular panniculitis (*see below*) and cutaneous polyarteritis (*see* p. 20).

Erythema nodosum is considered to be a type of allergic cutaneous vasculitis and may therefore result from a number of provocative stimuli. In Western countries it used to occur most usually with primary tuberculosis. This, however, is now an extremely rare cause in childhood and preceding streptococcal infection is more common. Erythema nodosum may also occur with fungal and other infections including *Yersinia, Leptospirosis* (Buckler, 1977) and cat-scratch fever as well as with regional enteritis (O'Donoghue and Dawson, 1977) and ulcerative colitis, where it can be the presenting feature. In contrast to adults, in children it is rarely due to sarcoidosis. The prognosis for the episode is excellent, recovery usually occurring in four to 12 weeks, symptomatic treatment being all that is required. There may be recurrences, however, and if one occurs a re-check for streptococcal infection should be initiated. If this proves negative, investigation for ulcerative colitis and regional enteritis should be instituted.

RELAPSING NODULAR NON-SUPPURATIVE PANNICULITIS

This is a rare condition and probably does not represent a single disease entity. Histologically there are foci of degeneration and inflammation in the subcutaneous fat. Clinically, crops of subcutaneous nodules develop on any part of the body (*Figure 8.3*), thighs, abdomen, arms as well as legs and buttocks. When these develop they are associated with pain, redness and warmth of the skin. They regress in days to weeks and may leave no scarring or pigmented depression. As crops are appearing, arthralgia and myalgia are not uncommon and there is frequently a raised ESR. Very occasionally there appears to be a close association with streptococcal or other intercurrent infection. In appearance the lesions mimic erythema nodosum but are usually somewhat smaller, more widespread and tend to recur over months and years (Hendricks *et al.*, 1978). If they are associated with streptococcal infection it is wise to consider prophylactic antibiotics. However,

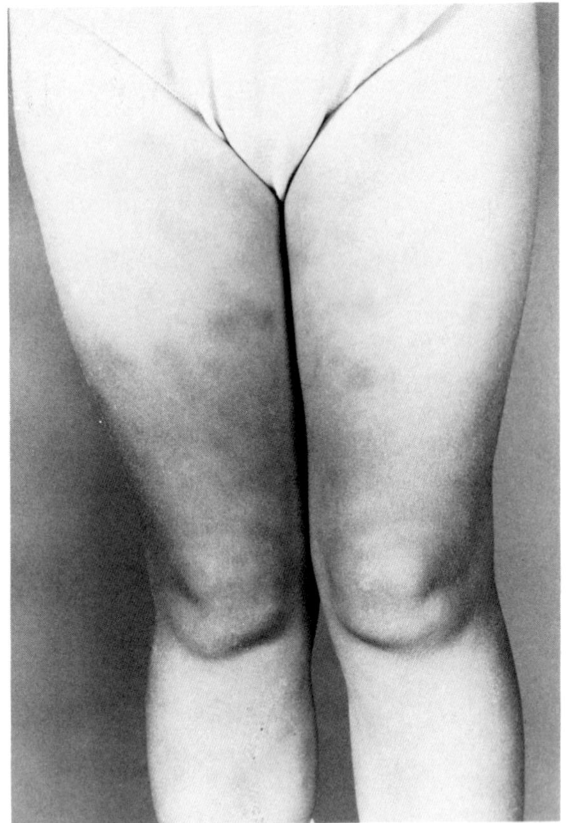

Figure 8.3. Panniculitis in a four year old girl, characterised by recurrent nodules over the whole of the legs, arms and body; regression of the lesions has not left scarring

as the majority are not, it is often considered necessary, from time to time, to give low-dose corticosteroid therapy on an alternate-day regime to control the quite severe discomfort as well as the fever that may occur.

LIPODYSTROPHIC SYNDROMES

The relationship between the various lipodystrophic syndromes and autoimmune disorders is currently of particular interest. In congenital generalised lipodystrophy there is a paucity of subcutaneous fat noticed early in infancy, with hypertrichosis, acanthosis nigricans, prominent superficial veins and muscles, hepatomegaly and often mental retardation. This is thought to be a genetic disorder as there is often a high incidence of consanguinity of parents and siblings are also affected. In some series hypertriglycidaemia has been noted in infancy (Najjar *et al.*, 1975). In later cases insulin resistance and abnormalities of human growth hormone are recorded. It is considered that a diencephalic disturbance is the most likely cause (Seip, 1971).

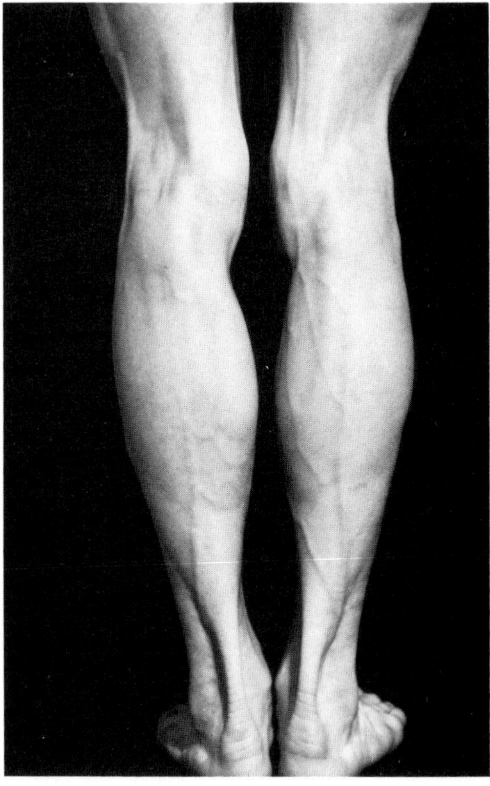

Figure 8.4. Lipodystrophy in a 13 year old girl who developed her first episode of pain and redness one year earlier after an injury to the heel. Biopsy showed panniculitis. The present picture shows the loss of fat that had occurred on subsidence of these areas of redness. At this time she had a raised ESR, antibodies to thyroid cytoplasm and immune complexes by the $C1_q$ technique. Two years later she developed thyrotoxicosis

Partial lipodystrophy is not uncommon; the relationship of the various syndromes to complement abnormalities (Sissons *et al.*, 1976) and antibodies to membrane receptors is of particular interest.

In the rheumatological field the child presents with areas of panniculitis which may be large, suggesting infection often associated with a raised ESR. On the decline of the inflammation, loss of fatty tissue is obvious (*Figure 8.4*); this may be associated with the later development of other autoimmune diseases. Thus in the case illustrated in *Figure 8.4* thyrotoxicosis first developed four years after the onset of episodes of acute lipodystrophy. A number of such cases have been reported, one of which had her first symptoms at the age of 11 years and over the next 25 years developed a multiplicity of autoimmune diseases (Wilson *et al.*, 1978). In the case described by Ipp *et al.* (1976) lipodystrophy was noted at nine years of age, followed by diabetes, then at 15, the sicca syndrome, with marked hyperreactivity of the humeral immune system and suppression of cell mediated immunity.

Other cases may more closely mimic polyarteritis nodosa; large nodules constantly recur and look just like erythema nodosum but on regression they leave fat atrophy. These, too, are frequently associated with immune complexes in the serum and a very high ESR, but do not necessarily have auto-antibodies at presentation. They respond well to systemic corticosteroid therapy. As yet, two children under my surveillance with this type of disorder have not developed evidence of other autoimmune disorders.

ARTHROGRYPHOSIS

Arthrogryphosis is the name given to a symptom complex characterised by stiffness and contractures of joints at birth. The majority of cases are sporadic, but concordance has been recorded in monozygotic twins, and, very occasionally, a suggestion that, in a particular family, it has been inherited as an autosomal recessive (Wynn-Davies, 1973). It is thought to result from immobility of the fetus *in utero*, which can be myogenic, neurogenic, or even purely mechanical; the possibility of drug therapy in the mother causing a peripheral neuropathy must also be considered.

Clinical features

The deformities are present at birth. Arthrogryphosis can affect both upper and lower limbs (50 per cent), lower limbs only (40 per

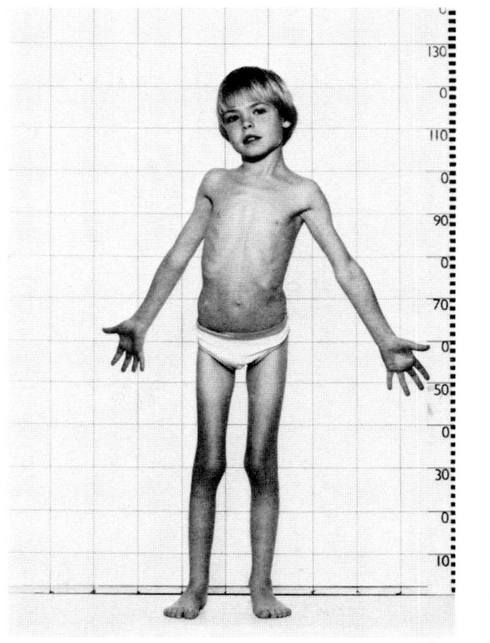

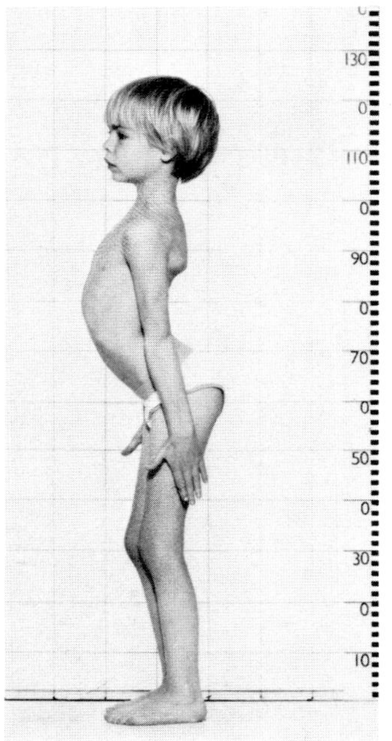

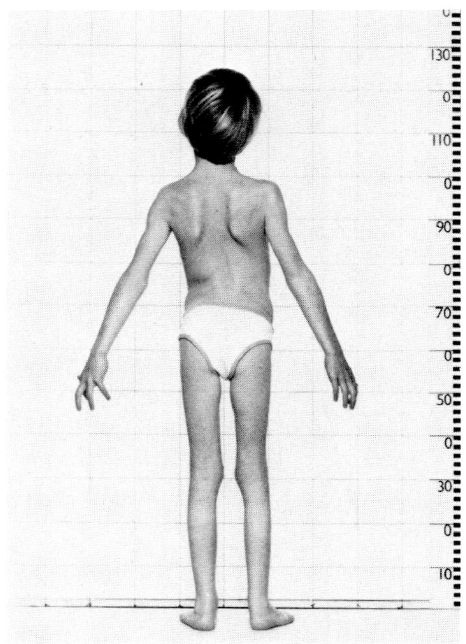

Figure 8.5. Localised arthrogryphosis in a boy of eight years. Note the marked lumbar lordosis with scoliosis, contracture of the hips and slight contractures at the knees, loss of soft tissue around the knee

cent) and upper limbs only (10 per cent). The distal joints are often severely affected, with talipes equinovarus and flexion deformity of the wrist being common; these are often associated with flexion contractures of the knees and fixed extended elbows (Lloyd-Roberts and Lettin, 1970). The normal contours of the joints are lost, as are the skin creases over them; there is absence or underdevelopment of surrounding muscles. The rigidity of the joints is thought to be due to fibrosis. There is little difficulty in recognising complete forms, which may also present with other congenital defects, particularly of the skeleton. There are, however, a number of children who appear to have isolated limitation of movement, particularly flexion at hips, knees or elbows, and it is these patients who are most usually referred for appraisal for a possible rheumatic aetiology (*Figure 8.5*).

Management

A marked degree of improvement can be achieved with manipulation and splinting, while soft tissue release of ligaments and tendons around joints can help the fixed deformities. This needs to be followed by intensive physiotherapy to improve bulk and function of remaining muscular tissue.

CONGENITAL CONTRACTURAL ARACHNODACTYLY

Congenital contractural arachnodactyly needs to be differentiated from arthrogryphosis. Although superficially resembling Marfan's disease, instead of joint laxity there are contractures and in the early stages the cardiovascular and eye complications do not occur; in addition, there is a characteristic deformity of the external ear. Contractures of the proximal interphalangeal joints, elbows, and knees are present at birth and tend to improve as the child grows. The hands and feet are long and the affected children tend to grow tall. The disorder appears to be inherited as an autosomal dominant (Mirise and Shear, 1979).

ALGODYSTROPHY (REFLEX NEUROMUSCULAR DYSTROPHY)

The importance of recognising this condition in childhood has been stressed by Bernstein and his colleagues (1978) from Los Angeles, who, when reviewing 21 children, noted the frequency of late referral and the deleterious effects of immobilisation in plaster.

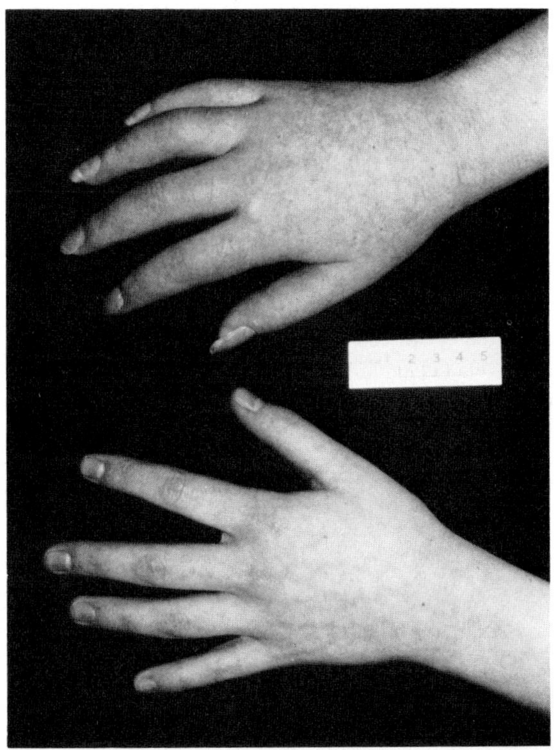

(a)

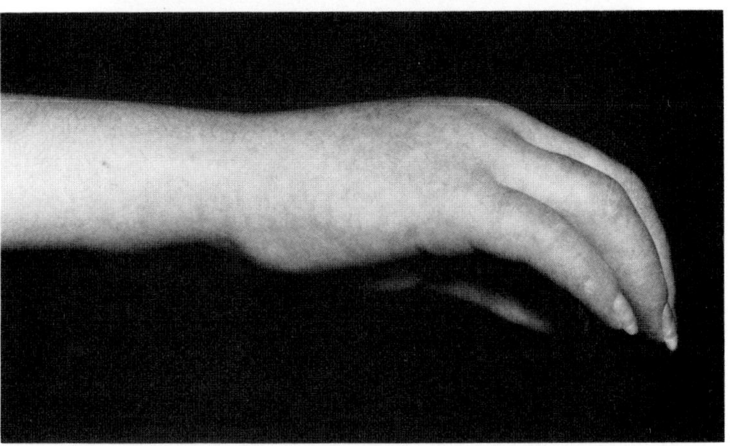

(b)

Figure 8.6. Algodystrophy in a 16 year old girl. (a) Note the mottled skin and oedema with difficulty in extending the fingers which is particularly obvious in (b) the lateral view

Clinical features

Both sexes can be affected, and the disorder usually occurs in older children, i.e. ten years and upwards. The presenting feature is pain, often intense, with hyperaesthesia; this is associated with vasomotor changes, usually vascular dilatation, oedema and disturbance of sweating. It is thought that any part of the locomotor system can be involved, but in all the juveniles I have seen it has been either a hand (*Figure 8.6*) or a foot.

After a few weeks a cold cyanosis develops and the skin becomes smooth and shiny. If movement is not encouraged, eventually the soft tissues waste, the sweat glands atrophy, and, radiologically, severe osteoporosis develops. In most patients there is some antecedent injury, usually minor, before the onset of symptoms, but this can be anything from days to months earlier.

The aetiology is unknown but there is little doubt that, as in adults, psychological factors are important. In the majority of such children there is often longstanding family conflict and it is important that this aspect is adequately investigated at the first interview.

Management consists of intensive physiotherapy, including mandatory graduated increased weightbearing if the foot is affected and, for both hand and foot, active exercises of the extremity. In general, analgesics and careful handling are all that are required. Occasionally, corticosteroids are employed and similarly sympathetic ganglion blocks; in one young patient a lumbar sympathectomy had already been carried out prior to referral. These last two treatments usually give only transient benefit if attention is not paid to the background of the illness and to improving function by physical and psychological measures.

FIBROUS DYSPLASIA OSSIFICANS PROGRESSIVA (MYOSITIS OSSIFICANS PROGRESSIVA)

In this condition there is progressive calcification and then ossification of fascia, aponeuroses and other fibrous structures. It is said to be sporadic but it is just possible that there is some form of inheritance link (Wynn-Davies, 1973).

Clinical aspects

The disorder affects males more often than females and usually begins before the age of ten years. Localised, often very painful,

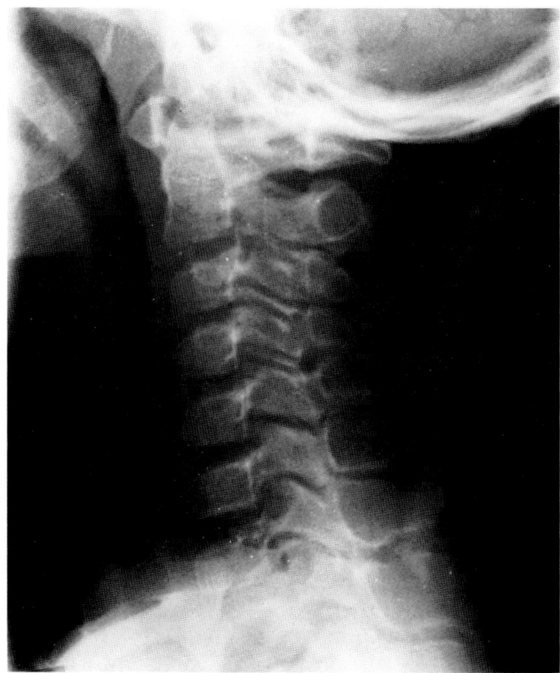

Figure 8.7. Fibrous dysplasia ossificans progressiva. This nine year old boy had presented with severe pain in the neck and marked loss of cervical extension. Note the calcification extending almost from the skull to the thoracic spine

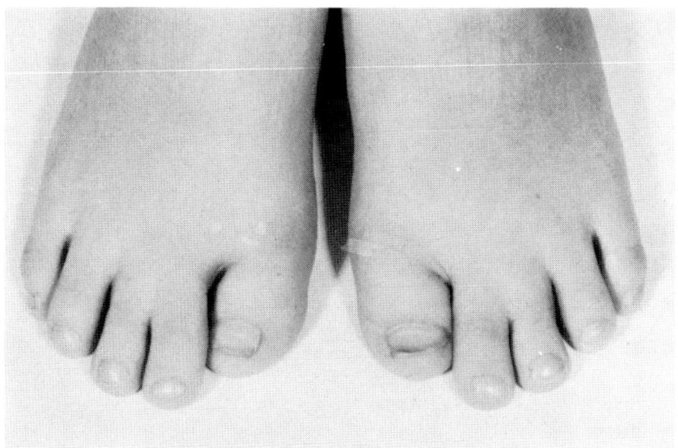

Figure 8.8. Fibrous dysplasia ossificans progressiva. A growth anomaly of the great toes present from birth in the case shown in Figure 8.7

swellings develop first at the back of the neck and limit movement; this is followed by involvement of the muscles of the back. Subsequently the proximal muscles of the limbs are involved; all muscles can be affected as well as the palmar and plantar fascia. Although exacerbations and remissions occur, the condition tends to be slowly progressive. Bridges of bone develop between adjacent muscle groups (*Figure 8.7*) causing severe restriction of movement and ultimately bony ankylosis of joints (Hentzer *et al.*, 1977). Calcium, phosphate and alkaline phosphatase are all normal (Hentzer *et al.*, 1977).

An associated feature is shortening of the great toes (*Figure 8.8*) and occasionally the thumb. This feature is present at birth and antedates overt calcification; indeed, it is a valuable diagnostic clue when the child presents with neck pain.

There is no therapy (including chelating agents) that has been shown to control the process satisfactorily (Smith *et al.*, 1976).

ANEURALGIC AMYOTROPHY

The typical picture of aneuralgic amyotrophy is of acute pain in the shoulder region with tenderness around the insertion of the deltoid and the scapular muscles, followed by weakness and varying degrees of wasting: it is occasionally bilateral. There is often a history of non-specific infection or vaccination, e.g. against influenza, just prior to the onset of symptoms.

The disorder is distinguished from shoulder arthritis by the amount of local wasting present; by the fact that the shoulder can be passively moved through a full range of movement; by the absence of any overt symptoms of synovitis either in the shoulders or elsewhere; and from the beginning of fibrous dysplasia ossificans progressiva by the patient's age. It tends to occur in children aged 11 and upwards and the neck itself is not involved. Electromyography shows patchy demyelination (Lane and Dewar, 1978).

Once pain has subsided, active exercises are required. Recovery is slow but is usually complete over six to 12 months.

THE MUCOPOLYSACCHARIDOSES

These inborn errors of mucopolysaccharide metabolism, which are of recessive inheritance, and are characterised by specific enzyme defects, are all associated with skeletal dysplasia, particularly of the hands (Fisher *et al.*, 1974), hips and vertebrae. It is important to be aware that some of these syndromes may present as joint problems in order to recognise the disorder early. This is particularly important in Hurler's and Hunter's syndrome so that one can perform a prenatal diagnosis of other sibs. Ultimately, when the features are fully developed in Hurler's disease, with dwarfism, coarse facies, clouding of cornea and progressive mental retardation, stiffening of the joints is but one aspect. However, this whole syndrome takes some 18 months to two years to be obvious, so that suspicion due to flexion deformity of fingers, will allow early recognition (*Table 8.1*). Similarly, in the Hunter/Scheie syndrome, stiff shoulders associated with some degree of dwarfism may be the presenting feature.

In Scheie's syndrome there is no dwarfing and there is normal mentality. The progressive stiffening of joints which begins in the hands and spreads to affect elbows and knees, can easily be

TABLE 8.1
Mucopolysaccharidoses

	Type	*Urinary excretion*	*Enzyme deficiency*
I H	Hurler's	Dermatan sulphate Heparan sulphate	αL-Iduronidase
I S	Scheie's	Dermatan sulphate	αL-Iduronidase
I H/S	Hurler/Scheie	Dermatan sulphate Heparan sulphate	
II	Hunter's	Dermatan sulphate Heparan sulphate	Sulphoiduromidase Sulphatase
II	Hunter/Scheie	Dermatan sulphate Heparan sulphate	
III	Sanfilippo A B	Heparan sulphate	x-Acetyl-glucosaminidase
IV	Morquio– Brailsford	Keratan sulphate Chondroitin-6-sulphate	Hexosamine-6-sulphatase
VI	Maroteaux– Lamy	Dermatan sulphate	Aryl-sulphatase B

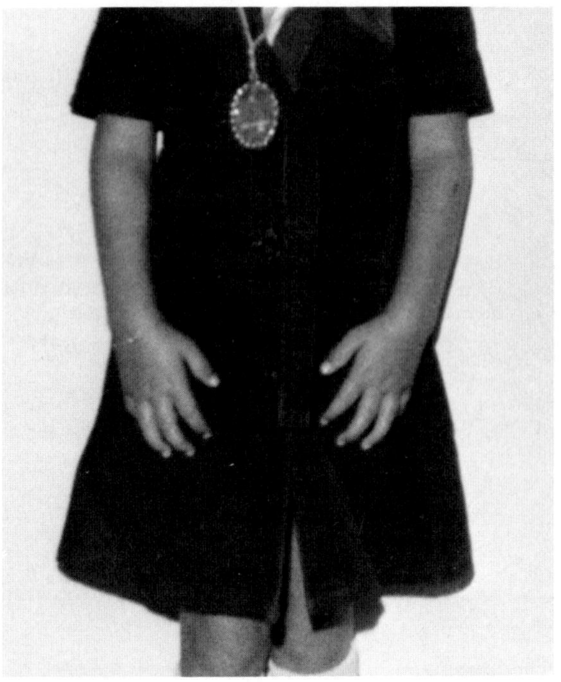

Figure 8.9. Scheie's syndrome in a six year old girl who presented with progressive contractures of the fingers and knees

mistaken for juvenile chronic arthritis (*Figure 8.9*). There is, however, an absence of soft tissue swelling and pain. The ESR and haemoglobin are normal while rheumatoid factors and antinuclear antibodies are absent. Corneal clouding, which can sometimes be mistaken for chronic iridocyclitis, and the presence of dermatan sulphate in the urine, will support the diagnosis of Scheie's syndrome. It is important to recognise this in order to protect the child against unnecessary therapy with drugs such as gold or penicillamine.

The skeletal abnormalities and dwarfing in type IV (Morquio–Brailsford) can also suggest juvenile chronic arthritis. There is a waddling gait, valgus deformity at the knees and contracting small hands. In addition, joint laxity and protrusion of the sternum are usual. Radiology is of help as the pelvis shows poorly developed acetabulae and dysplastic hips as well as characteristic spinal changes (Gordon and Ross, 1977).

REFERENCES

Bernstein, B., Singsen, B. H., Kent, J. T., Kornreich, H., King, K., Hicks, R. and Hanson, V. (1978). Reflex neurovascular dystrophy in childhood. *Journal of Pediatrics*, **93**, 211

Buckler, J. M. H. (1977). Leptospirosis presenting with erythema nodosum. *Archives of Disease of Childhood*, **52**, 418

Burrington, J. D. (1970). ‚Pseudorheumatoid' nodules in children; report of 10 cases. *Pediatrics*, **45**, 473

Fassbender, H. G. (1975). *Pathology of rheumatic diseases*, p. 146. Berlin, Heidelberg, New York; Springer Verlag

Fisher, R. C., Horner, R. L. and Wood, V. E. (1974). The hand in mucopolysaccharide disorders. *Clinical Orthopaedics and Related Research*, **104**, 191

Gordon, I. R. S. and Ross, F. G. M. (1977). *Diagnostic Radiology in Paediatrics*. London; Butterworths

Hendricks, W. M., Ahmad, M. and Gratz, E. (1978). Weber-Christian syndrome in infancy. *British Journal of Dermatology*, **98**, 175

Hentzer, B., Jacobsen, H. H. and Asboe-Hansen, G. (1977). Fibrous dysplasia ossificans progressiva. *Scandinavian Journal of Rheumatology*, **6**, 161

Ipp, M. M., Howard, N. J., Tervo, R. C. and Gelfand, E. W. (1976). Sicca syndrome and total lipodystrophy; a case in a 15-year-old female patient. *Annals of Internal Medicine*, **85**, 443

Lane, R. J. M. and Dewar, J. A. (1978). Bilateral neuralgic amyotrophy. *British Medical Journal*, **1**, 895

Lloyd-Roberts, G. C. and Lettin, A. W. F. (1970). Arthrogryphosis multiplex congenita. *Journal of Bone and Joint Surgery*, **52B**, 494

Mirise, R. T. and Shear, S. (1979). Congenital contractural arachnodactyly; description of a new kindred. *Arthritis and Rheumatism*, **22**, 542

Najjar, S. E., Salem, G. M. and Idriss, Z. H. (1975). Congenital generalized lipodystrophy. *Acta Paediatrica Scandinavia*, **64**, 273

O'Donoghue, D. P. and Dawson, A. M. (1977). Crohn's disease in childhood. *Archives of Disease of Childhood*, **52**, 627

Seip, M. (1971). Generalized lipodystrophy. *Ergebnisse der Inneren Medizin und Kinderheilkunde*, **31**, 59

Sissons, J. G. P., West, R. J., Fallows, J., Williams, D. G., Boucher, B. J., Amos, N. and Peters, D. K. (1976). The complement abnormalities of lipodystrophy. *New England Journal of Medicine*, **294**, 461

Smith, R., Russell, R. G. G. and Woods, C. G. (1976). Myositis ossificans progressiva; clinical features of eight patients and their response to treatment. *Journal of Bone and Joint Surgery*, **58B**, 48

Wilson, W. A., Sissons, J. G. P. and Morgan, O. S. (1978). Multiple autoimmune diseases with bilateral optic atrophy and lipodystrophy. *Annals of Internal Medicine*, **89**, 72

Wynn-Davies, R. (1973). *Heritable disorders in orthopaedic practice*. Oxford; Blackwell Scientific Publication

CHAPTER 9

Some Skeletal Disorders Mimicking Arthritis

In this chapter a wide variety of skeletal disorders which mimic, or are associated with arthritis are discussed. No attempt has been made to cover every possibility; only those conditions which have, at times, given rise to confusion either in rheumatic outpatients or in a combined rheumatological/orthopaedic clinic have been described. In addition to well recognised syndromes, several oddities that, as yet, defy diagnosis have been included.

DIAPHYSEAL ACLASIS

This condition is also known as hereditary multiple exostoses. It is a rare inherited condition in which exostoses arise alongside the epiphyseal plates, producing bony swelling adjacent to joints and affecting the normal growth of the involved bone. This can result in local bone deformity, particularly valgus deformity of the lower leg and bowing or deviation of the forearm (Gordon and Ross, 1977).

PROGRESSIVE DIAPHYSEAL DYSPLASIA

In this condition, which affects children usually between the age of three and five years, there is progressive thickening of the cortex of the diaphyses of long bones, usually of the lower extremities, accompanied by muscular pain and weakness. Clinically, there may be a history of failure to thrive but, in general, the presentation is with pain and weakness spreading down the whole of the lower limbs. The alkaline phosphatase may be raised but diagnosis is based on the radiological change of a thickened diaphysis with a normal epiphysis and metaphysis (Gordon and Ross, 1977).

ENCHONDROMATOSIS

Enchondromatosis, also known as Ollier's disease, is another rare developmental disease in which cartilage islands remain in the metaphysis and diaphysis of the long bones, usually of the digits, often adjacent to the epiphyseal plate, so growth is disturbed producing shortening and deformities. As the most commonly affected sites are hands and feet, the swelling may initially be mistaken for arthritis. However, radiologically lucent chondromata are seen expanding the shafts of the affected bones. Associated haemangiomatous malformation may also be present – then the condition is known as Maffucci's syndrome (Johnson *et al.*, 1960).

ACRO-OSTEOLYSIS (DISAPPEARING BONE DISEASE)

Destruction and disappearance of bone as a primary condition is rare; a number of different types have been described (Brown *et al.*, 1976).

Hereditary osteolysis is inherited as an autosomal dominant. It is seen in children of both sexes, usually beginning at about the age of three. It affects the bones of the carpus and tarsus particularly, to a lesser extent the hands and feet, as well as bones adjacent to the elbows and knees. The presentation with tender, swollen, limited wrists and ankles mimics juvenile chronic arthritis but there is no evidence of synovitis, and the ESR is normal (Beals and Bird, 1975). Initially the x-rays are normal but after a few years there is porosis of carpal and tarsal bones, followed by localised destruction and finally complete disappearance of bone (*Figure 9.1a, b* and *c*). The condition tends to stabilise spontaneously in early adult life.

Osteolysis with nephropathy (Shurtleff *et al.*, 1964) is a non-hereditary condition which closely resembles hereditary osteolysis, but is associated with progressive, and ultimately, fatal renal lesions.

Phantom bone disease (Gorham's disease) (Gorham and Stout, 1955) another non-hereditary form, usually occurs somewhat later

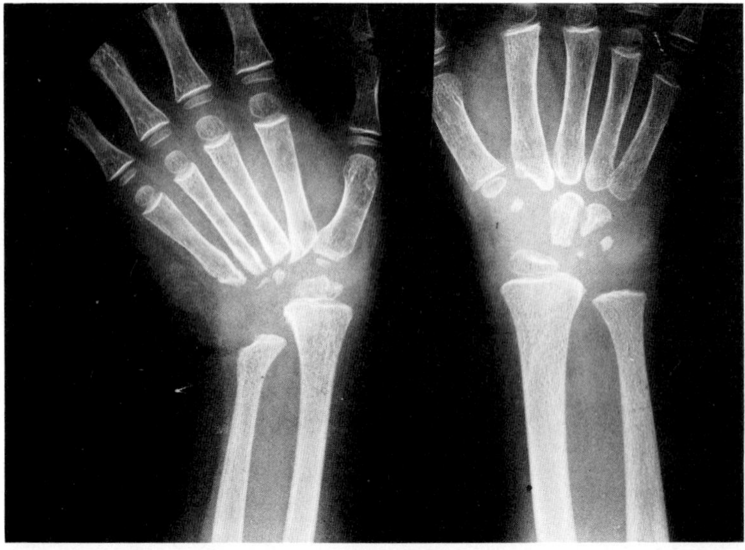

(a)

(b)

Figure 9.1. Acro-osteolysis. (a) Pain and deformity of the left wrist followed by the right, commenced at the age of 18 months. One year later the radial epiphyses and the left ulna are being absorbed and carpal changes are obvious. (b) Two years later progressive changes in the ulni, radii and carpi have occurred as well as now, involvement of the bases of the metacarpals. Elbows and knees are now similarly affected

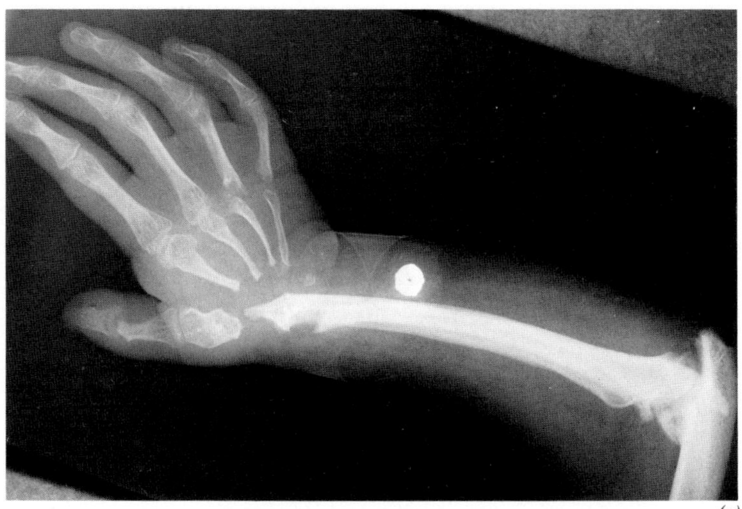

(c)

Figure 9.1(c). This shows state of the wrists, carpi and metacarpals on the right together with the elbow shortly before death from renal failure at the age of 16. Proteinuria had first been noted at aged ten; the renal biopsy showed interstitial fibrosis

between five and ten years of age. Any bone may be affected but there are usually multiple sites which are asymmetrical in distribution. Histologically, there is proliferation of thin-walled blood vessels. *Distal osteolysis*, thought to be inherited as an autosomal dominant, is characterised by progressive osteolysis of phalanges, metatarsals or metacarpals and recurrent ulceration of the hands and feet. This disease also tends to occur in somewhat older children (eight or nine) and tends to heal spontaneously although some fingers or toes may be lost (Elias *et al.*, 1978).

HISTIOCYTOSIS X

This represents a group of disorders characterised by lesions which histologically have the appearance of granulomata with histiocyte proliferation. In one study 17 of 42 patients with histiocytosis X presented with bone pain particularly affecting the long bones, usually the humerus, femur and tibia (Sims, 1977). There is variation in presentation, the most benign form being eosinophilic granuloma of bone which may be single or multiple. A more serious form of histiocytosis is the Hand–Schuller–Christian disease which is usually seen in children under the age of three and characterised by widespread bony lesions, lymphadenopathy, hepatomegaly, skin rashes and exophthalmos: this very rarely has to be differentiated from systemic juvenile chronic arthritis. The most severe form is Letterer–Siwe disease, where there is widespread skin and visceral involvement; here, generalised features predominate over those due to bony involvement and very occasionally this disease needs to be differentiated from systemic juvenile chronic arthritis. Diagnosis is based on histology of lymph glands, bone lesion or skin.

PSEUDO-HYPERTROPHIC OSTEOARTHROPATHY (PACHYDERMOPERIOSTITIS)

The presence of finger clubbing or more generalised clubbing of digits (*Figure 9.2*) should remind one of pseudo-hypertrophic/osteoarthropathy. As a primary condition this is uncommon in childhood (Vogl and Goldfischer, 1962). It is more usually

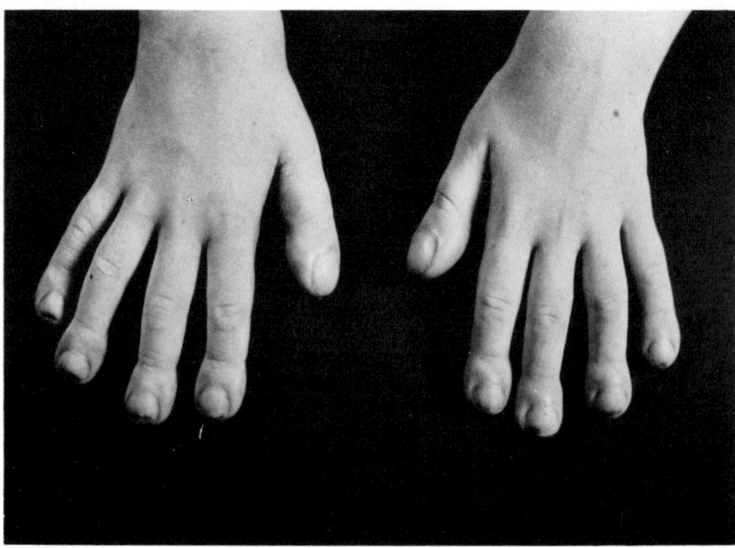

Figure 9.2. Primary pseudo-hypertrophic osteoarthropathy. Generalised enlargement of the finger ends in a boy of seven whose father also suffers from the same condition

seen in adolescence, when it is characterised by soft tissue swelling aroung large joints, particularly knees and wrists, associated with restriction in movement. There may be a mild synovitis. Radiologically there is diffuse periostitis (*Figure 9.3*). The condition can be

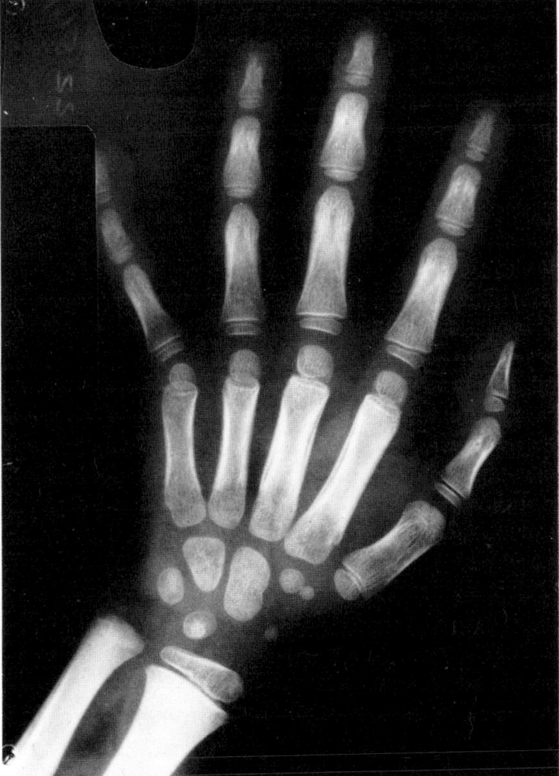

Figure 9.3. Primary pseudo-hypertrophic osteoarthropathy. The x-ray of another case showing periostitis along the shafts of the second and third metacarpals and the ulna

familial; in one family we observed that the father and all three male children were affected, with marked thickening of the forehead occurring late. The secondary form can occur at any age, and may be seen in association with cyanotic congenital heart disease, bowel disorders such as ulcerative colitis and Crohn's disease but it is most usually associated with pulmonary metastases secondary to osteogenic sarcoma (Petty *et al.*, 1976).

OTHER BONE ODDITIES

Aneurysmal bone cyst

This is most commonly seen in adolescence but can occur at any age. The aetiology is unknown, but not uncommonly there is a history of trauma. The most usual complaint is of discomfort; the most common sites are the metaphyses of long bones or the spine. The x-ray shows a cystic lesion with an expanded cortex and periosteal reaction. Exploration will reveal a haemorrhagic multilocular cyst with fibrous tissue and spicules of bone. Histologically there is a network of communicating blood-filled spaces and giant cells. Evacuation usually leads to a cure although there can be recurrences (Pullen *et al.*, 1978).

Bone tumours

In general, malignant bone tumours rarely cause confusion, as although pain may be related to a limb or joint, the radiological appearance allows early diagnosis. Thus in chondrosarcoma, which is probably the most common bone tumour, there is radiological expansion of the bone with sub-periosteal spiculation and sometimes calcification within the tumour shown as localised densities, while osteosarcoma is very much more aggressive. Occasionally osteosarcoma is present in multiple sites, when arthritis can be simulated (*Figure 9.4*).

Acute transient osteoporosis

This is a rare condition and, although in adults it has been reported in a number of sites, to date, I have only seen the hip affected in juveniles; these have been older children, ten and upwards. There has usually been a history of preceding trauma (such as falling off a horse without apparent injury), then some weeks later severe pain has occurred in the hip, often with marked loss of movement. The acute phase tends to last for several weeks (Lequesne *et al.*, 1977). Histology of the synovial membrane in one such case showed no evidence of synovitis. Recalcification of the area proceeds slowly; at times there appears to be some loss of joint space as a sequel to this. The ESR is usually normal and the general health is unaffected. The most important differential diagnosis is from osteoid osteoma (p. 34).

Osseous lesions and pancreatitis

An uncommon complication of acute and chronic pancreatitis and pancreatic pseudocysts is disseminated fat necrosis. The patients

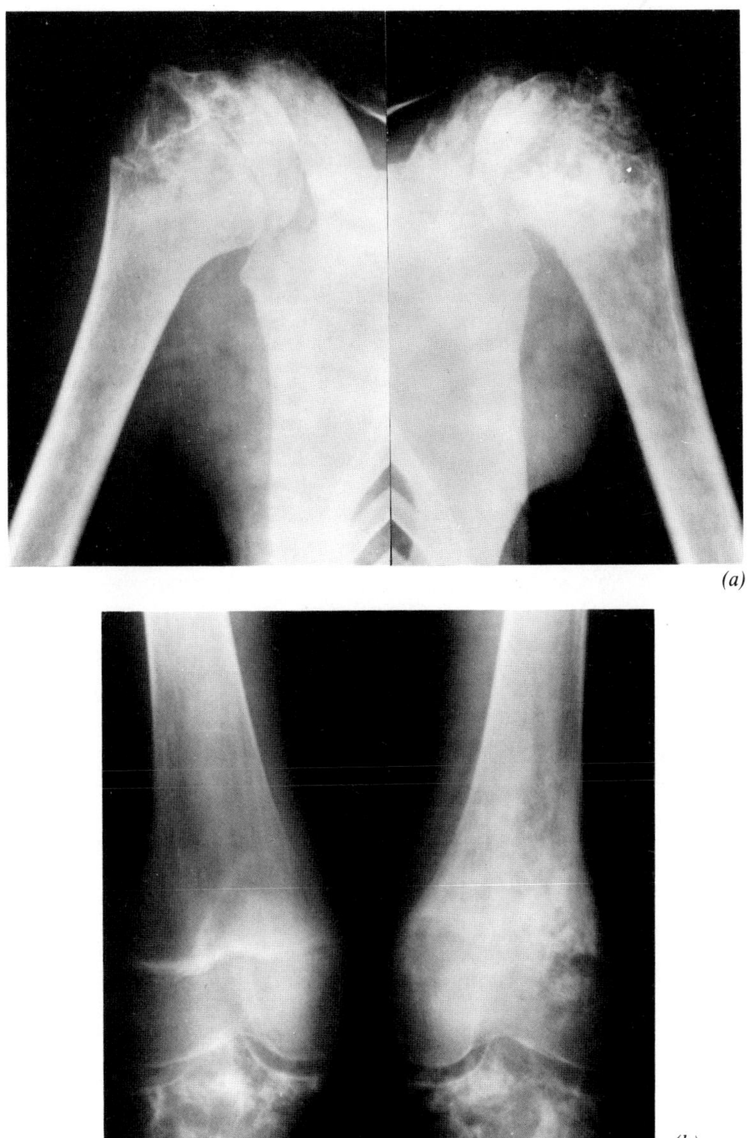

(a)

(b)

Figure 9.4. Multiple bone tumours. A 13 year old boy who had presented with a polyarthritis 12 months before with pain in numerous sites (a) shoulders, (b) knees. The biopsy showed sheets of small closely packed round or oval cells with trabeculae of osteoid tissue and new bone formation suggesting osteosarcoma

may present with fever associated with tender, erythematous subcutaneous nodules, soft tissue swelling of digits suggesting polyarthritis and raised ESR. The osteolytic lesions are frequently multiple, sometimes silent but tend to be painful and affect the small bones of the hands and feet. They may regress very quickly and spontaneously (Shackleford, 1977) (*Figure 9.5*). These lesions

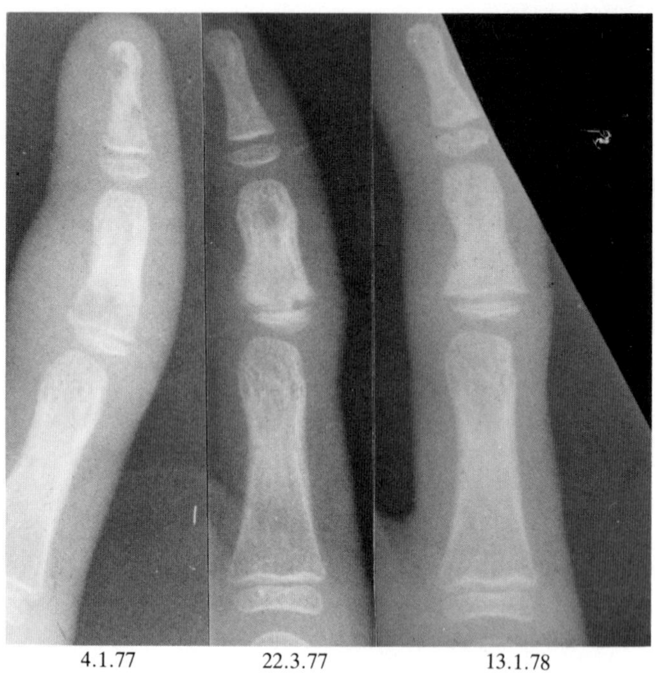

Figure 9.5. This seven year old girl presented with painful swelling of a toe and finger. Previous episodes had occurred over the preceding three years. X-rays showed lytic lesions of terminal phalanx and proximal phalanx which have regressed over one year. Later that year, she underwent removal of a pancreatic cyst

have to be differentiated from infection, sickle cell anaemia and leukaemia. Biopsy of a nodule will reveal fat necrosis. The clue to diagnosis is suspicion so that levels of serum lipase and amylase can be measured: these will be raised. A previous history of trauma to the abdomen, e.g. fall from a bicycle, may be helpful. Pancreatitis in childhood is being recognised with increasing frequency (Buntain *et al.*, 1978).

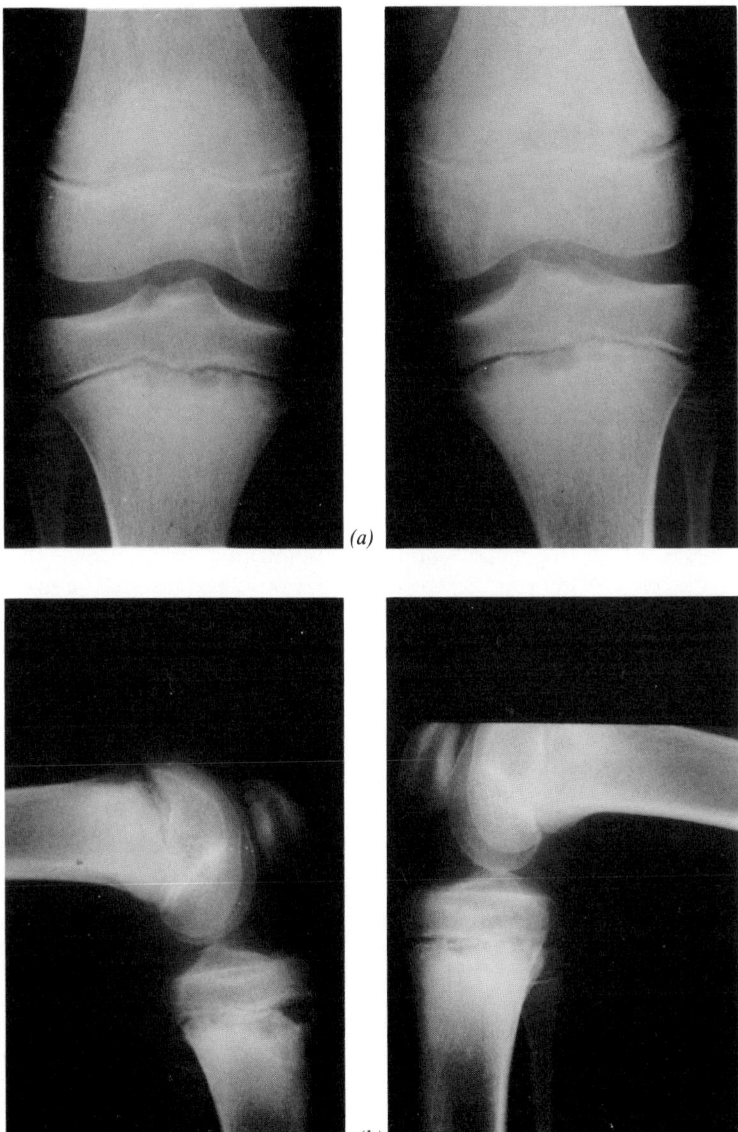

Figure 9.6(a) and (b). Bony infiltration below the epiphyses of both knees in a girl aged ten who had presented with pain in the ankle following an injury at hockey. Biopsy revealed chronic granulation tissue – with no growth on culture. Her white cells functioned normally – there was no evidence of any immunological disturbance. The lesions have regressed spontaneously

Chronic granulomatous disease

In this condition children are usually infected with *Staphylococcus aureus* or Gram-negative organisms. However, fungal infections particularly unusual ones, are becoming more common (Bujak *et al.*, 1974). It is the intracellular reaction which provokes the granulomatous reaction. In addition to overt changes, chronic lesions are becoming increasingly recognised. The x-rays shown in *Figure 9.6* were so diagnosed; however, no evidence of infection or anomaly in host response could be detected in our patient.

Primary protrusio acetabuli

During the past six years five cases similar to the one described by D'Arcy *et al.* (1978) have been referred for an opinion of their hip pain and, in particular, as to whether they were suffering from juvenile chronic arthritis. There were two boys and three girls. While they may have noticed a slight limp before, they have all presented with acute symptoms mimicking an irritable hip syndrome. A minor strain or injury has occurred just before these acute symptoms. Although presenting with pain in one hip the other hip is usually found to be limited at first examination which will immediately suggest to the examiner that this is not a simple irritable hip. In all except one of our cases, by the time of presentation, marked protrusio was obvious radiologically (*Figure 9.7*). Idiopathic protrusio is a well recognised condition, as is its

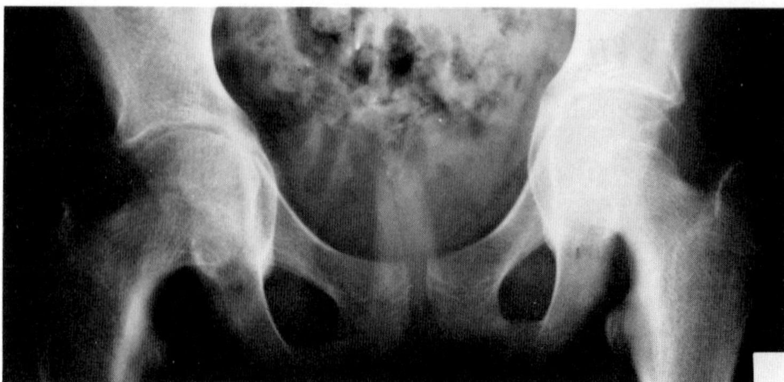

Figure 9.7. Primary protrusio acetabuli. The radiograph of a 13 year old girl who had been noticed to have a slight limp for two years. After prolonged squatting while potato picking she developed acute pain in the right hip, and required admission. Note that even at this time there is evidence of severe protrusio

familial nature, but presentation with severe pain and the rapid development of flexion contractures in this small group of young patients appears to constitute a real problem in terms of both diagnosis and management.

Management

Management is very unsatisfactory. The acute symptoms will usually subside on traction and some movement will be retained by physiotherapy. Only one of our six patients has maintained a reasonable functional state into her twenties; she has required several periods of prolonged traction and intensive physiotherapy and now still has poor movement in both hips but with only very minor flexor contractures. One young patient has undergone soft tissue release followed by traction and physiotherapy at an early stage but it is, as yet, too soon to know how far we have influenced the progression. To date, bilateral total replacement arthroplasty has been carried out in four of our patients while they were still in their teens.

SOME EPIPHYSEAL ODDITIES

Thieman's disease

Thieman's disease tends to commence at about the age of ten or 11 years. It is characterised by progressive enlargement of the proximal interphalangeal joints of the hands, the interphalangeal joints of the great toes and occasionally other toes, followed by flexion of the enlarged joints. Clinically this disease appears as a bony swelling with no evidence of soft tissue swelling, the ESR is normal, and radiologically there is irregularity of the epiphyses of the phalanges (Molloy and Hamilton, 1978). It tends to be familial (Allison and Blumberg, 1958) and has no sinister significance.

Osteochondritis dissecans

While osteochondritis dissecans usually affects a single joint (p. 36) multiple sites, usually knees, elbows and ankles, can be affected. There may be a positive family history (Stougard, 1964) and very occasionally it is associated with dwarfism (White, 1957)

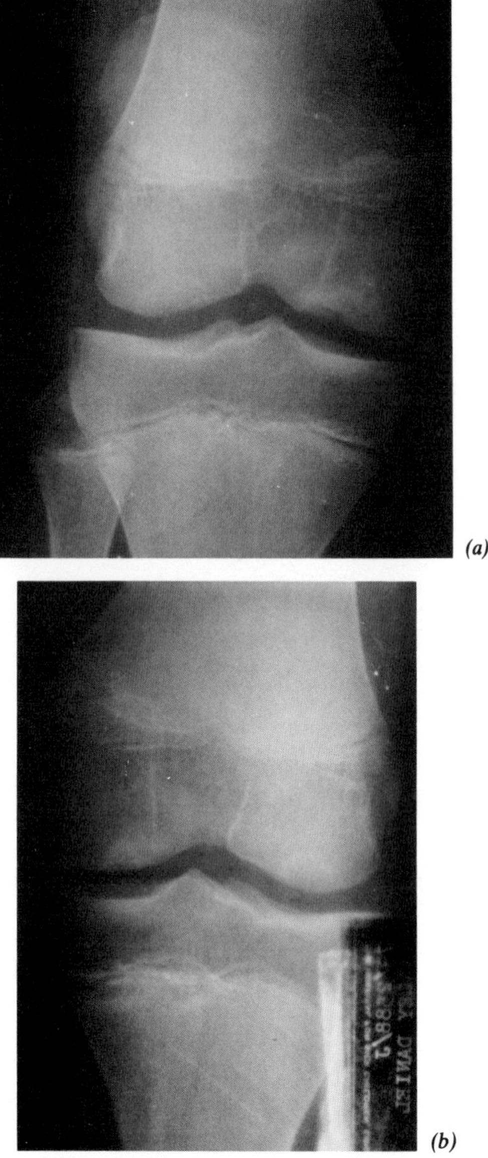

Figure 9.8. Multiple osteochondritis dissecans. This boy now aged 14 had first developed episodes of pain and some swelling of the knees and elbows at the age of nine. He was of short stature as was his father who had had similar symptoms as a teenager

(*Figure 9.8*). Symptoms arise in adolescence and consist of joint pain with episodes of swelling, particularly after marked physical activity (Robinson *et al.*, 1978). While the knees are the most common site, it can present in elbows or ankles. The ESR is usually normal. Synovial histology and radiology confirms the diagnosis.

Multiple epiphyseal dysplasia

This term probably includes a group of disorders in which the main finding is disordered growth in a number of epiphyses with metaphyses normal (Wynn-Davies, 1973). One type certainly appears to be of autosomal dominant inheritance and there seems to be a similarity of distribution of lesions within one family. The condition usually becomes apparent in early childhood. When the lesions are confined to the lower limbs, where it is principally the hip joints that are affected, the child may present with a limp or even discomfort after sport. Severe dwarfing is not a feature of this condition although the child may be on the shorter side of normal. The spine is not significantly affected.

Spondylo-ephiphyseal dysplasia

In this form, in addition to epiphyseal dysplasia, there is involvement of the vertebral bodies and dwarfism usually becomes evident shortly after birth. Some flattening of the face may also be noted (*Figure 9.9a*). At times there appear to be episodes of pain and limitation of movement at joints and, indeed, it was loss of movement at the metacarpophalangeal joints which caused referral of the boy shown in *Figure 9.9*. At this time there were only epiphyseal changes in the hips (*Figure 9.9b*). This form is sometimes known as the pseudo-achondroplastic type (Gordon and Ross, 1977).

Other epiphyseal problems

Other epiphyseal oddities have also given rise to confusion. The patient shown in *Figure 9.10a* was referred, on account of increasing deformity of his elbows, as a possible case of juvenile chronic arthritis. However, there had been no evidence of synovitis at any time. Elbow deformity on the left had been noted

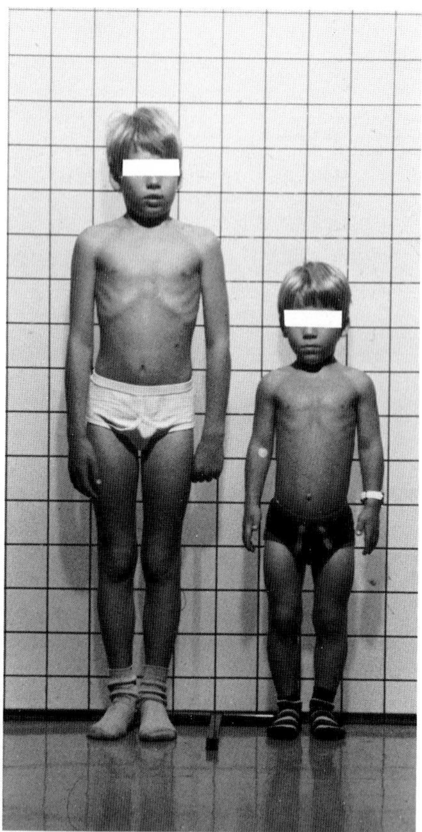

(a)

Figure 9.9. Spondylo-epiphyseal dysplasia. (a) Patient on the right aged eight with normal nine year old brother. There was no family history. (b) X-ray of the patient's hips showing the fragmented state of the femoral epiphyses. (It is just possible that he is suffering from Leri's pleonosteosis)

at the time he started school and had steadily progressed. The right side had become affected while his knees and ankles were now showing some loss of movement. The only possibly relevant point in his history was that the mother had had mumps in the early part of her pregnancy. Initially, there was bony enlargement and some loss of movement of the elbows particularly, but also loss of movement at the wrists and knees, while radiologically (*Figure 9.10b*) the elbows show a gross disturbance of epiphyseal development with irregular overgrowth and premature fusion. Other sites were similarly, but less severely, involved; these included the ankles, knees, feet and hands (*Figure 9.10c*).

Familial epiphyseal damage with constitutional symptoms

A family in whom there were epiphyseal anomalies associated with severe general illness has already been described by us (Ansell *et al.*, 1975). Our index case was a boy who, we too thought, had Still's disease initially. He had presented with a rash immediately after his premature birth; this was followed some time later by fever, hepatosplenomegaly, lymphadenopathy and towards the end of the first year, when he tried to stand, he suddenly became unable to do so and appeared to have arthritis of his knees. His sister, born nine years later, and also premature, was noted to have a similar rash, but rather more severe, on the second day of life (*Figure 9.11a*). Since that time a number of other such children have been drawn to our attention.

The features appear to be a severe systemic illness commencing very early in life, usually on the first or second day, with a rash somewhat similar to Still's disease, followed by a febrile illness, lymphadenopathy, hepatosplenomegaly, a high ESR, leucocytosis and anaemia. Biopsy of a lymph gland has shown merely reactive hyperplasia. There appears to be general enlargement of the head with frontal bossing (*Figure 9.11a*); mental retardation of some degree has been present in most children and this tends to be progressive. At times, the children complain of headaches and two, at least, have had a high protein level in their CSF. Joint manifestations start at about the age of one and consist of acutely painful swelling in a number of joints with the knees and elbows the most common sites (*Figures 9.11b, c* and *d* and *9.12a* and *b*), but we have also seen wrists (*Figure 9.12c* and *d*) and ankles affected. The joints are held in flexion and any attempt to straighten them is associated with intense pain and resistance on the part of the child. Ultimately, the epiphyseal alteration shown is

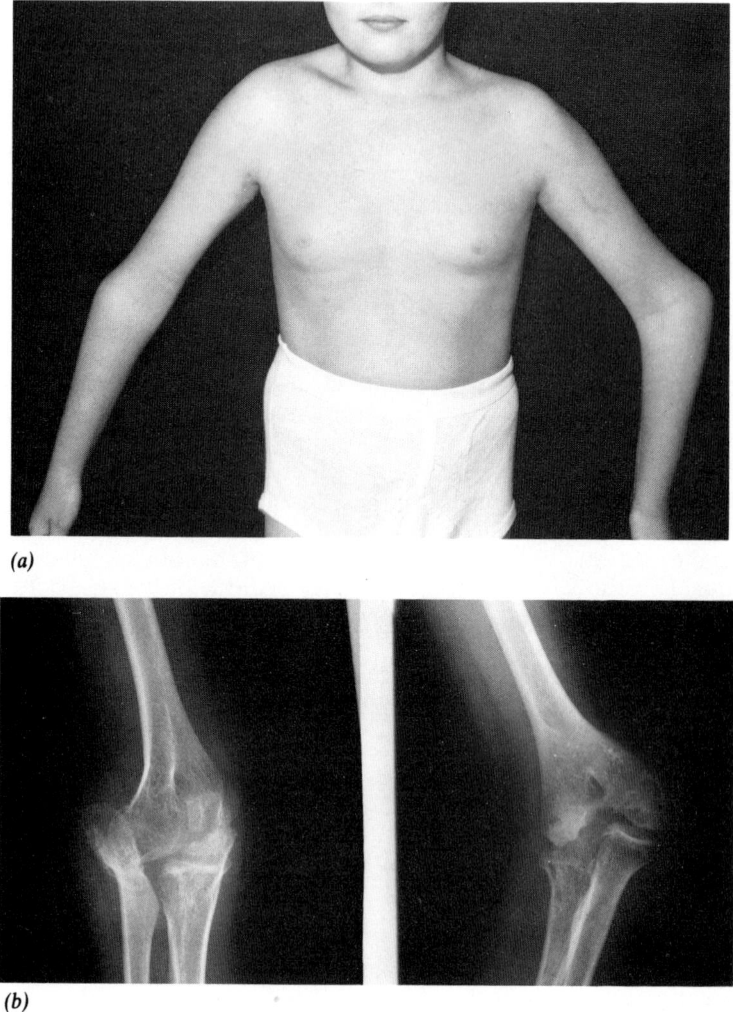

(a)

(b)

Figure 9.10. Multiple epiphyseal abnormalities of unknown type. (a) Bony enlargement and loss of extension of elbows, at 13 years; the deformity having commenced aged five. (b) Elbow x-rays showing already overgrowth premature fusion of epiphyses together with distortion

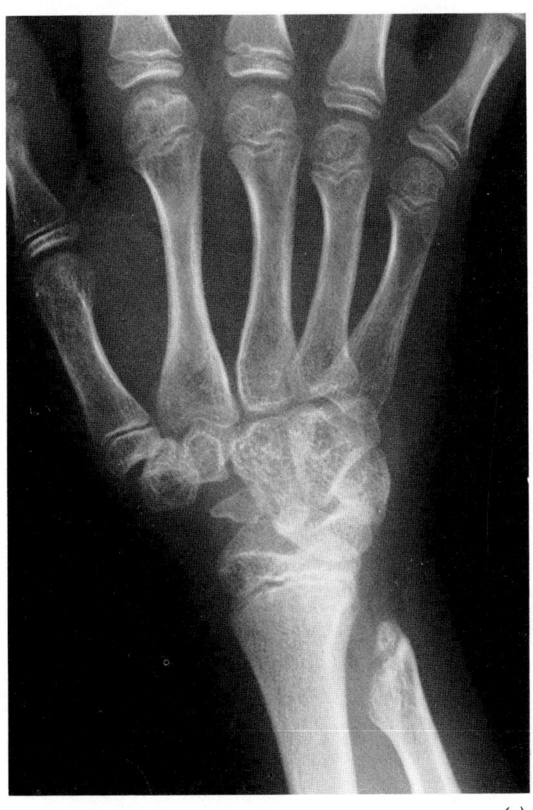

(c)

Figure 9.10(c). X-ray of hands showing growth anomaly of the ulna, crowding and alteration in carpal shape and minor changes in the metacarpal epiphyses

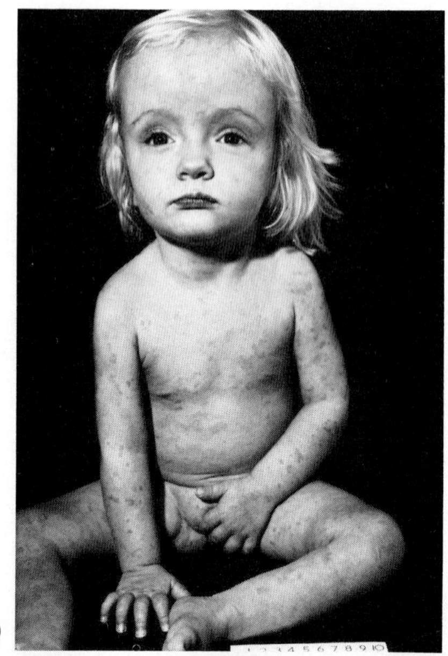

(a)

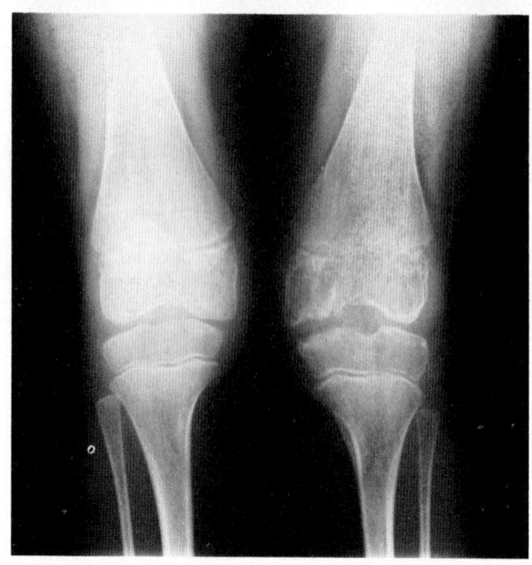

(b)

Figure 9.11. Bizarre epiphyseal anomalies associated with constitutional symptoms. (a) Child aged 18 months with prominent forehead and extensive rash. (b) Knees of child aged six showing the epiphyseal anomalies

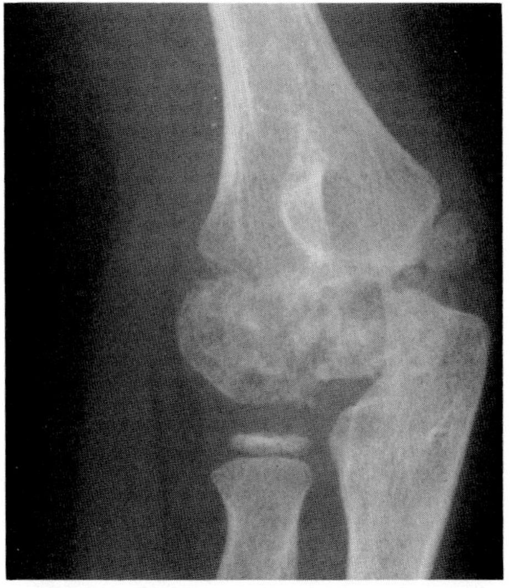

(c)

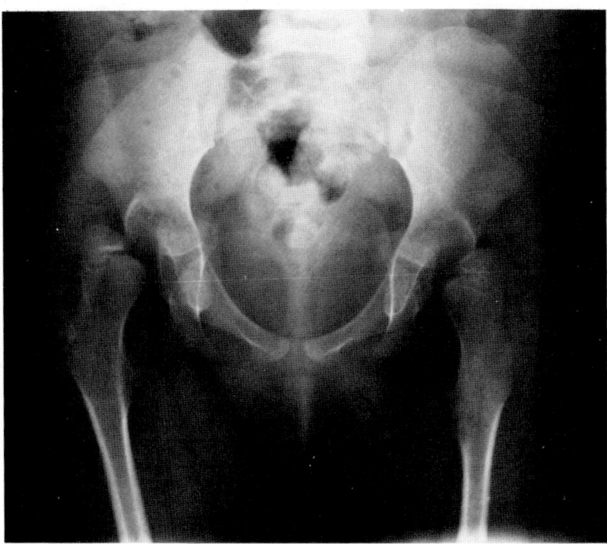

(d)

Figure 9.11(c). Elbow of child aged seven again showing epiphyseal change. (d) Pelvis of child aged seven showing no abnormality of the epiphysis but failure of development and subluxation presumably because the severe pain in the knees had prevented walking

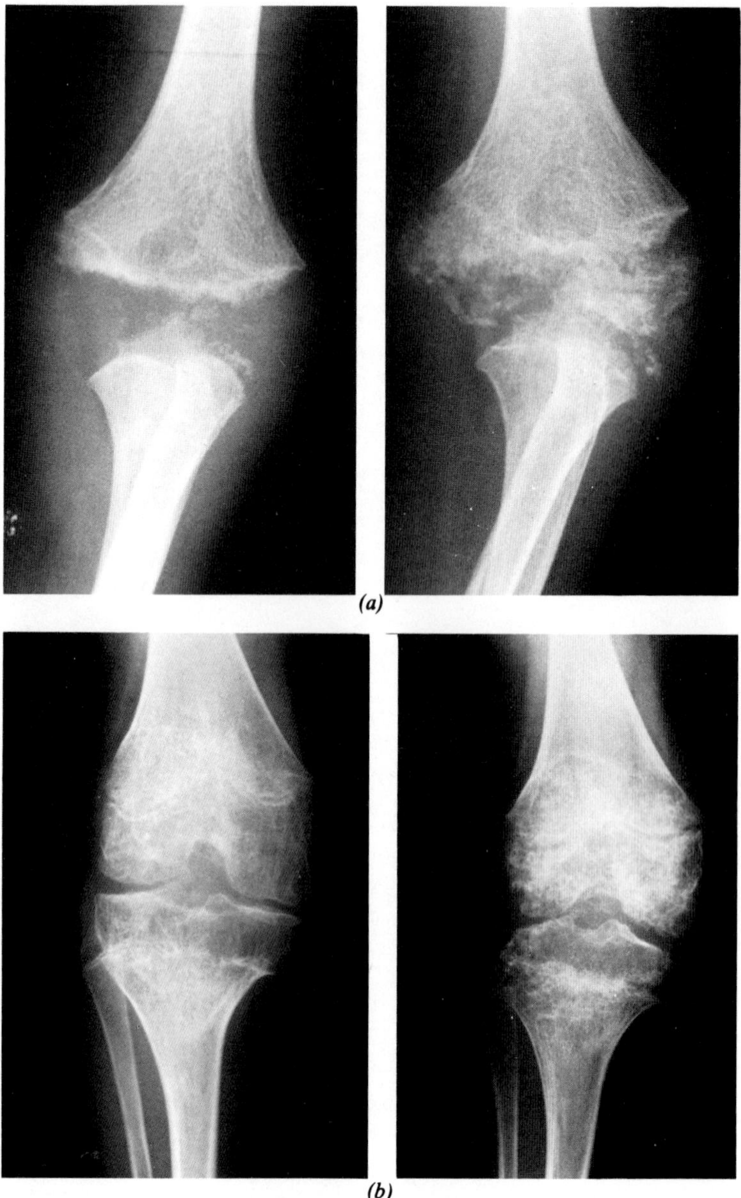

Figure 9.12. X-rays of brother of case demonstrated in Figure 9.11. (a) Knee epiphyses aged eight and 11. (b) Lateral view to show patellar enlargement when aged nine

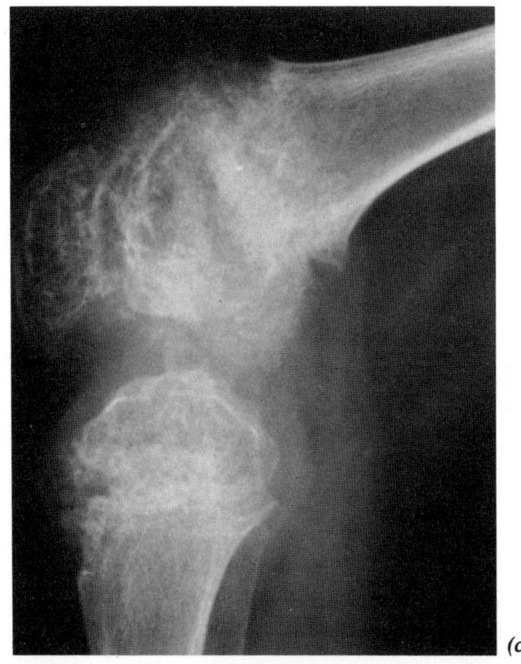

(c)

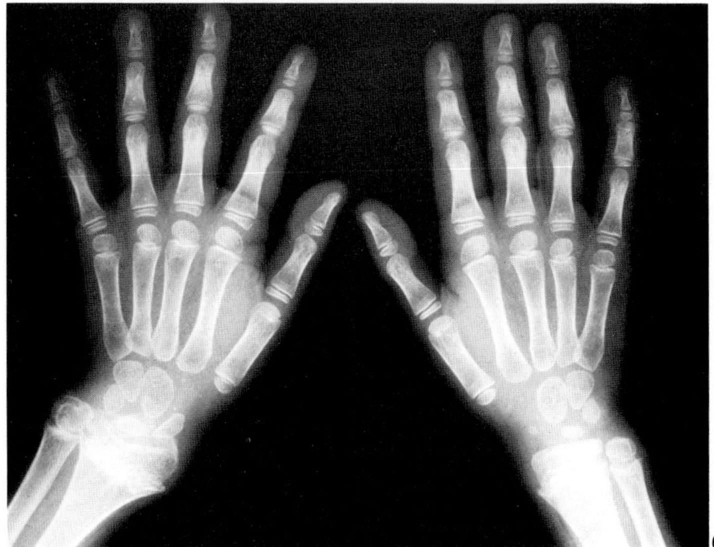

(d)

Figure 9.12(c). Elbow epiphyses when aged six. (d) Hands when aged nine

noted. Full screening of the originally reported family has failed to reveal any evidence of a mucopolysaccharidosis or anomaly of complement metabolism. Current studies are in progress in consideration of a congenital viral infection. It may well be that there are incomplete syndromes as suggested by the child in *Figure 9.13*.

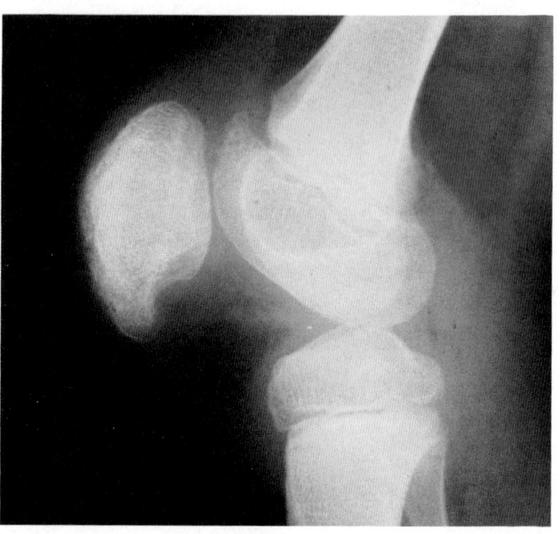

Figure 9.13. Lateral view of knees to show bony enlargement of patella in an unrelated boy aged eight who had presented with rash at birth followed by fever, lymphadenopathy and bilateral painful knees from aged 18 months

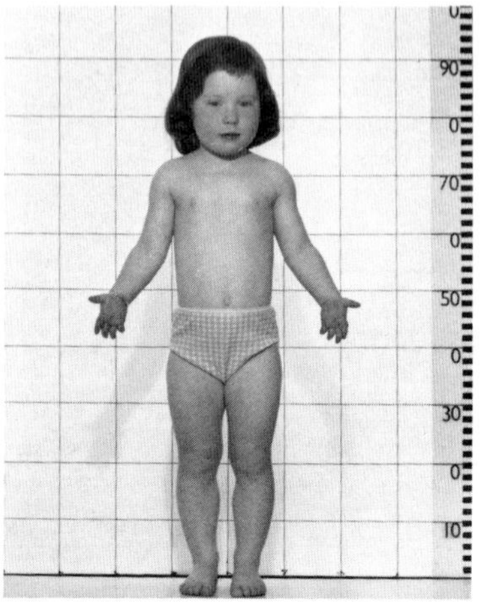

(a)

Figure 9.14. Moore–Federman syndrome (a) Girl of seven and a half who was of normal birth weight but had failed to grow. Aged three difficulty in bending the fingers noted – note size and lack of extension of elbows

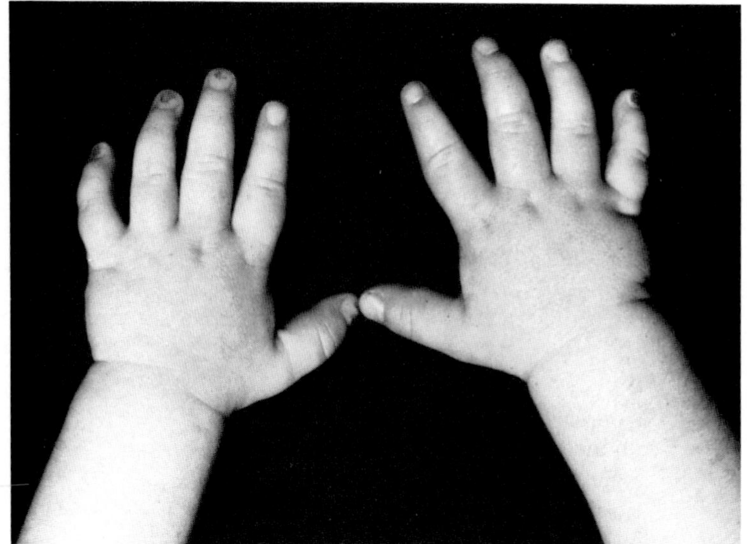

(b)

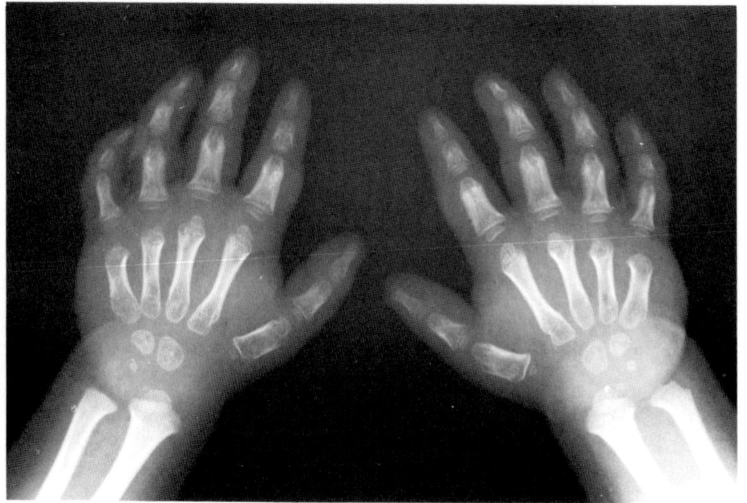

(c)

Figure 9.14(b). Hands at 4 years 10 months showing short stubby fingers tending to bend and (c) x-ray at the same time with widening of phalanges and radii and ulnae with poor epiphyseal development

Brachydactyly

Arthritis or, indeed, disorders such as sickle cell disease and tumours, particularly exostoses, as well as trauma can give rise to various types of brachydactyly. These may need to be distinguished from the many types of congenital hand anomalies (Pozsnanski, 1974). They can be single entities but at other times may be associated with congenital anomalies. Occasionally the small short hands with which the patient has difficulty in bending the fingers may be confused with juvenile chronic arthritis. In the Moore–Federman syndrome (1965) short hands are noted early followed by developing contractures at other joints (*Figure 9.14a, b* and *c*).

Hypervitaminosis

Chronic ingestion of vitamin A causes pain in the limbs associated with a general irritability, apathy and loss of hair and, after some time, growth alterations (Pease, 1962). Radiologically, there is cortical hyperostosis involving the ulna and metatarsals classically, but other bones can be involved; periosteal elevation and damage to the epiphyseal plate are occasionally seen. Overdosage with vitamin D in childhood (this may not need to be more than the continuous ingestion of 500 000 units) is also thought to be associated with pain and sclerosis of bone (Christensen *et al.*, 1951). It is, however, difficult to know how much of the changes described are in fact due to hypervitaminosis A.

REFERENCES

Allison, A. C. and Blumberg, B. S. (1958). Familial osteoarthropathy of the fingers. *Journal of Bone and Joint Surgery*, **40B**, 538

Ansell, B. M., Bywaters, E. G. L. and Elderkin, F. M. (1975). Familial arthropathy with rash, uveitis and mental retardation. *Proceedings of the Royal Society of Medicine*, **68**, 584

Beals, R. K. (1977). Hereditary arthro-ophthalmopathy (the Stickler Syndrome); report of a kindred with protrusio acetabuli. *Clinical Orthopaedics and Related Research*, **125**, 32

Beals, R. K. and Bird, C. B. (1975). Carpal and tarsal osteolysis; a case report and review of the literature. *Journal of Bone and Joint Surgery*, **57A**, 681

Brown, D. M., Bradford, D. S., Gorlin, R. J., Desnick, R. J., Langer, L. O., Jowsey, J. J. and Sauk, J. J. (1976). The acro-osteolysis syndrome; morphologic and biochemical studies. *Journal of Pediatrics*, **88**, 573

Bujak, J. S., Kwon-Chung, K. J. and Chusid, M. J. (1974). Osteomyelitis and pneumonia in a boy with chronic granulomatous disease of childhood caused by a mutant strain of *Aspergillus nidulans*. *American Journal of Clinical Pathology*, **61**, 361

Buntain, W. L., Wood, J. B. and Woolley, M. M. (1978). Pancreatitis in childhood. *Journal of Pediatric Surgery*, **13**, 143

Christensen, W. R., Liebman, C. and Sosman, M. C. (1951). Skeletal and periarticular manifestations of hypervitaminosis. *American Journal Roentgenology*, **65**, 27

D'Arcy, K., Ansell, B. M. and Bywaters, E. G. L. (1978). A family with primary protrusio acetabuli. *Annals of Rheumatic Diseases*, **37**, 53

Elias, A. N., Pinals, R. S., Anderson, H. C., Gould, L. V. and Streeten, D. H. P. (1978). Hereditary osteodysplasia with acro-osteolysis (the Hajdu-Cheney syndrome). *American Journal of Medicine*, **65**, 627

Gordon, I. H. S. and Ross, F. G. M. (1977). *Diagnostic radiology in paediatrics*. London; Butterworths

Gorham, L. W. and Stout, A. P. (1955). Massive osteolysis (acute spontaneous absorption of bone, phantom bone, disappearing bone); its relationship to hemangiomatosis. *Journal of Bone and Joint Surgery*, **37A**, 985

Johnson, J. L., Webster, J. R. and Sippy, H. Y. (1960). Maffucci's syndrome (dyschondroplasia with hemangiomas). *American Journal of Medicine*, **28**, 864

Lequesne, M., Kerboull, M., Bensasson, M., Perez, C., Dreiser, R. and Forest, A. (1977). Partial transient osteoporosis. *Skeletal Radiology*, **2**, 1

Maudsley, R. H. (1955). Dysplasia epiphysialis multiplex; a report of fourteen cases in three families. *Journal of Bone and Joint Surgery*, **37B**, 228

Molloy, M. G. and Hamilton, E. B. D. (1978). Thiemann's disease. *Rheumatology and Rehabilitation*, **17**, 179

Moore, W. T. and Federman, D. D. (1965). Familial dwarfism and 'stiff joints'. *Archives of Internal Medicine*, **115**, 398

Pease, C. N. (1962). Focal retardation and arrestment of growth of bones due to vitamin A intoxication. *Journal of the American Medical Association*, **182**, 980

Petty, R. E., Cassidy, J., Heyn, R., Kenien, A. G. and Washburn, R. L. (1976). Secondary hypertrophic osteo-arthropathy; an unusual case of arthritis in childhood. *Arthritis and Rheumatism*, **19**, 902

Poznanski, A. K. (1974). *The hand in radiologic diagnosis*. Philadelphia; W. B. Saunders & Co

Pullan, C. R., Alexander, F. W. and Halse, P. E. (1978). Aneurysmal bone cyst; a report of three cases. *Archives of Disease in Childhood*, **53**, 899

Robinson, R. P., Franck, W. A., Carey, E. J. Jr. and Goldberg, E. B. (1978). Familial polyarticular osteochondritis dissecans masquerading as juvenile rheumatoid arthritis. *Journal of Rheumatology*, **5**, 190

Shackleford, P. G. (1977). Osseous lesions and pancreatitis. *American Journal of Diseases of Children*, **131**, 731

Shurtleff, D. B., Sparkes, R. S. and Clawson, D. K. (1964). Hereditary osteolysis with hypertension and nephropathy. *Journal of the American Medical Association,* **188,** 363

Sims, D. G. (1977). Histiocytosis X; follow-up of 43 cases. *Archives of Disease in Childhood*, **52**, 433

Stougaard, J. (1964). Familial occurrence of osteochondritis dissecans. *Journal of Bone and Joint Surgery*, **46B**, 542

Vogl, A. and Goldfischer, S. (1962). Pachydermoperiostosis; primary or idiopathic hypertrophic osteoarthropathy. *American Journal of Medicine*, **33**, 166

White, J. (1957). Osteochondritis dissecans in association with dwarfism. *Journal of Bone and Joint Surgery*, **39B**, 261

Wynn-Davies, R. (1973). *Heritable Disorders in Orthopaedic Practice*. Oxford; Blackwell Scientific Publications

Wynn-Davies, R. and Fairbank, T. J. (1976). *Fairbank's Atlas of General Affections of the Skeleton*. Edinburgh; Churchill Livingstone

APPENDIX

Laboratory Tests

The purpose of this short appendix is to indicate the tests in current use together with some of the problems. This is a developing field with new techniques and tests being evolved. It is essential that the reader checks the accepted values in the laboratories that he himself uses.

BLOOD

ESR

The Westergren test is the most useful. The upper limit of normal is 10 mm/h. (Plump adolescents and menstruating teenagers tend to have raised levels.)

Acute phase reactants

C-reactive protein and other proteins such as orosomucoids, α2-macroglobulin, haptoglobins, etc. may be estimated as part of a research programme.

Plasma viscosity

Plasma viscosity is measured in some laboratories instead of the ESR, but does not correlate as well with disease activity in rheumatic disorders.

IgM rheumatoid factor

Not standardised.

	Significant titres
Sheep cell agglutination titre (SCAT)	1 : 32 or above
Differential agglutination titre (DAT)	1 : 16 or above
Rheumatoid arthritis haemagglutination (RAHA)	1 : 80 or above
Latex agglutination	1 : 20 or above

IgG rheumatoid factor

Not routine (Hay and Nineham, 1979).

Lupus erythematous cell

Detection depends on method and duration of search; errors in interpretation of phagocytosed nuclear material are common. This test is tedious to perform and rarely used except for special reasons, e.g. a specific research project.

Nuclear antibodies (ANA)

WHO International Standard Reference Serum available.

With WHO's reference the significant level is 25 μg/ml or above on a composite block of liver, kidney or stomach. Not all laboratories are using this standard, and in such instances the results will be given as positive or by titre. Note also the fluorescent pattern – homogeneous, speckled or nucleolar.

In general
- Systemic lupus erythematosus – homogeneous or speckled at high levels (1600 μg/ml or more)
- Dermatomyositis – homogeneous
- Scleroderma – speckled, homogeneous or nucleolar
- Mixed connective tissue syndrome – speckled
- Juvenile chronic arthritis – homogeneous
- Juvenile rheumatoid arthritis – homogeneous
- Sjögrens – homogeneous.

Granulocyte antinuclear antibodies (Rosenberg *et al.*, 1975)

Primarily of research interest.

Antibodies to DNA

Not yet standardised (Holborow, 1978).

Levels vary with laboratories and technique.
Radio-immune assay (Farr technique).
Passive haemagglutination (Fjuizoki test).
Crithidia lucillae (under investigation).

High levels of double stranded DNA suggest systemic lupus erythematosus.

Immunoglobulins

The usual techniques are:

Mancini (radial immune diffusion)
Laurell–Rocket immuno-electrophoresis
Nephelometric

The levels vary with age and sex as well as disease states.

Enzyme estimations

Not yet standardised.

Values depend on the technique employed and temperature at which it is carried out.
Creatine phosphokinase – raised in inflammation of muscle in some 80 per cent.

Transaminase Transpeptidases Lactate dehydrogenase	} May be raised in disease of muscle, or liver problems, particularly drug induced.

Alkaline phosphatase – this varies with age and is particularly high during adolescence (Salz *et al.*, 1973).

Extractable nuclear antigen (ENA)

Not yet routine.

Haemagglutination test aginst calf thymus nuclei.
Counter immuno-electrophoresis.
Detects ribonuclear protein which when RN-ase sensitive is said to be specific for MCTD (mixed connective tissue disease) (Sharp, 1975).

Anticytoplasmic antibodies

Not yet routine (Homberg *et al.*, 1974).

Lymphocytotoxins

Not yet routine (DeHoratius and Messner, 1975).

Immune complexes

Many different techniques available. Not yet standardised (Maini and Holborow, 1977; Lambert, 1979).
The one in most common use is $C1_q$.
Found in sero-positive rheumatoid arthritis, systemic juvenile chronic arthritis, systemic lupus erythematosus, arteritis of all types and indeed, any form of immune complex disease.

Complement

CH_{50}, C_3, C_4 — Detect overall complement level and utilisation.

Deposition of complement components

Deposition of complement components in fresh tissue section may be detected by fluorescent microscopy using appropriate anti-sera. Readily available anti-sera include $C1_q$, C_4, C_3, properdin and factor B.

SYNOVIAL FLUID

The volume, viscosity, colour, turbidity as well as blood staining should be noted.

For cell count and differential, 2 ml synovial fluid should be mixed with EDTA. (RBC indicate a traumatic tap or haemarthrosis.)
For microscopy and culture, 1 ml synovial fluid in a sterile container unless unusual organisms, e.g. *Gonococcus*, when a special culture medium is indicated.
When estimation of protein required, mix with hyaluronidase.

Non-inflammatory synovial fluid

Viscous
Light yellow
Clear
WBC less than $1.0 \times 10^9/l$
Glucose normal
Protein 1 g/l
Culture sterile

Inflammatory synovial fluid (Gardner, 1972)

Non-viscous
Turbid in varying degree according to WBC
WBC Juvenile chronic arthritis $30–100 \times 10^9/l$ predominantly polymorphs
Viral arthritis $5–20 \times 10^9/l$ often mononuclear
Traumatic $1–2 \times 10^9/l$ often mononuclear
Septic $100 \times 10^9/l$ polymorphs
Glucose low
Protein 20–40 g/l

Special studies

Bilirubin
Identification of crystals, e.g. urate, calcium pyrophosphate
Complement levels
Immune complexes
Rheumatoid factor.

REFERENCES

Dehoratius, R. J. and Messner, R. P. (1975). Lymphocytotoxic antibodies in family members of patients with systemic lupus erythematosus. *Journal of Clinical Investigation*, **55**, 1254

Gardner, G. L. (1972). *Synovial Fluid in the Pathology of Rheumatic Disease*. Chapter 8, p. 84–89. London; Arnold

Hay, F. C. and Nineham, L. J. (1979). Standardisation of assays for rheumatoid factor and antiglobulins. *Laboratory Tests in Rheumatic Diseases*, Chapter 12, p. 101. Editors D. C. Dumonde and M. W. Steward. Lancaster; MTP Press Ltd.

Holborow, E. J. (1978). The serology of connective tissue disorders. *British Journal of Hospital Medicine*, **00**, 250

Homberg, J.-C., Rizzetto, M. and Doniach, D. (1974). Ribosomal antibodies detected by immunofluorescence in systemic lupus erythematosus and other collagenoses. *Clinical and Experimental Immunology*, **17**, 617

Lambert, P. H. (1979). Standardization of assays for the measurement of immune complexes. In *Laboratory Tests in Rheumatic Diseases,* p. 107. Edited by Dumonde, D. C. and Steward, M. H. Lancaster; MTP Press Ltd

Maini, R. N. and Holborow, E. J. (1977). Detection and measurement of circulating soluble antigen-antibody complexes and anti-DNA antibodies. *Annals of the Rheumatic Diseases*, 77, supplement 1

Rosenberg, J. N., Johnson, G. D., Holborow, E. J. and Bywaters, E. G. L. (1975). Eosinophil-specific and other granulocyte-specific antinuclear antibodies in juvenile chronic polyarthritis and adult rheumatoid arthritis. *Annals of the Rheumatic Diseases*, **34**, 350

Salz, J. L., Daum, F. and Cohen, M. I. (1973). Serum alkaline phosphatase activity during adolescence. *Journal of Pediatrics*, **82**, 536

Sharp, G. C. (1975). Mixed connective tissue disease. *Bulletin on Rheumatic Diseases*, **25**, 828

Index